Cardiac CT

Marc Dewey

Cardiac CT

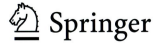 Springer

Privatdozent Dr. Marc Dewey
Charité - Universitätsmedizin Berlin
Humboldt-Universität zu Berlin
Freie Universität Berlin
Institut für Radiologie
Charitéplatz 1
10117 Berlin
Germany
marc.dewey@charite.de

ISBN 978-3-642-14021-1   e-ISBN 978-3-642-14022-8
DOI 10.1007/978-3-642-14022-8
Springer Heidelberg Dordrecht London New York

Library of Congress Control Number: 2010930076

Cover design: eStudioCalamar, Figueres/Berlin

Printed on acid-free paper

Springer is part of Springer Science+Business Media (www.springer.com)

Foreword

Computed tomography has been going through a dramatic evolution of technology in the past years. The increased spatial and temporal resolution directly translate into improved image quality and more versatile applications. Indeed, entirely new areas of clinical application have emerged, one of the most prominent being the recent advent of cardiac computed tomography. Especially CT angiography of the coronary arteries – often referred to as coronary CT angiography – has received tremendous interest and is currently entering the clinical arena. In fact, it has the potential to greatly alter the way in which many patients with suspected coronary artery disease will be worked up. However, the technique is still relatively new to the medical community. Furthermore, in the recent past several developments – such as substantial further improvement of scanner technology and the extensive use of low-dose acquisition protocols – have been introduced and will influence the utilization of cardiac CT. At this stage, it is crucial that all those potentially involved in the new imaging technology – those who perform and interpret the scan and also those who order a cardiac CT and advise their patients as to whether a CT examination might be the right test for them – are well informed about the technology and answers it can provide, about its limitations and problems, and about how to best apply it in a given clinical situation.

This is why the textbook edited by Dr. Dewey is most welcome. With ample illustrations, it provides the technological background and principles of scan acquisition and interpretation as well as outlines the range of clinical applications of cardiac CT. May it be a useful resource to its readers and may it contribute towards the further development of this exciting field.

Erlangen, Germany   Stephan Achenbach
Baltimore MD, USA   Elliot K Fishman
April 2010

Acknowledgments

We thank our patients, without whom we would not be able to conduct our clinical work and studies to continuously increase our understanding of the clinical utility of cardiac CT.

We are indebted to our technicians, assistants, and nurses at the Department of Radiology of the Charité – Universitätsmedizin Berlin for their contributions to the success of our clinical cardiovascular imaging program. Without their support, this book would not have been possible. The editorial assistance of Bettina Herwig and Deborah McClellan has been instrumental in writing this book. Stephanie Kreutzer has created beautiful artwork to illustrate essential concepts and approaches.

The excellent collaboration with the Department of Cardiology and Angiology at the Charité (Chairman: Professor Gert Baumann, Vice Chairman: Professor Karl Stangl) has tremendously facilitated this work. We thank Professor Wolfgang Rutsch, who has headed the cardiac catheterization laboratory at the Charité (Campus Mitte) for several years, and his coworkers Dr. Adrian Borges, Dr. Hans-Peter Dübel, Dr. Michael Laule, Dr. Christoph Melzer, Professor Verena Stangl, and Professor Heinz Theres for providing the majority of the conventional invasive angiograms presented in this book.

I wholeheartedly thank Drs. Martina and Charles Dewey.

Berlin, Germany
June 2010

Marc Dewey

Contents

Contributors

Marc Dewey, PD Dr. med.
CharitéCentrum 06 für diagnostische und
interventionelle Radiologie und Nuklearmedizin
Institut für Radiologie
CCM, Charitéplatz 1, 10117 Berlin
Germany
Email: dewey@charite.de

Gerd Adam, Prof. Dr. med.
Universitätsklinikum Hamburg-Eppendorf
Diagnostikzentrum Klinik und
Poliklinik für Diagnostische und
Interventionelle Radiologie
20246 Hamburg
Germany
Email: g.adam@uke.uni-hamburg.de

Katharina Anders, Dr. med.
Universitätsklinikum Erlangen
Radiologisches Institut
Maximiliansplatz 1, 91054 Erlangen
Germany
E-mail: katharina.anders@uk-erlangen.de

Raoul Arnold, Dr.med.
Universitätsklinikum Freiburg, Zentrum für
Kinderheilkunde und Jugendmedizin
Klinik III: Angeborene Herzfehler/Pädiatrische
Kardiologie, Mathildenstr. 1, 79106 Freiburg
Germany
Email: raoul.arnold@uniklinik-freiburg.de

Philipp G.C. Begemann, PD Dr. med.
Röntgeninstitut Düsseldorf
Kaiserswerther Strasse 89
40476 Düsseldorf, Germany
Email: p.begemann@roentgeninstitut.de

Adrian Constantin Borges, PD Dr. med.
HELIOS Klinikum Emil von Behring – Klinik für
Innere Medizin I Kardiologie und Diabetologie
Walterhöferstr. 11, 14165 Berlin
Germany
Email: adrian.borges@helios-kliniken.de

Gudrun Feuchtner, Ao. Univ.-Prof. Dr. med.
Institut für Radiologie II
Medizinische Universität Innsbruck
Anichstr. 35, A-6020 Innsbruck
Austria
Email: Gudrun.Feuchtner@i-med.ac.at

Jacob Geleijns, PhD
Leids Universitair Medisch Centrum
Afdeling Radiologie, Postbus 9600
2300 RC Leiden
The Netherlands
Email: k.geleijns@lumc.nl

Thomas Gerber, MD, PhD
Division of Cardiovascular Diseases
Mayo Clinic, 4500 San Pablo Road
Jacksonville, FL 32224
USA
Email: gerber.thomas@mayo.edu

Maria Grigoryev, Dr. med.
CharitéCentrum 06 für diagnostische und
interventionelle Radiologie und Nuklearmedizin
Institut für Radiologie, CCM, Charitéplatz 1
10117 Berlin
Germany
Email: maria.grigoryev@charite.de

Bernd Hamm, Prof. Dr. med.
CharitéCentrum 06 für diagnostische und
interventionelle Radiologie und Nuklearmedizin
Institut für Radiologie, CCM
Charitéplatz 1, 10117 Berlin
Germany
Email: bernd.hamm@charite.de

Martin K. Hoffmann, Prof. Dr. med.
Klinik für Diagnostische und interventionelle
Radiologie, Universitätsklinikum Ulm
Steinhövelstraße 9, 89075 Ulm
Germany
Email: martin.hoffmann@uniklinik-ulm.de

Oliver Klass, Dr. med.
Klinik für Diagnostische und
Interventionelle Radiologie
Universitätsklinikum Ulm
Steinhövelstraße 9, 89075 Ulm
Germany
Email: oliver.klass@uniklinik-ulm.de

Christian Klessen, Dr. med.
CharitéCentrum 06 für diagnostische und
Interventionelle Radiologie und Nuklearmedizin
Institut für Radiologie
CCM Charitéplatz 1
10117 Berlin
Germany
Email: christian@klessen.net

Lucia J.M. Kroft, Dr.
Leids Universitair Medisch Centrum
Afdeling Radiologie, Postbus 9600
2300 RC Leiden
The Netherlands
Email: L.J.M.Kroft@lumc.nl

Lukas Lehmkuhl, Dr. med.
Universität Leipzig - Herzzentrum
Diagnostische und Interventionelle Radiologie
Strümpellstrasse 39
04289 Leipzig
Germany
Email: lukas.lehmkuhl@med.uni-leipzig.de

Sebastian Ley, PD Dr. med.
Diagnostische und Interventionelle Radiologie
Universitätsklinik Heidelberg
Im Neuenheimer Feld 430
69120 Heidelberg
Germany
Email: ley@gmx.net

Gunnar Lund, PD Dr. med.
Universitätsklinikum Hamburg-Eppendorf
Diagnostikzentrum Klinik und Poliklinik für
Diagnostische und Interventionelle Radiologie
20246 Hamburg
Germany
Email: g.lund@uke.uni-hamburg.de

Eugenio Martuscelli
University of Rome "Tor Vergata"
Department of Internal Medicine
Division of Cardiology
Viale Oxford 81, 00133 Rome
Italy
Email: e.martuscelli@libero.it

Koen Nieman, MD, PhD
Erasmus Medical Center
Departments of Cardiology and Radiology
Thoraxcenter Bd 434, Dr Molewaterplein 40
30 15 GC Rotterdam
The Netherlands
Email: koennieman@hotmail.com

Hiroyuki Niinuma, MD, PhD
Iwate Medical University, Memorial Heart Center
1-2-1 ChuoDori, Morioka
Iwate, 020-8505
Japan
Email: h_niinuma@imu.ncvc.go.jp

Paul Schoenhagen, MD
Division of Radiology, Cardiovascular Imaging
and Department of Cardiovascular Medicine
The Cleveland Clinic Foundation
9500 Euclid Cleveland, OH44195
USA
Email: schoenp1@ccf.org

Karl Stangl, Prof. Dr. med.
CharitéCentrum 13 für Innere Medizin
mit Kardiologie, Gastroenterologie
Nephrologie
Medizinische Klinik mit Schwerpunkt
Kardiologie und Angiologie
CCM, Charitéplatz 1
10117 Berlin
Germany
Email: karl.stangl@charite.de

Florian Wolf, Dr. med.
Medizinische Universität Wien, Universitätsklinik für
Radiodiagnostik, Abteilung für Kardiovaskuläre und
Interventionelle Radiologie
Währinger Gürtel 18-20
A-1090 Wien
Austria
Email: florian.wolf@meduniwien.ac.at

Elke Zimmermann, Dr. med.
CharitéCentrum 06 für diagnostische und
interventionelle Radiologie und Nuklearmedizin
Institut für Radiologie
CCM, Charitéplatz 1
10117 Berlin
Germany
Email: elke.zimmermann@charite.de

Introduction

B. Hamm

The advent of multislice computed tomography was a quantum leap for CT technology. When this technical innovation was first introduced, the radiological community was faced with the task of putting its advantages to use for diagnostic patient management and optimizing its clinical applications. One of the major clinical challenges was to develop this new tool for noninvasive cardiac imaging applications ranging from coronary angiography, to ventricular function analysis, to cardiac valve evaluation.

Marc Dewey and the authors of the book have closely followed the development of this new generation of CT scanners in the clinical setting, in scientific studies, and in experimental investigations. The team of authors has gained a wealth of experience spanning CT from 16-row technology to the most recent generation of 320-row CT scanners. In their scientific investigations, the authors have always placed great emphasis on a critical appraisal of this emerging imaging modality in comparison to well-established diagnostic tests such as coronary angiography, magnetic resonance imaging, and echocardiography, also including the socioeconomic perspective. The close cooperation with the Departments of Cardiology and Cardiac Surgery of the Charité – Universitätsmedizin Berlin was pivotal for obtaining valid results in both clinical examinations and scientific studies and also led to many improvements of the diagnostic workflow.

This book focuses on how to integrate cardiac CT into routine practice. Readers will learn how to perform noninvasive imaging of the heart using CT and how to interpret the images. A clear overview of the essentials is given, and numerous clinical cardiac CT cases are presented for illustration.

All steps involved in cardiac CT examination are described in detail, including patient preparation, the actual examination, and analysis and interpretation of the findings. *Cardiac CT* is based on an earlier book – *Coronary CT Angiography* – but also updates all chapters of this book and includes completely new chapters on radiation exposure, clinical practice, coronary artery stents, bypass grafts, coronary anomalies, and congenital heart disease. Separate chapters discuss upcoming clinical applications of cardiac CT – plaque imaging and assessment of cardiac functions and valves. Another asset of the book in terms of practical clinical application is that the authors present and discuss the specific features of the CT scanners from all four major vendors as they relate to cardiac imaging. In a final chapter, an outlook is given on conceivable future technical and clinical developments.

I congratulate the team of authors on an excellent book that focuses on the practical clinical aspects of cardiac CT and offers its readers an easy to follow introduction to this promising new diagnostic tool. However, the book also provides useful tips and tricks for those already familiar with this imaging modality, which will help them further improve their diagnostic strategy for the benefit of their patients.

M. Dewey, *Cardiac CT*,
DOI: 10.1007/978-3-642-14022-8_1, © Springer-Verlag Berlin Heidelberg 2011

Technical and Personnel Requirements

M. Dewey

List 2.1. Technical requirements for cardiac CT

1. CT scanner with at least 64 simultaneous rows
2. CT scanner with a gantry rotation time of below 400 ms
3. Adaptive multisegment reconstruction or dual-source CT
4. ECG for gating and triggering[a] of acquisitions
5. Dual-head contrast agent injector for saline flush
6. Workstation with automatic curved multiplanar reformation and three-dimensional data segmentation and analysis capabilities

---

[a] This refers to the acquisition method: retrospective (ECG gating) or prospective (ECG triggering). See Chap. 8 for details on radiation exposure reduction using ECG triggering

Abstract

In this chapter, we summarize the requirements for setting up a cardiac CT practice.

2.1 Technical Requirements

Noninvasive coronary angiography is an ascending clinical application that requires very high spatial and temporal resolution. Thus, CT scanners with multiple detector rows (multislice CT [MSCT]), short gantry rotation times, and thin-slice collimation are essential for establishing a successful cardiac CT imaging center. Because 64-row CT is superior to 16-row CT in terms of image quality and diagnostic accuracy, we believe that (at least) 64-row technology should be used for noninvasive coronary angiography (**List 2.1**). CT with 64-row technology not only increases the quality of the images (**Figs. 2.1–2.3**) but also improves the workflow because scanning and breath-hold times are shorter (**Table 2.1**). Even greater improvements can be achieved with imaging during a single heartbeat (**Table 2.1** and **Fig. 2.2**), which is feasible with 320-row volume CT and second-generation dual-source CT (Chaps. 10a and 10b). The shorter breath-hold time of 64-row CT and single-beat imaging is also very relevant for patients after coronary bypass grafting (**Fig. 2.4**, Chap. 12). The faster gantry rotation speed of recent CT scanners (**List 2.1**) improves temporal resolution and dramatically reduces the likelihood of relevant motion artifacts.

Temporal resolution can be significantly improved by using two simultaneous X-ray sources (dual-source CT, Siemens) and adaptive multisegment reconstruction (Toshiba and Philips). We believe that one of these two approaches should be implemented on cardiac CT scanners to reduce the influence of heart rate on image quality (**List 2.1**). In addition to these technical improvements, beta blocker administration should be used whenever possible to lower the heart rate to below approximately 65 beats per min, because slowing the heart rate to this level further improves both the image quality and the diagnostic accuracy (Chaps. 7 and 9) while also reducing radiation exposure because ECG triggering can be used (Chap. 8). Finally, an ECG, a dual-head contrast agent injector, and an automatic three-dimensional analysis workstation are required for cardiac CT (**List 2.1**).

M. Dewey, *Cardiac CT*,
DOI: 10.1007/978-3-642-14022-8_2, © Springer-Verlag Berlin Heidelberg 2011

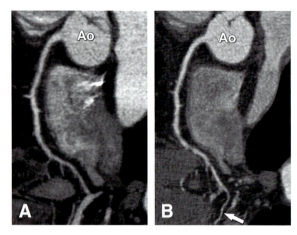

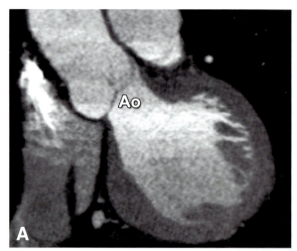

Fig. 2.1 Comparison of 16-row (**Panel A**) and 64-row CT coronary angiography (**Panel B**) of the right coronary artery (curved multiplanar reformation) in a 61-year-old male patient. 64-row CT shows longer vessel segments, especially in the periphery (*arrow*). This enhanced performance can be explained by fewer motion artifacts (due to breathing, extrasystoles, or variations in the length of the cardiac cycle) and the better contrast between arteries and veins resulting from the faster scan and consequently better depiction of the arterial phase. The improved depiction of the arterial phase using 64-row CT is also demonstrated in **Fig. 2.2**. **Panel B** also illustrates the slightly higher image noise with 64-row CT, which can be compensated for by the better depiction of the arterial phase and the higher intravascular density. *Ao* aorta

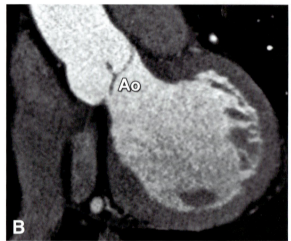

Fig. 2.2 The improved depiction of the arterial phase using 64-row CT (**Panel B**) and even further using 320-row CT (**Panel C**) when compared with 16-row CT (**Panel A**) is illustrated by a double-oblique coronal slice along the left ventricular outflow tract, with the aortic valve nicely depicted (Ao). In the craniocaudal direction, the density in the aorta and left ventricle shows less variation and decline when 64 simultaneous detector rows are used (**Panel B**) and almost no difference with 320-row CT acquired during a single heartbeat. Use of 64- and 320-row CT thus improves image quality and facilitates the application of automatic coronary vessel and cardiac function analysis tools

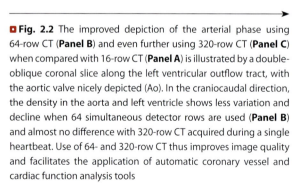

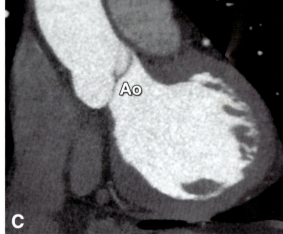

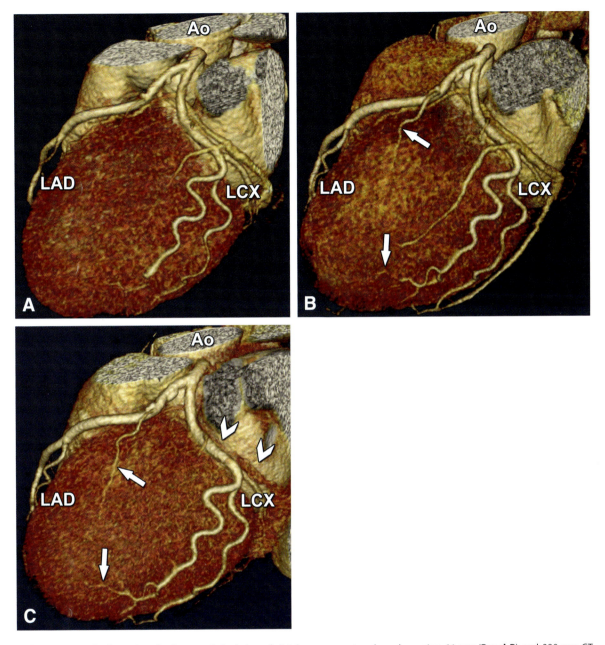

⬛ **Fig. 2.3** Example illustrating the improved depiction of distal coronary artery branches using 64-row (**Panel B**) and 320-row CT (**Panel C**) in a 58-year-old female patient. Three-dimensional volume-rendered reconstructions of the left coronary artery with the left anterior descending (LAD) and left circumflex coronary artery (LCX) examined using 16-row (**Panel A**), 64-row (**Panel B**), and 320-row CT coronary angiography (**Panel C**). Note the improved depiction of smaller side branches with the 64-row (*arrows* in **Panel B**) and 320-row technology (*arrows* in **Panel C**) when compared with the same segments in 16-row CT (**Panel A**). Also, there is best depiction of the arterial phase (with less venous overlap, *arrowheads* in **Panel C**) using 320-row CT. Single-beat imaging using 320-row CT or second-generation dual-source CT with a fast prospective spiral also greatly reduces radiation exposure (Chap. 8). *Ao* aorta

2

□ **Table 2.1** Typical characteristics of 16- and 64-row as well as single-heartbeat CT scanners

	16-row	64-row	Single heart beat CT[a]
Slice collimation			
Coronary arteries	0.5–0.75 mm	0.5–0.75 mm	0.5–0.6 mm
Coronary bypass grafts	0.5–1.25 mm	0.5–0.75 mm	0.5–0.6 mm
Gantry rotation time			
Coronary angiography	0.4–0.6 s	0.27–0.4 s	0.28–0.35 s
Scan length			
Coronary arteries	9–13 cm	Increase by 15%[b]	9–13 cm
Coronary bypass grafts	12.5–22 cm	Increased by 5–10%	12.5–22 cm[c]
Effective radiation dose			
Coronary arteries	5–15 mSv	10–20 mSv[d]	1–5 mSv
Coronary bypass grafts	10–30 mSv	20–40 mSv[d]	2–10 mSv
Contrast-to-noise ratio			
Coronary angiography	15–25	Similar	Similar
Vessel lengths free of motion			
Coronary angiography		Improved by 10–30%[e]	Further improvements expected
Breath-hold time[f]			
Coronary arteries	25–30 s	8–12 s	3 s
Coronary bypass grafts	40–50 s	12–15 s	5 s
Contrast agent amount			
Coronary arteries	90–130 ml	60–90 ml	40–70 ml
Coronary bypass grafts	130–160 ml	80–110 ml	50–80 ml

[a] CT of the heart during a single beat can be performed using 320-row volume CT (Chap. 10a) and second-generation dual-source CT with a fast spiral acquisition (Chap. 10b)

[b] This increase is due to the larger overranging effect of 64-row CT, which in turn also increases radiation exposure by 15%

[c] Bypass grafts are scanned with 320-row CT in two heartbeats and with dual-source CT in the caudocranial direction with the proximal parts of the bypass grafts covered during the next R-wave and early systole of the next beat

[d] The values given here are for retrospectively acquired data. The increase in effective dose with 64-row CT can be explained by the larger over-ranging effect, the fact that scanning cannot be stopped as abruptly once the lower border of the heart has been reached because of the faster table speed, and the higher mA settings necessary (because of the increased scattered radiation and noise with 64-row CT). Using prospectively acquired data with 64-row CT, effective dose can be drastically reduced to below 5 mSv in nearly all patients with stable and low heart rates (<65 beats per minute). See Chap. 8

[e] The increase in the visible vessel length free of motion that can be obtained for the three coronary arteries with 64-row CT scanners is approximately 10% for the left anterior descending, 20% for the left circumflex, and 30% for the right coronary. Most notably, in more than one-third of all cases, the length of the right coronary free of motion is increased by more than 5 cm when 64-row CT is used

[f] This includes a 2–3 s wait period after the breathing command before scanning to assure normalization of heart rate after inspiration

least 64-row technology is clearly needed. The decision to purchase a scanner from any particular manufacturer not only depends on its meeting the relevant technical criteria, such as those mentioned earlier, but will definitely also be influenced by local pricing policies and, more important, by the quality of the maintenance and service support (**List 2.2**). How to perform cardiac CT exams using scanners from the four main vendors is explained in Chap. 10.

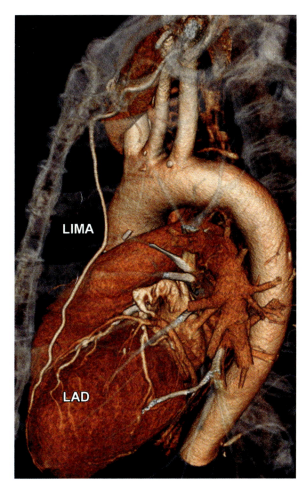

◻ Fig. 2.4 Arterial bypass graft (left internal mammary artery, LIMA), which extends all the way down to the LAD and was scanned in less than 15 s, using a 64-row CT scanner. With this technology, preoxygenation is no longer necessary for bypass imaging. With 16-row technology, the scanning took an average of 40–50 s, and preoxygenation was almost always required. Note that CT nicely depicts the distance between the sternum and coronary bypass graft, which can be of relevance if repeat cardiac surgery is considered. Bypass imaging time can be further shortened with 320-row CT and second-generation dual-source CT (**Table 2.1**)

> **List 2.2. Factors to consider in deciding to purchase a particular CT scanner**
>
> 1. Local situation and mixture of different examination types
> 2. Quality of technical and maintenance support
> 3. Availability of high temporal and spatial resolution
> 4. Quality and durability of the application support
> 5. Integration into existing picture archiving and communication systems
> 6. Local pricing policies

Multislice CT has a variety of other applications in addition to cardiac imaging, and CT scanners used solely for cardiac applications are very unlikely to reach the break-even point. Thus, we believe that a mixture of different CT applications is a prerequisite for clinical and economic success. In the US, the Center for Medicare and Medicaid Services (CMS) recently decided after an extensive review that no Medicare national coverage of coronary CT angiography is appropriate at this time. In the decision memo, it is concluded that no adequately powered study has established that improved health outcomes can be causally attributed to coronary CT angiography for any well-defined clinical indication. Thus, coverage will be determined by local contractors through the local coverage determination process or case-by-case adjudication. Effective January 1, 2010, the American Medical Association (AMA) released the new Current Procedural Terminology (CPT) Category I codes for cardiac CT with four new codes. These replace the previous Category III CPT codes for cardiac CT, which listed cardiac CT examinations as "emerging technology." Chapter 5 discusses cardiac CT in clinical practice and Chap. 6 presents clinically most relevant indications for cardiac CT.

2.2 Purchasing a Scanner

The purchase costs of CT scanners still differ enormously. For applications other than cardiac imaging, 16-row CT scanners are clearly sufficient to answer the vast majority of clinical questions. For cardiac applications, however, at

2

2.3   Personnel Requirements

Having well-trained technicians who are knowledgeable in cardiac CT applications is a prerequisite for success (**List 2.3**). It is better to have a limited number of specialized technicians who perform cardiac CT than to have all technicians perform this test. On the one hand, having specialized staff members can ensure a consistently high level of image quality, and these experienced technicians can assist in further educating other coworkers about the entire scanning and reconstruction procedure. On the other hand, if more technicians are involved in performing cardiac CT, coronary CT angiography can easily be offered at night; doing so, however, also requires a physician trained in reading the images 24 by 7. What we consider most helpful in terms of training is to give constant feedback to the technicians about good as well as bad examinations. This approach ensures that a high level of quality is maintained, and small mistakes are prevented from creeping in. Moreover, providing positive feedback about high-quality examinations is very motivating.

List 2.3. Personnel requirements for cardiac CT

1. Well-trained and experienced CT technicians
2. Physician knowledgeable in CT and radiation exposure
3. Physician knowledgeable in cardiac anatomy and pathophysiology
4. Team focused on quality assurance

There are two major prerequisites for physicians, in addition to good anatomical, technical (incl. radiation issues), and clinical knowledge: (1) a clear understanding of the entire examination procedure, and (2) the ability to independently interpret three-dimensional cardiac CT datasets on workstations.

Chapters 7 and 9 will discuss how to prepare the patient for cardiac CT and how to perform the procedure. Being present during examinations is the key to understanding the work of the technicians and the special requirements of cardiac CT. It is also enlightening for physicians to perform examinations themselves, because doing so can yield important insights into the procedural steps and problems that can be encountered during scanning. This hands-on training also strengthens the position of the physician as an educator of other physicians or technicians. In larger centers, it is good to identify two to three doctors who will be considered the primary contacts for cardiac CT imaging for the technicians as well as the referring physicians.

Competence in image interpretation is best achieved by correlating conventional coronary angiograms with CT angiography results. How to read and interpret cardiac CT scans is explained in Chap. 11. To understand and gain skill in using the workstations, physicians should practice operating them without time pressure. The time necessary to feel comfortable with the workstations will depend on an individual's general computer skills, but 2–4 continuous weeks should be sufficient, and attending one of the true hands-on courses is a good way to begin the learning process. Such workshops should ideally offer direct comparison of CT findings (on interactive workstations) with conventional coronary angiography or the results of cardiac stress tests. This is the only way of acquiring a thorough understanding of coronary and cardiac pathology. Good cardiac CT courses and fellowships also offer active participation in patient preparation and scanning. Nevertheless, the learning curve for centers with some prior experience has been shown to last at least 6 months before the diagnostic accuracy stabilizes, and the learning curve of individuals with little prior exposure is considerable (at least about 12 months).

Moreover, learning does not stop after a few weeks of intensive familiarization with the workstations or a short course: Even in a team of experienced readers, certain coronary lesions will sometimes be misinterpreted (overcalled or even overlooked). Thus, continuous learning efforts with comparison of CT to the invasive coronary angiography findings, e.g., in joint interdisciplinary conferences, are necessary to maintain high quality.

There is also a formal accreditation of the physicians' skills and knowledge. The American College of Radiology (ACR) and the American College of Cardiology (ACC) have established guidelines for assessing clinical competence in performing and interpreting cardiac CT. These guidelines play an increasing role in obtaining certification and claiming reimbursement in the US. Those outside the US may find it useful to study these guidelines as a basis for starting discussions about certification of cardiac CT readers and centers in their own countries.

In Germany, for instance, the law requires that every physician performing CT (of any organ) hold the *Fachkunde* ("technical qualification") for CT, which requires having conducted 1,000 examinations over a period of at least 12 months and participating in a course on radiation protection. Such regulations offer promise for reducing patient radiation exposure and they emphasize the relevance of the ongoing discussion on requirements for cardiac CT.

2.3.1 Guidelines of the ACR

Several ACR guidelines are relevant to coronary CT angiography. Most important is the "ACR Practice Guideline for the Performance and Interpretation of Cardiac Computed Tomography" (http://www.acr.org/ SecondaryMainMenuCategories/quality_safety/guidelines/dx/cardio/ct_cardiac.aspx). Other important guidelines are the "ACR Clinical Statement on Noninvasive Cardiac Imaging," "ACR Practice Guideline for the Performance and Interpretation of CT Angiography," and the "ACR Practice Guideline for Performing and Interpreting Diagnostic Computed Tomography." Later we briefly outline and discuss the recommendations arising from the guidelines that directly relate to coronary CT angiography.

The ACR defines cardiac CT as a chest CT performed primarily for the evaluation of the heart (including the cardiac chambers, valves, myocardium, aorta, central pulmonary vessels, pericardium, coronary arteries, and veins). However, noncardiac structures are included and must be evaluated by a trained physician. Trained physicians are defined in the "ACR Practice Guideline for Performing and Interpreting Diagnostic Computed Tomography" as board-certified radiologists who have interpreted and reported at least 100 CT examinations over each of the past 3 years and interpret and report at least 100 CT examinations per year to maintain competence. These physicians can achieve competence in the performance and interpretation of coronary CT angiography by at least 30 h of CME in cardiac anatomy, physiology, pathology, and cardiac CT, plus the interpretation, reporting, and/or supervised review of at least 50 cardiac CT examinations during the past 3 years (**Table 2.2**). Physicians who are not defined in this guideline as trained physicians in diagnostic CT can achieve competence in the performance and interpretation of coronary CT angiography by at least 200 h of CME in the performance and interpretation of cardiac CT, plus the interpretation, reporting, and/or supervised review of at least 500 chest CT examinations (including 50 cardiac CT examinations) during the past 3 years (**Table 2.2**). The ACR stresses that all physicians performing cardiac CT need to be knowledgeable about the administration, risks, and contraindications of beta blockers and nitroglycerin.

2.3.2 Guidelines of the ACC

The "ACC Clinical Competence Statement on Cardiac Imaging with Computed Tomography and Magnetic Resonance" (http://www.cbcct.org/resources/ CT_CMRcompetency.pdf) states that it is intended to be complementary to the recommendations of the ACR on

◻ Table 2.2 ACR physician requirements for coronary CT angiography

	Not trained in general or thoracic CT	Board-certified radiologists[a]
CME (category I)	Completion of an ACGME approved training program in the specialty practiced	Training in cardiac CT in an ACGME approved training program
	200 h in cardiac CT[b]	30 h in cardiac anatomy, physiology, pathology, and cardiac CT
Interpretation, reporting, and/or supervised review[c]	500 CT examinations[d]	50 cardiac CT examinations
Maintaining competence	75 contrast-enhanced cardiac CT examinations every 3 years 150 h of CME every 3 years	

ACGME Accreditation Council for Graduate Medical Education

[a] In addition, at least 100 CT examinations are required during each of the past 3 years, as also at least 100 CT examinations per year to maintain competence according to the ACR practice guideline for performing and interpreting diagnostic CT

[b] Including at least 30 h in cardiac anatomy, physiology, pathology, and cardiac CT

[c] Examinations (noncontrast examinations do not count) in a supervised environment during the past 3 years; supervising physician needs to meet the ACR requirements

[d] At least 100 must be a combination of thoracic CT or thoracic CT angiography (exclusive of calcium scoring exams). At least 50 contrast-enhanced cardiac CT examinations must also be included

2

◘ **Table 2.3** ACC physician requirements for coronary CT angiography

	Level 2[a]	Level 3[b]
CME (category I)	20 h in cardiac CT	40 h in cardiac CT
Training[c]	8 weeks	6 months
Interpretation, reporting, and/or supervised review	50 noncontrast and 150 contrast-enhanced cardiac CT examinations[d]	100 noncontrast and 300 contrast-enhanced cardiac CT examinations[d]
Maintaining competence	50 contrast-enhanced cardiac CT examinations every year, 20 h of CME in cardiac CT every 3 years	100 contrast-enhanced cardiac CT examinations every year, 40 h of CME in cardiac CT every 3 years

[a] Allows independent performance and interpretation of cardiac CT

[b] Allows serving as a director of an independent cardiac CT center

[c] Training must be conducted under the supervision of a level 3 physician. Each week consists of at least 35 h. The time commitment does not go into effect until July 2010

[d] Physically present and involved in the acquisition, performance, and interpretation of 50 (level 2) or 100 (level 3) contrast-enhanced cardiac CT examinations. The noncontrast examinations can be performed in the same patients who undergo contrast-enhanced CT

noninvasive cardiac imaging. Cardiac CT is defined in this guideline as the imaging of anatomy, function, coronary calcium, noncalcified plaque, and congenital heart disease. The guideline defines three levels of competence in coronary CT angiography, of which two are relevant here. Level 2 allows independent performance and interpretation of cardiac CT and requires 8 weeks (each consisting of at least 35 h) of cumulative training in a clinical cardiac CT laboratory plus 150 contrast-enhanced and 50 noncontrast cardiac CT examinations. A physician willing to achieve level 2 competence needs to be physically present and involved in the acquisition and performance of 50 of the 150 contrast-enhanced cardiac CT examinations (**Table 2.3**). Level 3 allows serving as a director of an independent cardiac CT center and requires 6 months of cumulative training in a clinical cardiac CT laboratory plus 300 contrast-enhanced and 100 noncontrast cardiac CT examinations. A physician willing to achieve level 3 competence needs to be physically present and involved in the acquisition and performance of 100 of the 300 contrast-enhanced cardiac CT examinations (**Table 2.3**). An additional recommendation for "Training in Advanced Cardiovascular Imaging (Computed Tomography)" has been released by the ACC. The ACC stresses that all physicians performing cardiac CT need to be knowledgeable about radiation risks and noncardiac findings on coronary CT angiography. Interestingly, Pugliese et al. have recently shown that it may take more than 12 months of full-time training in cardiac CT for a novice to acquire moderate expertise

and they conclude that the levels of training suggested by the ACC may thus be insufficient to become an independent practitioner of cardiac CT. However, the debate is ongoing and further recommendations are expected.

Recommended Reading

1   Achenbach S, Chandrashekhar Y, Narula J (2008) Computed tomographic angiography and the Atlantic. JACC Cardiovasc Imaging 1:817–819

2   Budoff MJ, Achenbach S, Berman DS et al (2008) Task force 13: training in advanced cardiovascular imaging (computed tomography) endorsed by the American Society of Nuclear Cardiology, Society of Atherosclerosis Imaging and Prevention, Society for Cardiovascular Angiography and Interventions, and Society of Cardiovascular Computed Tomography. J Am Coll Cardiol 51:409–414

3   Budoff MJ, Cohen MC, Garcia MJ et al (2005) ACCF/AHA clinical competence statement on cardiac imaging with computed tomography and magnetic resonance. J Am Coll Cardiol 46:383–402

4   Chin S, Ong T, Chan W et al (2006) 64 row multi-detector computed tomography coronary image from a centre with early experience: first illustration of learning curve. J Geriatric Cardiol 3:29–34

5   Dewey M, Hamm B (2007) Cost effectiveness of coronary angiography and calcium scoring using CT and stress MRI for diagnosis of coronary artery disease. Eur Radiol 17:1301–1309

6   Dewey M, Hoffmann H, Hamm B (2007) CT coronary angiography using 16 and 64 simultaneous detector rows: intraindividual comparison. Fortschr Röntgenstr 179:581–586

7   Hamon M, Morello R, Riddell JW (2007) Coronary arteries: diagnostic performance of 16- versus 64-section spiral CT compared with invasive coronary angiography–meta-analysis. Radiology 245: 720–731

8   Hausleiter J, Meyer T, Hadamitzky M et al (2007) Non-invasive coronary computed tomographic angiography for patients with suspected coronary artery disease: the Coronary Angiography by Computed Tomography with the Use of a Submillimeter resolution (CACTUS) trial. Eur Heart J 28:3034–3041

9   Jacobs JE, Boxt LM, Desjardins B, Fishman EK, Larson PA, Schoepf J (2006) ACR practice guideline for the performance and interpretation of cardiac computed tomography (CT). J Am Coll Radiol 3:677–685

10   Pannu HK, Alvarez W Jr, Fishman EK (2006) Beta-blockers for cardiac CT: a primer for the radiologist. AJR Am J Roentgenol 186:S341–S345

11   Pugliese F, Hunink MG, Gruszczynska K et al (2009) Learning curve for coronary CT angiography: what constitutes sufficient training? Radiology 251:359–368

12   Weinreb JC, Larson PA, Woodard PK et al (2005) ACR clinical statement on noninvasive cardiac imaging. J Am Coll Radiol 2:471–477

The ACR practice guideline for the performance and interpretation of cardiac CT (Jacobs et al.) can be accessed at:
http://www.acr.org/SecondaryMainMenuCategories/quality_safety/guidelines/dx/cardio/ct_cardiac.aspx
The guideline of the ACC (Budoff et al.) can be accessed at:
http://www.cbcct.org/resources/CT_CMRcompetency.pdf
http://www.escr.org
http://www.nasci.org
http://www.scct.org

Anatomy

M. Dewey and L.J.M. Kroft

Abstract

This chapter reviews coronary and myocardial anatomy and stresses its relevance to cardiac CT.

3.1 Coronary Arteries

The major coronary arteries, together with their second-order branches, can usually be well-visualized by CT. Third-order branches may be visualized, but smaller branches are generally not visible because of their small size and the limitations of the scanner with regard to spatial and temporal resolution.

In the normal situation, the coronary arteries arise from the proximal aorta. The right and left coronary arteries arise from the right and left sinus of Valsalva, respectively. The noncoronary sinus of Valsalva is usually the posterior one. The main coronary artery segments run in the left and right atrioventricular grooves between the atria and ventricles, and then perpendicularly in the anterior and posterior interventricular grooves between the left and right ventricles (**Fig. 3.1**). The coronary arteries and their side branches vary greatly in terms of their presence or absence and their size, shape, and length. A pragmatic approach that can help understand the relationship between the heart and the three-dimensional coronary artery anatomy uses the demonstrator's left and right hand for illustration (**Fig. 3.2**).

The right coronary artery (RCA) arises from the aorta at the right sinus of Valsalva and courses in the right atrioventricular groove. Along its course, it first gives off the conus artery (in 50% of all individuals; in the other 50%, the conus artery arises directly from the aorta). It then gives off the sinoatrial node artery (in roughly 60%; in the remaining individuals, it arises from the left circumflex coronary artery [LCX]). Acute marginal branches arise from the mid-segment and posterior right ventricular branches from the distal segment. In case of a right-dominant circulation, the RCA gives rise to the posterior descending artery (PDA) at or near the crux cordis (where the left and right atrioventricular groove and posterior interventricular groove join), from where it courses in the posterior interventricular groove, and the RCA gives rise to posterolateral artery branches as it continues in the left atrioventicular groove beyond the crux. In case of a left-dominant circulation, the LCX gives rise to the PDA. The RCA supplies both the myocardium of the right atrium and ventricle and posterior portions of the left ventricle and interventricular septum.

The left main coronary artery (LM) arises from the aorta at the left sinus of Valsalva and has a length that varies from 0 to 15 mm. The LM usually bifurcates into the left anterior descending coronary artery (LAD) and LCX; however, in a third of the population, the LM ends as a trifurcation with an intermediate branch (IMB, also called ramus medianus) arising between the LAD and the LCX (**Fig. 3.3**). An IMB can be regarded as a diagonal branch or as an obtuse marginal branch, depending on its course along the left ventricle. In about 1% of the population, the LM is absent, and there are separate ostia for the LAD and LCX (**Fig. 3.3**).

The LAD courses in the anterior interventricular groove. The major branches of the LAD are the septal branches that pass downward into the interventricular septum and the diagonal branches (usually one to three are present) that pass over the anterolateral aspect of the heart. The LAD and its side branches supply the anterior

M. Dewey, *Cardiac CT*,
DOI: 10.1007/978-3-642-14022-8_3, © Springer-Verlag Berlin Heidelberg 2011

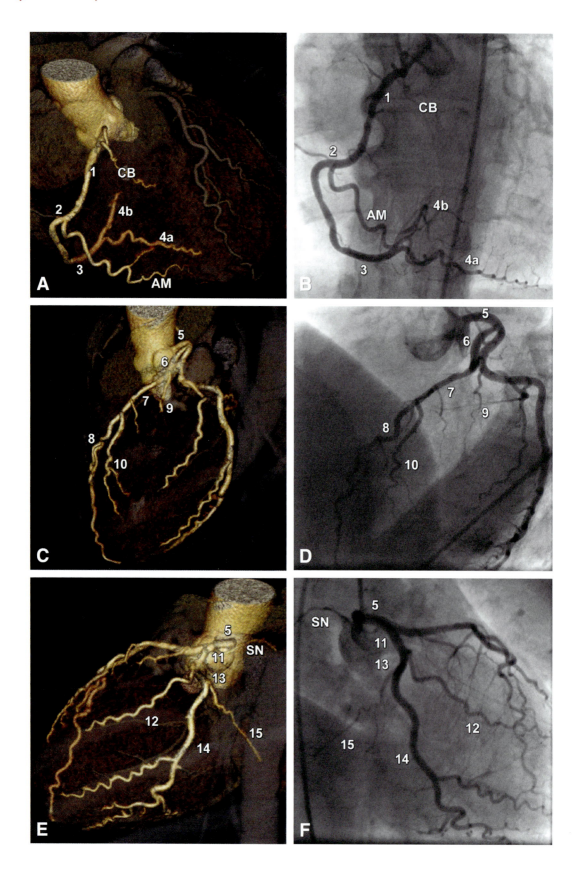

Fig. 3.1 Direct comparison of segmental coronary artery anatomy, as depicted by CT (*left panels*, three-dimensional reconstructions) and conventional coronary angiography (*right panels*). If an intermediate branch is present (about 30% of patients) this segmentation model consists of 17 segments. The RCA with its 5 segments is shown in **Panels A** and **B**, and the left coronary artery with its two main branches – the left anterior descending and the left circumflex – in **Panels C–F**. The RCA (**Panels A** and **B**) is composed of segments 1–4, with the distal segment (4) being further subdivided into 4a (posterior descending artery, PDA) and 4b (right posterolateral branch). The left main coronary artery (**Panels C–F**) is referred to as segment 5, and the left anterior descending coronary artery (**Panels C** and **D**) is composed of segments 6–10, with the two diagonal branches being segments 9 and 10. The LCX (**Panels E** and **F**) is composed of segments 11–15, with the two (obtuse) marginal branches being segments 12 and 14. Note that the distal left circumflex (segment 15) is rather small in this patient with a right-dominant coronary circulation. The sinus node artery (SN) is the first branch of the LCX in this patient (**Panels E** and **F**) but is more commonly one of the first branches of the RCA. *AM* acute marginal branch; *CB* conus branch. **Table 3.1** gives an overview of all coronary artery segment numbers and names

Table 3.1 Coronary artery anatomy using a 17-segment model[a]

Segment no.	Vessel name	Segment name
1	Right coronary artery (RCA)	Proximal right coronary
2		Mid right coronary
3		Distal right coronary
4a		Posterior descending artery[b]
4b		Right posterolateral branch[b]
5	Left main coronary artery (LM)	Left main coronary artery
6	Left anterior descending artery (LAD)	Proximal left anterior descending
7		Mid left anterior descending
8		Distal left anterior descending
9		First diagonal branch
10		Second diagonal branch
11	Left circumflex artery (LCX)	Proximal left circumflex
12		First (obtuse) marginal
13		Mid left circumflex
14		Second (obtuse) marginal
15		Distal left circumflex[b]
16	Intermediate branch[c]	Intermediate branch[c]

[a] This segmentation is based on the AHA segmentation published in 1975 by Austen et al.

[b] In case of RCA dominance, at least one right posterolateral branch (segment 4b) is present and supplies the inferolateral myocardial segments. If the left coronary artery is dominant, the distal LCX ends as the posterior descending coronary artery (segment 4a). In case of codominance, segment 4a is part of the RCA, and the distal left circumflex ends as a posterolateral branch after giving off two marginal branches

[c] An intermediate branch (ramus intermedius) is present in approximately 30% of patients and is the 17th segment in this model (note that the RCA has five segments with segment 4 being subdivided into 4a and 4b)

3

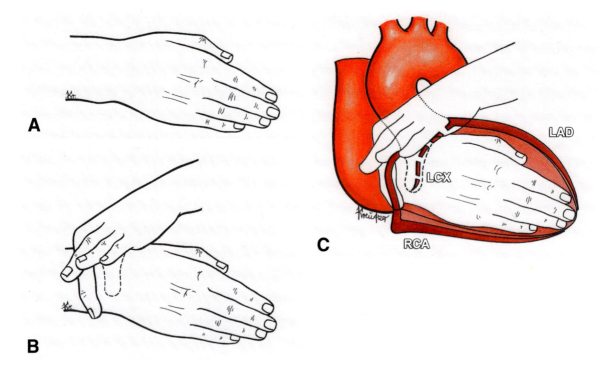

▫ **Fig. 3.2** Simple method of teaching three-dimensional coronary artery anatomy. The technique utilizes the concept of two imaginary circles around the interventricular and atrioventricular grooves, which are indicated by the position of the demonstrator's right and left hand, respectively. **Panel A** shows the right hand which demonstrates the position of the interventricular septum with its margins, the posterior and anterior interventricular groove. In **Panel B** the atrioventricular groove is represented by the thumb and index finger of the added left hand, which encircle the right wrist. The superimposed cardiac structures with the coronary arteries are shown in **Panel C**. *LAD* left anterior descending artery; *LCX* left circumflex coronary artery; *RCA* right coronary artery. Adapted from Sos and Sniderman Radiology 1980

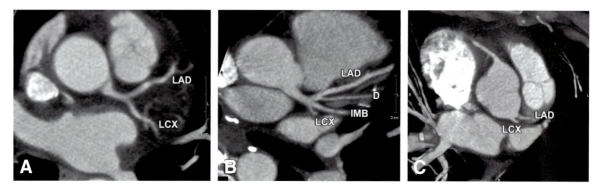

Fig. 3.3 Different types of left main coronary artery bifurcation. Oblique transverse thin-slab maximum-intensity projection images. The left main coronary artery is shown bifurcating into the left anterior descending coronary artery (LAD) and LCX (**Panel A**), the left main with trifurcation into the LAD and the LCX, and in between an intermediate branch (IMB, **Panel B**). Note the high diagonal branch (D) from the LAD (**Panel B**). An absent left main coronary artery, with separate origins for the LAD and LCX (**Panel C**)

as well as the anteroseptal and anterolateral left ventricular segments. The septal branches, in particular, serve as important collateral pathways.

The LCX courses in the left atrioventricular groove, where the major side branches are the obtuse marginal branches (usually one to three are present) that supply the lateral free wall of the left ventricle. The left atrial circumflex branches that supply the lateral and posterior aspect of the left atrium also arise from the LCX.

3.1.1   Coronary Artery Dominance

The circulation is right-dominant in about 60–85% of the population (the RCA gives rise to the posterior descending and at least one posterolateral branch). Left coronary dominance (the LCX gives rise to the PDA) is found in 7–20% of the population, whereas a balanced (or co-dominant) distribution is seen in 7–20% (the RCA gives rise to the PDA, and the LCX gives rise to posterolateral branches). In the case of a left-dominant circulation, the RCA is small and does not supply blood to the left ventricular myocardium. Recognizing the dominancy of the circulation is important, so as to avoid confusing this situation with branch occlusion (e.g., a short RCA in a left-dominant circulation, **Fig. 3.4**). Although it is the RCA that is typically dominant, it is usually the left coronary artery that supplies the major part of the left ventricular myocardium as well as the anterior and mid portions of the interventricular septum.

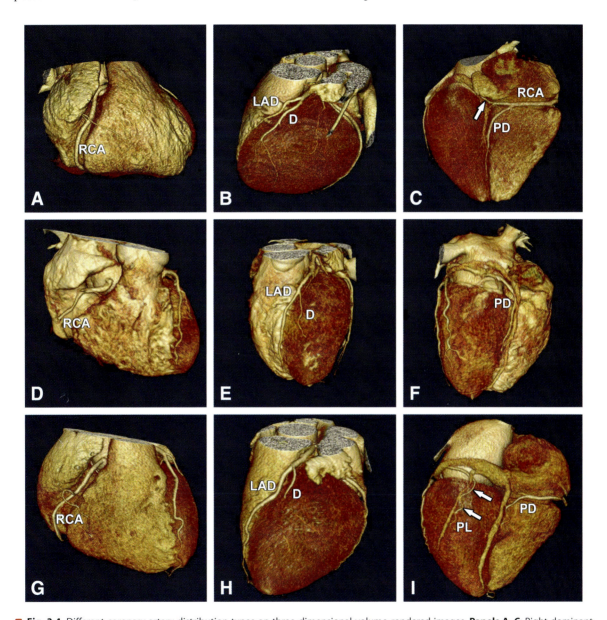

■ **Fig. 3.4** Different coronary artery distribution types on three-dimensional volume-rendered images. **Panels A–C**: Right-dominant circulation. The RCA is dominant and gives rise to the posterior descending artery (PD), and also continues in the left atrioventricular groove (*arrow* in **Panel C**). **Panels D–F**: Left-dominant circulation. The LCX is dominant and gives rise to the posterior descending artery (PD in **Panel F**). Note the small RCA in the left-dominant coronary artery system (**Panel D**). **Panels G–I**: Balanced circulation (codominant circulation), where the RCA gives rise to the PD and the LCX gives rise to a posterolateral branch (PL in **Panel I**). *D* diagonal branch; *LAD* left anterior descending artery

3

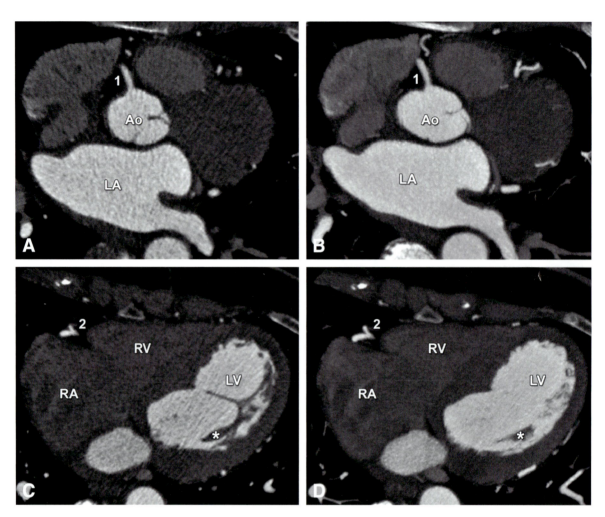

◨ **Fig. 3.5** The RCA with all its segments in axial slices (*left panels*), and the corresponding maximum-intensity projections of 5-mm thickness in the axial orientation for comparison (*right panels*). The proximal segment of the RCA (1) comes off the aorta, arising from the right sinus of Valsalva (**Panels A** and **B**). It first moves anteriorly and then (as segment 2) caudally in the right atrioventricular sulcus (**Panels C** and **D**) to the posterior surface of the heart (**Panels E** and **F**), where it again moves in the horizontal plane on the diaphragmatic face of the heart as segment 3

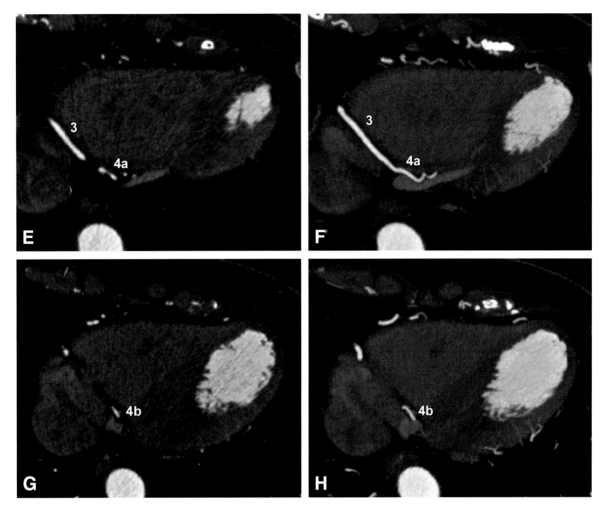

◘ **Fig. 3.5** (continued) At the crux cordis, segment 3 bifurcates into the posterior descending artery (4a) and the right posterolateral branch (4b in **Panels G** and **H**). In cases of dominance of the RCA (as in this case), segments 4a and b are side branches of the RCA. In case of left coronary artery dominance, the posterior descending artery (4a) is part of the LCX. *Ao* aorta; *Asterisk* papillary muscles; *LA* left atrium; *LV* left ventricle; *RA* right atrium; *RV* right ventricle

3.1.2   Coronary Artery Segments

The coronary arteries with their side branches can be further subdivided and classified (**Figs. 3.1, 3.5–3.7** and **Table 3.1**). These segments are of tremendous importance in describing the location of significant coronary stenoses found on noninvasive imaging and correlating them with possible myocardial ischemia, as well as for accurately guiding subsequent revascularization. Use of the 17-segment model further described in **Table 3.1** and **Figs. 3.1, 3.5–3.7** is recommended for this purpose; in the case of pathology (i.e., the presence of stenoses), it is recommended that the location be reported either by segment name or by number. The 17-segment model has several advantages over its competitor segmentation schemes, the foremost being its simplicity and conciseness.

3

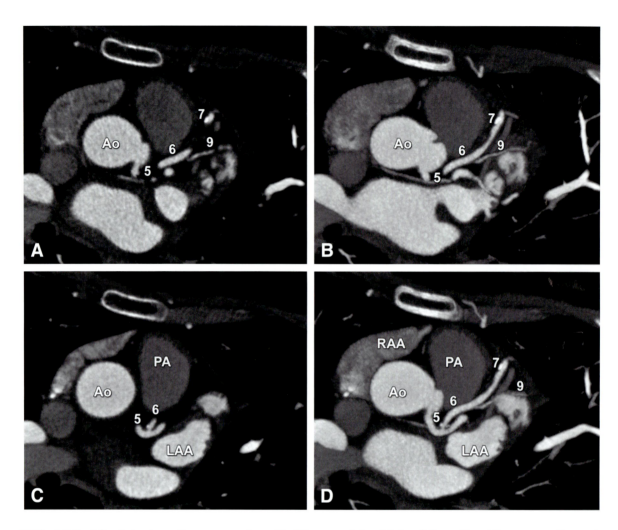

☐ **Fig. 3.6** The left anterior descending coronary artery with all its segments in axial slices (*left panels*), and the corresponding maximum-intensity projections of 5-mm thickness in the axial orientation for comparison (*right panels*). The proximal left anterior descending coronary artery segment (6) is the anterior branch of the left main coronary artery (5, **Panels A–D**). Segment 6 of the left anterior descending coronary artery then bifurcates into the mid-left anterior descending (7) and the first diagonal branch (9, **Panels A–D**)

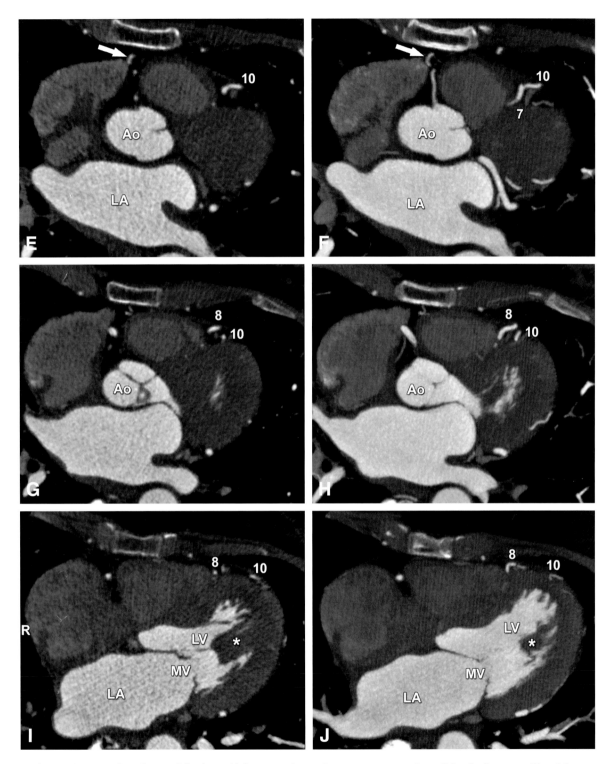

☐ **Fig. 3.6** (continued) Further caudally, the mid-left anterior descending coronary artery gives off the distal segment (8) and the second diagonal (10, **Panels E–J**) In **Panels E** and **F**, the conus branch (*arrows*, first side branch of the RCA), which travels cranial to the proximal RCA segment, is also visible. *Ao* aorta; *Asterisk* papillary muscles; *LAA* left atrial appendage; *LA* left atrium; *LV* left ventricle; *MV* mitral valve; *PA* pulmonary artery; *RAA* right atrial appendage

3

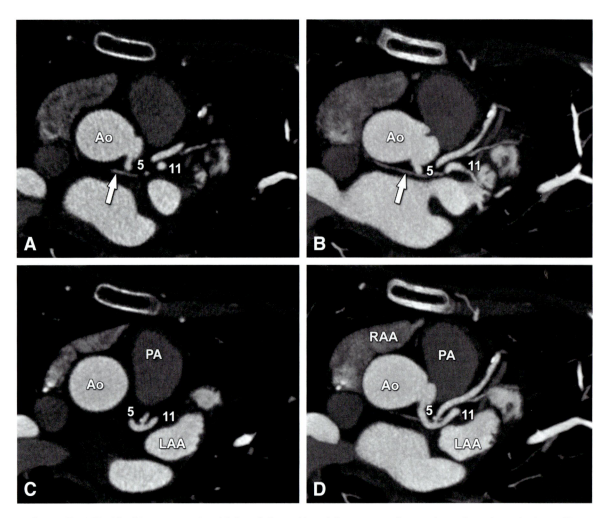

■ **Fig. 3.7** The LCX with all its segments in axial slices (*left panels*), and the corresponding maximum-intensity projections of 5-mm thickness in the axial orientation for comparison (*right panels*). The proximal LCX segment (11) is the posterior branch of the left main coronary artery (5, **Panels A–D**)

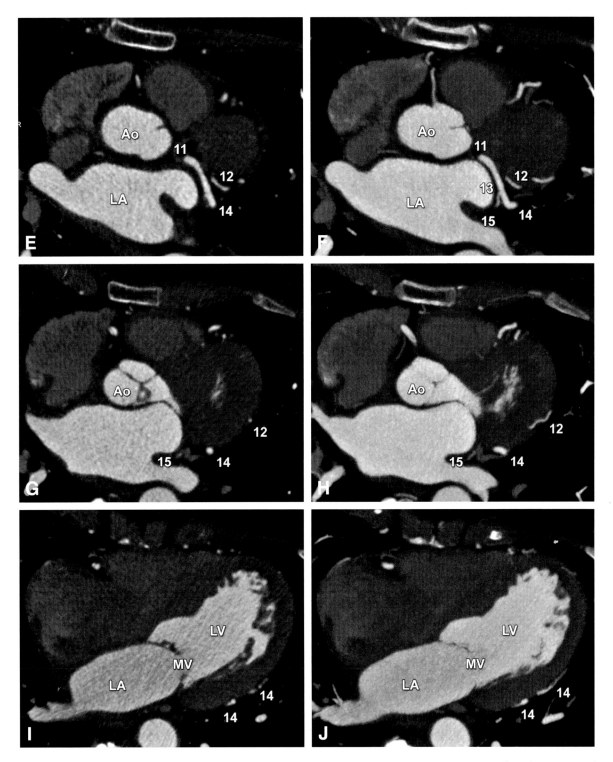

Fig. 3.7 (continued) Further down, the proximal left circumflex splits into the mid-left circumflex (13) and the first (obtuse) marginal branch (12, **Panels E–H**). The mid-left circumflex (13) then gives off the distal left circumflex (15, **Panels F–H**) (obtuse) marginal branches (14, **Panels E–J**), which supply the inferolateral myocardial segments. In the case of left coronary artery dominance, the distal circumflex (15) ends as the posterior descending artery (4a), whereas in right coronary dominance, as in this case, the RCA gives rise to the posterior descending and at least one posterolateral branch. The sinus node artery (*arrow* in **Panels A** and **B**) is the first branch of the LCX in this patient.

Ao aorta; *LAA* left atrial appendage; *LA* left atrium; *LV* left ventricle; *MV* mitral valve; *PA* pulmonary artery; *RAA* right atrial appendage

3.1.3   Frequent Coronary Artery Variants

In addition to the variation in normal anatomy caused by left or right dominance, there are other variations, such as myocardial bridging and anomalous origin, as well as variability in the course of the coronary arteries.

In less than 5% of patients, interventional coronary angiography identifies myocardial bridging. This term refers to the descent of a portion of the coronary artery into the myocardium (**Fig. 3.8**). Because of the improved imaging of myocardial tissue that can be achieved with cardiac CT, myocardial bridging can be observed in about 25–30% of patients when this technique is used, a figure that is consistent with most pathological reports. Myocardial bridging is usually confined to the LAD, diagonal or IM branches. At systole, the overlying bridge of myocardial tissue contracts and may cause systolic compression of the coronary artery segment. At diastole, the caliber is generally normal. Because most of the flow through the coronary arteries occurs at diastole, myocardial bridging does not usually cause symptoms. Thus, myocardial bridging should not be considered an anomaly but a variant. However, incidental cases have been associated with ischemia (Chap. 18).

The anomalous origin or course of a coronary artery is less frequently encountered (<1%). The existence of separate origins for the LAD and LCX has already been discussed. The two most frequent other anomalies are an RCA with an anomalous origin from the LM or the left sinus of Valsalva, and an LCX with an anomalous origin from the RCA or the right sinus of Valsalva.

In the case of an anomalous origin of the RCA from the left sinus of Valsalva or LM, the RCA commonly courses anteriorly between the aorta and the pulmonary trunk (**Fig. 3.9**). This inter-arterial course is also called "malignant course," because these patients have a high risk for exercise-induced ischemia and sudden death. At exercise, more blood is present in the aorta and pulmonary artery, causing the anomalous segment to be squeezed between these large arteries and potentially inducing ischemia. Also, the anomalous artery is usually somewhat narrowed at the origin and forms an acute angle with the aorta that may be pinched off by exercise. Other (left coronary artery) anomalies with an inter-arterial course between the aorta and pulmonary trunk can also cause ischemia.

The most frequent LCX anomaly is an LCX having its origin from the RCA or right sinus of Valsalva, where the LCX courses posterior to the aorta to enter its normal location in the left atrioventricular groove (**Fig. 3.10**).

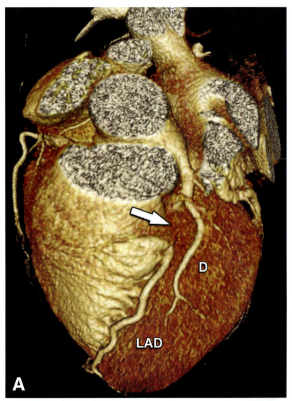

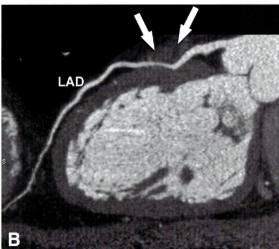

◘ Fig. 3.8 Myocardial bridging of a proximal left anterior descending coronary artery (LAD) segment (*arrows*). Three-dimensional volume-rendered image (**Panel A**) and curved multiplanar reformation (**Panel B**). Note the bridge of myocardial tissue overlying the LAD segment (*arrows*, **Panel B**). *D* diagonal branch

This is a benign condition that is not associated with ischemia. For details on coronary artery anomalies see Chap. 17.

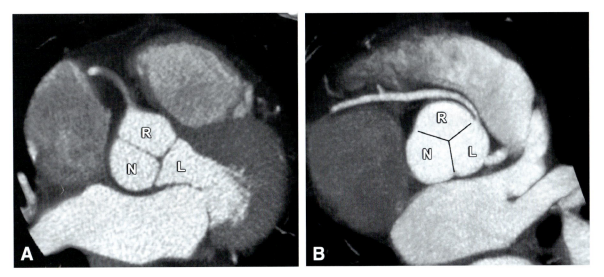

🔲 **Fig. 3.9** Normal origin of the RCA, arising from the right sinus of Valsalva (**Panel A**), in an oblique transverse thin-slab maximum-intensity projection image. Anomalous origin of the RCA, arising from the left sinus of Valsalva, with an inter-arterial course between the aorta and pulmonary trunk (**Panel B**). *L* left sinus of Valsalva; *R* right sinus of Valsalva; *N* non-coronary sinus

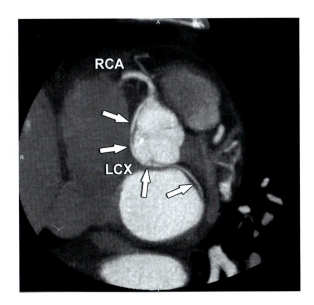

🔲 **Fig. 3.10** LCX with an anomalous origin, arising at the origin of the RCA, as shown in an oblique transverse thin-slab maximum-intensity projection image. The LCX follows a retro-aortic course to its normal position in the left atrioventricular groove (*arrows*). This is a benign variant that is not associated with ischemia

3

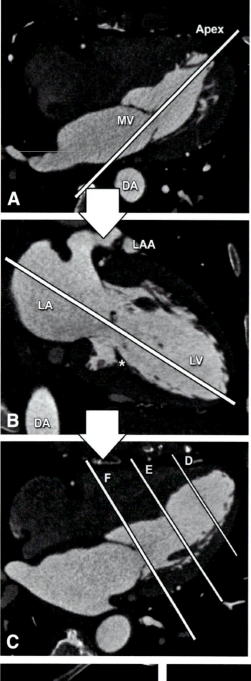

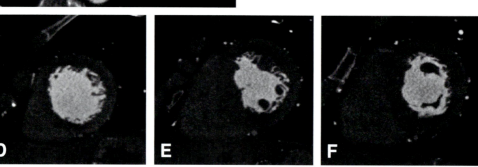

☐ **Fig. 3.11** Generating short and long-axis views for cardiac function analysis. On the basis of an axial CT slice (**Panel A**), a two-chamber view (**Panel B**) along the left ventricle (LV) and left atrium (LA) is created by connecting the apex of the left ventricle with the mitral valve (MV; white line in **Panel A**). From this two-chamber view, a four-chamber view is generated (**Panel C**) by again connecting the apex of the left ventricle with the mitral valve (MV). In this way, the individual double-oblique cardiac long axes can be identified. True cardiac short-axis slices are created by further reformations orthogonal to the interventricular septum (**Panels D–F**). In this way, apical (**Panel D**), mid-cavity (**Panel E**), and basal (**Panel F**) short-axis slices are created, for instance, to assess global and regional cardiac function; they can be viewed as cine loops throughout the cardiac cycle. *Asterisk* papillary muscles; *DA* descending aorta; *LAA* left atrial appendage; *LA* left atrium; *LV* left ventricle

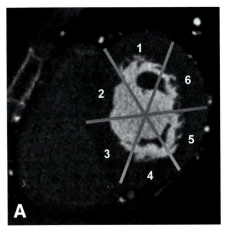

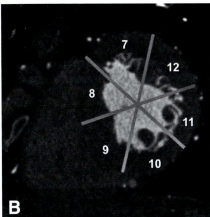

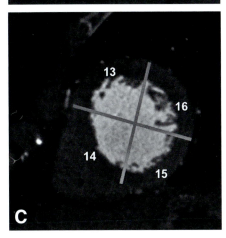

3.2   Myocardium

In addition to the coronary artery anatomy described in the previous section, a basic understanding of gross cardiac anatomy is necessary for reporting cardiac function analysis (Chap. 15) using CT. **Figure 3.11** describes how short and long axes orthogonal to the cardiac structures can be reconstructed from axial CT data sets. We recommend using the 17-segment model for reporting myocardial findings (**Fig. 3.12**), and for practical purposes it seems more convenient to use the myocardial segment names instead of the segment numbers (**Table 3.2**).

▫ **Table 3.2** Myocardial segmental anatomy[a]		
Segment no.	**Location**	**Segment name**
1	Basal	Anterior
2		Anteroseptal
3		Inferoseptal
4		Inferior
5		Inferolateral
6		Anterolateral
7	Mid-Cavity	Anterior
8		Anteroseptal
9		Inferoseptal
10		Inferior
11		Inferolateral
12		Anterolateral
13	Apical	Anterior
14		Septal
15		Inferior
16		Lateral
17	Apical	Apex

[a] AHA segmentation published in 2002 by Cerqueira et al.

▫ **Fig. 3.12** Segmental myocardial anatomy, as shown in true cardiac short-axis slices. The basal short axis is divided into segments 1–6, in counter-clockwise order (**Panel A**). The mid-cavity (**Panel B**) and apical segments (**Panel C**) are also numbered in counter-clockwise order with the numbers 7–12 and 13–17, respectively. Segment 17 is not displayed in the apical short-axis slice because it represents the apex, which is nicely seen in the long-axis views in **Panels B** and **C** of **Fig. 3.10**. The myocardial segment names and numbers are given in **Table 3.2**

Recommended Reading

1   Austen WG, Edwards JE, Frye RL et al (1975) A reporting system on patients evaluated for coronary artery disease. Report of the ad hoc committee for grading of coronary artery disease, council on cardiovascular surgery, American heart association. Circulation 51:5–40

2   Boxt LM (2005) CT anatomy of the heart. Int J Cardiovasc Imaging 21:13–27

3   Cerqueira MD, Weissman NJ, Dilsizian V et al (2002) Standardized myocardial segmentation and nomenclature for tomographic imaging of the heart: a statement for healthcare professionals from the cardiac imaging committee of the council on clinical cardiology of the American heart association. Circulation 105:539–542

4   Kini S, Bis KG, Weaver L (2007) Normal and variant coronary arterial and venous anatomy on high-resolution CT angiography. AJR Am J Roentgenol 188:1665–1674

5   Konen E, Goitein O, Sternik L, Eshet Y, Shemesh J, Di Segni E (2007) The prevalence and anatomical patterns of intramuscular coronary arteries: a coronary computed tomography angiographic study. J Am Coll Cardiol 49:587–593

6   Krakau I, Lapp H (2005) Das Herzkatheterbuch. Thieme, Stuttgart

7   Leschka S, Koepfli P, Husmann L et al (2008) Myocardial bridging: depiction rate and morphology at CT coronary angiography – comparison with conventional coronary angiography. Radiology 246:754–762

8   Levin DC, Harrington DP, Bettmann MA, Garnic JD, Davidoff A, Lois J (1982) Anatomic variations of the coronary arteries supplying the anterolateral aspect of the left ventricle: possible explanation for the "Unexplained" anterior aneurysm. Invest Radiol 17:458–462

9   O'Brien JP, Srichai MB, Hecht EM, Kim DC, Jacobs JE (2007) Anatomy of the heart at multidetector CT: what the radiologist needs to know. Radiographics 27:1569–1582

10   Popma J (2005) Coronary angiography and intravascular ultrasound imaging. In: Zipes DP (ed) Braunwald's heart disease: a textbook of cardiovascular medicine. Elsevier, Philadelphia

11   Saremi F, Abolhoda A, Ashikyan O et al (2008) Arterial supply to sinuatrial and atrioventricular nodes: imaging with multidetector CT. Radiology 246:99–107, discussion 08-9

12   Schmitt R, Froehner S, Brunn J et al (2005) Congenital anomalies of the coronary arteries: imaging with contrast-enhanced, multidetector computed tomography. Eur Radiol 15:1110–1121

13   Sos TA, Sniderman KW (1980) A simple method of teaching three-dimensional coronary artery anatomy. Radiology 134:605–606

14   Yamanaka O, Hobbs RE (1990) Coronary artery anomalies in 126, 595 patients undergoing coronary arteriography. Cathet Cardiovasc Diagn 21:28–40

15   Zimmermann E, Schnapauff D, Dewey M (2008) Cardiac and coronary anatomy in CT. Semin Ultrasound CT MR 29:176–181

CT in the Context of Cardiovascular Diagnosis and Management

A.C. Borges and K. Stangl

Abstract

Cardiac CT has emerged as a reliable diagnostic method for detecting significant coronary stenoses in selected patients.

4.1   CT as a Supplement to Other Noninvasive Imaging Tests

Echocardiography is the most important and the first-line noninvasive imaging method in cardiology and intensive care medicine, supplemented in special clinical situations by magnetic resonance imaging (MRI). There are a number of reasons for the first-line use of echocardiography: It offers a noninvasive approach, without radiation exposure; it does not involve renal clearance of the contrast medium; it is available in intensive care units, emergency and operating rooms; and extensive education and training in this technique is offered in most countries.

However, despite these advantages, echocardiography and MRI have recognized weaknesses in terms of calcium detection, plaque characterization, imaging of the pulmonary circulation, and direct visualization of the coronary arteries or bypass grafts. Multislice (multidetector-row) CT angiography is more sensitive and specific than MRI in the detection of significant ($\geq$50% diameter) stenoses of the coronary arteries. However, if many patients need invasive coronary angiography after positive coronary CT angiography, the additional contrast and radiation exposure incurred strongly argues against using CT (Chap. 6).

4.2   Role of CT in Clinical Cardiology

Assessing the clinical significance of stenotic lesions requires the integration of cardiac anatomy with the functional consequences of that anatomy (Chap. 3). Functional imaging is performed using nuclear cardiology (myocardial scintigraphy), stress echocardiography, and stress MRI. These imaging techniques detect stress-induced wall motion or perfusion abnormalities as markers of ischemia and have high diagnostic accuracy for detecting coronary artery disease (CAD). A normal study does not exclude coronary artery stenoses, but rather excludes lesions resulting in ischemia.

A variety of CT techniques are available for the evaluation of CAD. In addition to coronary artery calcium scoring, CT allows direct evaluation of the coronary arteries and the severity of stenosis. This diagnostic capability has attracted considerable attention because these CT techniques allow angiography to be performed noninvasively. Metaanalyses have demonstrated excellent diagnostic accuracy, with a mean per-patient sensitivity of 97% and specificity of 87% (Chap. 20). The high sensitivity reflects a high accuracy in excluding CAD, and recent studies have shown high negative predictive values of 95% on a per-patient basis. The introduction of 64-row and 320-row scanners has resulted in an increased accuracy in both the detection and exclusion of CAD. Although the high diagnostic accuracy of CT is well established, the most important question, clinically speaking, is: Which patients should undergo noninvasive coronary angiography with CT?

M. Dewey, *Cardiac CT*,
DOI: 10.1007/978-3-642-14022-8_4, © Springer-Verlag Berlin Heidelberg 2011

Much of the existing research is limited by preselection bias. Most of the studies thus far have been performed in patients with a high pretest likelihood of CAD. In the future, CT may serve as a *gatekeeper* or *filter* for invasive angiography: The higher accuracy of ≥64-row scanners virtually excludes false-negative CT studies. Thus, CT before valve surgery, for example, may be useful in ruling out significant stenoses, with an acceptable negative predictive value. Although CT seems to have limited value in most candidates for invasive coronary angiography, there is another important subset of patients to be considered: those with atypical angina pectoris. As previously demonstrated, negative results on CT angiography are associated with a posttest probability of CAD that is below 10% in patients with pretest probabilities of up to 70%. In patients with a pretest probability below 30% (i.e., in patients with unspecific chest pain and negative or equivocal results on noninvasive stress tests) CT achieves a posttest probability below 2% after a negative test. However, appropriate use of CT in such patients requires a careful clinical workup with functional tests because of the potentially rather low positive predictive value of CT (Chap. 6).

In addition to coronary angiography and plaque composition assessment (Chap. 14), other applications of CT that may be relevant are the evaluation of valvular and pericardial calcification, thickening, effusion, or cysts; and regional and global function assessment of the left and right ventricle (**Table 4.1**). Tracing of the left ventricular epicardial contour and the left ventricular cavity contour provides quantitative information about left ventricular wall motion as well as wall thickness and thickening (Chap. 15).

Patency vs. occlusion of coronary artery bypass grafts can be accurately assessed by CT (Chap. 12). However, the accuracy for detection of stenoses in the native vessels is reduced. Depiction of pulmonary vein anatomy may be important in many clinical situations (before and after electrophysiological testing or therapy).

◼ **Table 4.1** Main topics of interest

1. Frequently asked questions

Coronary calcium scoring for risk stratification

Anomalous coronary arteries

Coronary stenosis

Pulmonary embolism and aortic dissection

Cardiac masses and thrombi

Aortic aneurysm and dissection

Cardiac calcification (heart valves and pericardium)

Evaluation of bypass grafts (patency, stenosis, and age of occlusion)

Angiographic characterization of left and right internal mammarian artery

2. Future or seldomly asked questions

Influence of medical therapy (i.e., statins) on calcium score

Evaluation of coronary stents

Left and right ventricular volumes, ejection fraction, stroke volume, mass, and regional dyssynergy

Severity of aortic valve stenosis

Plaque characterization (plaque composition)

Coronary collaterals

Dilatation of superior and inferior vena cava and hepatic veins

Severity of mitral valve insufficiency

Possibility of grafting of distal coronary artery segments in case of proximal occlusion

Pulmonary veins before and after electrophysiological therapy (abnormalities, stenoses)

4.3   CT as a Screening Test: Indications in Asymptomatic Individuals?

Risk assessment in asymptomatic individuals is an unresolved issue of significant clinical importance: 88% of the patients with acute cardiac events were classified as low or intermediate-risk patients before, and 25–45% of the patients with acute myocardial infarction or acute cardiac death were asymptomatic before.

Only little information is available regarding the diagnostic accuracy of CT in predicting CAD in high-risk asymptomatic patient groups (i.e., diabetic patients). In asymptomatic patients with intermediate risk for CAD, noninvasive testing may be useful in providing more accurate risk assessment. However, head-to-head comparisons of different methods (stress echo, scintigraphy, stress MRI, and CT) are lacking, or only single-center results obtained in small numbers of patients are available. Negative stress tests have a high negative predictive value, with event rates below 1% within the next 5–10 years. The presence of coronary calcium is frequently associated with coronary atherosclerosis, and the amount of coronary calcium correlates with the "total coronary plaque burden" (except in the case of patients with chronic renal failure). The absence of coronary calcium virtually rules out coronary atherosclerosis and is associated with a very low risk of adverse coronary events.

Recent studies have shown that coronary calcium quantification is an independent predictor of adverse cardiac events and all-cause mortality. The European and other international societies on cardiovascular disease prevention state that "the calcium score is an important parameter to detect asymptomatic individuals at high risk for future cardiovascular events." However, calcium scanning cannot be recommended as a screening method for the unselected population, but it may play a role in individuals with intermediate risk, because a low calcium score may downgrade them to a low-risk group, or a high score may promote them to a high-risk group with the need for intensive risk-factor intervention.

4.4 Risk–Benefit of Cardiac CT: Economic and Biological Costs of Cardiac Imaging

Increased awareness of the economic, biological, and environmental costs of cardiac imaging will hopefully lead to greater appropriateness, wisdom, and prudence on the part of both the prescriber and the practitioner. The medical imaging market consists of several billion tests per year worldwide, with at least one-third being performed for cardiovascular indications. As each test incurs a cost and often involves a risk to the patient, we should consider every unnecessary and unjustifiable test one test too many. As clinical cardiologists, we want to know about the costs, risk, and radiation exposure associated with each available test. Radiation exposure is not a factor in echocardiography or MRI, but a sestamibi scan corresponds to 500 chest X-rays and a thallium scan to 1,150 chest X-rays. A recent study by Correia et al. showed

that more intense use of tests involving ionizing radiation is not associated with a higher awareness of its risks among professionals. Physicians working in a high-tech, tertiary-care referral center were described as being forgetful of the environmental impact, biorisks, dose exposure, and legal restrictions associated with the ionizing exams they prescribed or performed. This situation is complicated by the fact that in some instances the use of obscure or nonstandardized terminology can make it difficult for researchers and clinicians to really understand the dose and risks associated with different procedures.

In cardiac imaging, if we assume the average cost (not charges) of echocardiography to be 1, the cost of a CT is 3.1, that of myocardial scintigraphy 3.27, and that of MRI 5.51. Dewey and Hamm demonstrated that, from the perspective of society, coronary CT angiography is the most cost-effective modality for the diagnosis of CAD, up to a pretest likelihood of disease of 60% and invasive coronary angiography remains the most cost-effective modality in patients with a rather high likelihood of CAD (at least 60%).

Recommended Reading

1   Amis ES Jr, Butler PF, Applegate KE et al (2007) American college of radiology white paper on radiation dose in medicine. J Am Coll Radiol 4:272–284

2   Bax JJ, Schuijf JD (2005) Which role for multislice computed tomography in clinical cardiology? Am Heart J 149:960–961

3   Dewey M, Hamm B (2007) Cost effectiveness of coronary angiography and calcium scoring using CT and stress MRI for diagnosis of coronary artery disease. Eur Radiol 17:1301–1309

4   Dewey M, Teige F, Schnapauff D et al (2006) Noninvasive detection of coronary artery stenoses with multislice computed tomography or magnetic resonance imaging. Ann Intern Med 145:407–415

5   Genders TS, Meijboom WB, Meijs MF et al (2009) CT coronary angiography in patients suspected of having coronary artery disease: decision making from various perspectives in the face of uncertainty. Radiology 253:734–744

6   Picano E (2005) Economic and biological costs of cardiac imaging. Cardiovasc Ultrasound 3:13

7   Schuetz GM, Zacharopoulou NM, Schlattmann P, Dewey M (2010) Meta-analysis: noninvasive coronary angiography using computed tomography versus magnetic resonance imaging. Ann Intern Med 152:167–177

Cardiac CT in Clinical Practice

K. Nieman

Abstract

Cardiac CT applications include restratification of cardiovascular risk and rule-out of obstructive coronary artery disease in patients with stable, unstable, or atypical chest discomfort before, during, and after coronary revascularization.

5.1   Introduction

Over the past decade multislice computed tomography (CT) has seen an unparalleled technical development, which has enabled us to image the small coronary arteries. While there are many potential indications for noninvasive coronary imaging, investigation of its benefit compared with other techniques has not kept pace with the enthusiasm of its adoption into cardiovascular medicine. In this chapter we will discuss some of the most frequent applications of ECG-synchronized cardiac CT in clinical practice.

5.2   Cardiovascular Risk Refinement (in Asymptomatic Individuals)

Calcium detected by CT is a visible measure of coronary atherosclerosis. The amount of coronary calcium measured by CT correlates with the overall coronary plaque burden and predicts cardiovascular events. In routine clinical practice, cardiovascular risk is assessed using traditional risk factors and models derived from large population studies such as the Framingham Heart study or the European Systemic Coronary Risk Evaluation (SCORE). Coronary calcium scoring independently improves the prediction of adverse events and is incremental to the traditional risk factors. Whether performing a calcium scan is meaningful and will change a patient's medical management depends on the pretest cardiovascular risk estimated using the traditional risk factors (**Table 5.1**). Patients with a history of cardiovascular disease, diabetes mellitus, or a high estimated cardiovascular risk should receive the highest level of prevention (**Fig. 5.1**). A calcium scan is generally not recommended for patients at low risk, i.e., those who have no more than one risk factor, but may be useful in patients with an intermediate estimated risk of major adverse events (10–20% Framingham risk score) or cardiovascular mortality (SCORE 5–10%). A meta-analysis suggests that individuals with a low calcium score would have an event rate comparable to those at low risk by conventional risk assessment. A high calcium score is associated with an event rate comparable to that of patients in the highest conventional risk category. These patients might benefit from more intensive preventive measures, including medical treatment with statins, aspirin, and/or ACE inhibitors. Whether patients at

M. Dewey, *Cardiac CT*,
DOI: 10.1007/978-3-642-14022-8_5, © Springer-Verlag Berlin Heidelberg 2011

▫ **Table 5.1** Traditional cardiovascular risk estimation		
High CVD risk	**Intermediate CVD risk**	**Low CVD risk**
Estimated 10-year cardiovascular mortality (SCORE > 10%)	SCORE 5–10%	SCORE <5%
Established cardiovascular disease	Two or more risk factors (e.g., nicotine abuse, hypertension, low high-density lipoprotein cholesterol, family history of premature coronary artery disease, and age)	0–1 risk factors
Diabetes mellitus II		
Diabetes mellitus type I with microalbuminuria		
Markedly elevated single risk factor		

CVD cardiovascular disease; *SCORE* Systemic Coronary Risk Evaluation

5

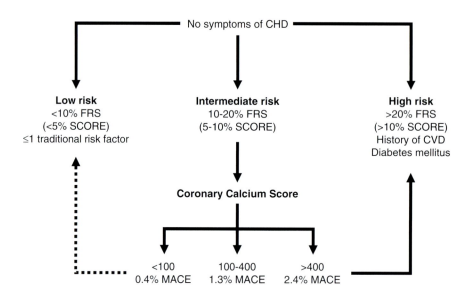

▫ **Fig. 5.1** Use of coronary calcium imaging in asymptomatic intermediate-risk individuals. Coronary calcium score can reclassify individuals at intermediate risk of coronary artery disease (10–20% 10-year risk by Framingham Risk Score, FRS) or cardiac death (5–10% 10-year by SCORE) into low, intermediate and high risk (major adverse cardiac events per year). While more intensive preventive measures are warranted in patients reclassified to high risk, there are no recommendations to decrease preventive measures in patients reclassified to low risk. This scheme follows the recommendations by Greenland et al. in the ACCF/AHA 2007 Expert Consensus Document. *CVD* cardiovascular disease; *MACE* major adverse cardiovascular events

intermediate risk and a negative calcium score should be managed as low risk is still debated. A substantial number of asymptomatic patients with a very high calcium score will have (silent) obstructive coronary artery disease. In these patients a low threshold to ischemia detection seems reasonable. Although calcium scoring in patients at intermediate risk seems reasonable, there is currently no data showing that this approach improves outcome (in a cost-effective manner).

Contrast-enhanced CT angiography is currently not recommended in patients who do not have symptoms.

While radiation exposure may become less of a concern with the development of low-dose scan protocols, there is still the need for intravenous injection of potentially harmful contrast media. Coronary CT angiography has the potential to identify patients with severe but noncalcified coronary artery disease, which would be missed by unenhanced CT. Finding severely obstructive disease is rare, and the overall prognosis of asymptomatic patients without detectable coronary calcium is excellent (<1% annual event rate). Although conceivable, there is no data with respect to the development of adverse events.

Whether identification of the small number of patients with significant noncalcified plaque justifies the higher radiation exposure and contrast agent administration is unclear and heavily debated.

5.3 Patients with Stable Chest Discomfort

In Europe exercise electrocardiography remains the most frequently used initial test in patients with suspected coronary artery disease, whereas in the USA single-photon emission computed tomography is most commonly used. Exercise electrocardiography has a high specificity but a low sensitivity. After correction for referral bias and exclusion of patients with prior myocardial infarction, the overall accuracy is only 68%, which means that every third test result is incorrect (**Fig. 5.2**). Myocardial perfusion imaging, using single-photon emission computed tomography, positron emission tomography, or magnetic resonance imaging (MRI), is more accurate but not considered cost-effective in comparison to exercise electrocardiography in the majority of patients (**Table 5.2**).

Coronary angiography by CT represents an attractive means to noninvasively assess patients with suspected coronary artery disease. The high sensitivity and negative predictive value of coronary CT angiography allow confident visual exclusion of coronary artery disease. Myocardial ischemia is extremely unlikely in the absence of obstructive coronary artery disease on CT. However, angiographic disease (by CT or catheter angiography) may exist without causing ischemia or symptoms and may not need revascularization. Additionally, stenosis severity cannot be assessed with the same level of accuracy as compared to conventional angiography and will often be overestimated when severe calcification is present. Therefore, coronary CT angiography appears most useful to exclude coronary artery disease in patients with a low-to-intermediate pretest likelihood of disease. Whether CT angiography should be used as the initial test in these patients or after an inconclusive stress test, is still under investigation. Most registries show a very low prevalence of significant obstructive disease in patients with stable chest symptoms without detectable calcium. Therefore, a calcium scan may be an appropriate first step and function as a gatekeeper to further testing, including contrast-enhanced CT angiography. To avoid unnecessary revascularization, we currently prefer to perform stress testing when CT shows moderate

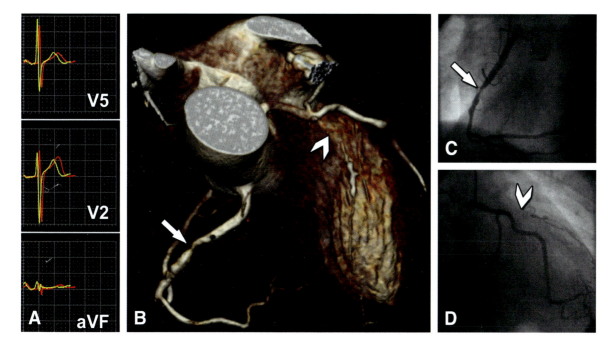

Fig. 5.2 False-negative exercise ECG and true-positive coronary CT angiography. Exercise ECG without significant ECG changes in a 57-year-old patient with stable angina symptoms (**Panel A**). Severely stenotic right coronary artery (*arrow*) and occluded left anterior descending coronary artery (*arrowhead*) on coronary CT angiography (**Panel B**), confirmed by conventional coronary angiography (**Panels C** and **D**)

◻ Table 5.2 Diagnostic accuracy for noninvasive detection of coronary artery disease

Modality	Diagnostic performance	
	Sensitivity (%)	Specificity (%)
Exercise electrocardiography	68	77
Exercise stress echocardiography	80–85	84–86
Dobutamine stress echocardiography	40–100	62–100
Vasodilator stress echocardiography	56–92	87–100
Exercise perfusion scintigraphy	85–90	70–75
Vasodilator perfusion scintigraphy	83–94	64–90
Dobutamine stress MRI	83 (79–88)	86 (81–91)
Vasodilator perfusion MRI	91 (88–94)	81 (77–85)
CT coronary calcium score (>0 threshold)	>95	≈50
≤16-row CT	95.6 (94.0–97.0)	84.7 (80.0–89.0)
>16-row CT	98.1 (97.0–99.0)	89.4 (86.0–92.0)

Reported diagnostic performance is derived from the 2006 ESC Guidelines on the management of stable angina, the ACCF/AHA 2007 Experts consensus document on calcium scoring, and Nandalur et al. (for MRI) and Schütz et al. (for coronary CT angiography). Numbers in parentheses give the 95% confidence intervals for CT and ranges for the other tests.

obstructive disease. As a matter of fact, if coronary CT angiography identifies obstructions of moderate severity at prognostically less important sites, a physician may be more confident in maintaining medical treatment rather than immediately sending the patient for revascularization.

In patients with suspected coronary anomalies, CT angiography is the most accurate imaging technique for assessment of the origin, course, and termination of abnormal coronary arteries in relation to surrounding structures (Chap. 17).

In conclusion, cardiac CT (including calcium scanning and CT angiography) has an emerging role in the assessment of suspected coronary artery disease. Whether the technique should be used as the initial test in low-to-intermediate risk patients followed by functional testing in patients with obstructive disease or secondary to functional tests that cannot be performed or produce equivocal results, is yet unresolved. Just as there are patients who are unsuitable to undergo stress testing, CT angiography should only be performed in patients in whom diagnostic image quality can be expected.

5.4   Acute Chest Pain

Cardiac CT may have various advantages over the current diagnostic approach in patients presenting to an emergency department with acute chest pain. Particularly when symptoms have subsided the ECG may be normal, while biomarkers could still take hours to convert in case of an acute coronary syndrome. Stress testing may exclude severe stenosis, but will neglect the presence and extent of coronary atherosclerosis. CT can visualize coronary artery atherosclerosis, identify severe obstructions, detect myocardial hypoperfusion (secondary to myocardial infarction), and allow detection of other potentially life-threatening conditions presenting with acute chest discomfort including aortic dissection, pulmonary emboli, pericardial effusions, and pulmonary disease.

A simple calcium scan may allow exclusion of severe disease in a substantial number of patients and is associated with excellent outcome. However, because of the potentially devastating consequences and the apparently higher incidence of noncalcified disease in patients with an acute presentation, many prefer contrast-enhanced CT angiography instead (**Fig. 5.3**). The limited data available shows that CT angiography can exclude an acute coronary syndrome with a similarly high negative predictive value, whereas the positive predictive value appears to be somewhat lower in acute patients. Also, the absence of coronary stenosis on CT does not entirely rule out an acute coronary stenosis. Nevertheless, CT could allow more patients to be discharged from the emergency without clinical follow-up and functional testing (**Fig. 5.4**). On the other hand, there is the danger of excessive use of cardiac CT in patients with a very low risk of acute coronary syndrome who would otherwise be discharged without further testing.

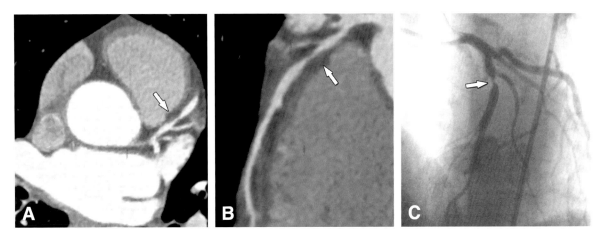

◘ **Fig. 5.3** Acute presentation of a 43-year-old man with progressive angina pectoris (without elevated troponin). Coronary CT angiography shows an outwardly (positively) remodeled, noncalcified, stenotic lesion (*arrow*) in the left anterior descending coronary artery (**Panel A**, axial image; **Panel B**, curved multiplanar reformation), confirmed on conventional coronary angiography (**Panel C**)

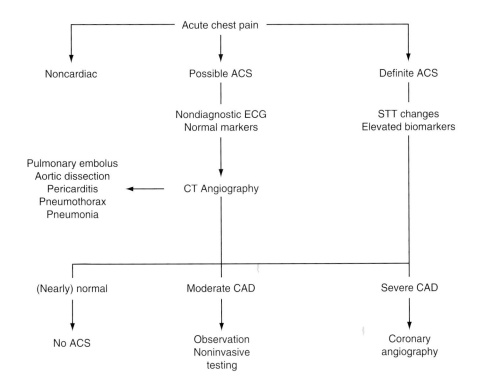

◘ **Fig. 5.4** Potential implementation of cardiac CT in patients with a suspected acute coronary syndrome. *ACS* acute coronary syndrome; *CAD* coronary artery disease; *STT* ST trace

When and how to use cardiac CT in the emergency room remains a matter of debate and proper recommendations will require further investigation of the incremental value of CT in comparison to the current standard of care. Use of cardiac CT in the emergency ward requires technicians and physicians experienced in coronary CT, a service few clinics can provide 24 by 7.

Routine performance of a triple rule-out scan for exclusion of myocardial infarction, pulmonary embolism, and aortic dissection is not recommended in patients with acute chest pain as this requires significantly more contrast agent and radiation and potentially degrades the quality in particular of the coronary arteries (Chap. 6).

5.5   Rule-Out of Coronary Artery Disease in Specific Situations

In certain clinical situations coronary artery disease needs to be excluded, even when concrete symptoms of ischemia are absent. Conventional coronary angiography is routinely performed in patients scheduled for (noncoronary) cardiac surgery, such as valve surgery. Except perhaps for patients with degenerative aortic valve disease, which is often associated with calcified coronary disease, coronary artery disease can be excluded in the majority of the presurgical patients using cardiac CT. In case of aortic valve endocarditis or aortic dissection, CT may in fact be preferred over manipulation of catheters in the affected region (Chap. 16). A small proportion of patients with heart failure, assumed to be nonischemic, will have obstructive coronary artery disease. Calcium scanning and/or CT angiography can be a useful alternative to rule out coronary arty disease in most of these patients.

5.6   Noninvasive Angiographic Follow-Up After Coronary Revascularization

Follow-up of patients after revascularization is more complicated than assessing patients without stents or bypass grafts, by any modality. Cardiac CT is limited by specific imaging complications of the stent material (Chap. 13), artifacts from surgical clips in the vicinity of grafts (Chap. 12), but mostly by the presence of (native) coronary artery disease, which is often diffuse. In particular the more abundant presence of calcified plaque reduces the reliability of cardiac CT angiography. Moreover, CT angiography does not have the ability to determine the hemodynamic significance of lesions, which may be unpredictable in the presence of collateral perfusion of the myocardium. This may be overcome with the development of stress myocardial perfusion CT or some kind of combination of coronary CT angiography and stress imaging.

After stenting, cardiac CT can be used to exclude in-stent obstruction of large-diameter stents in proximal coronary arteries. In-stent restenosis in an (unprotected) left main stent may have serious consequences. Because stress testing is considered less reliable, conventional coronary angiography is routinely performed after 3–6 months. Cardiac CT can exclude significant disease in the majority of these patients, thereby avoiding recatheterization in a substantial number of patients, particularly when "simple" stenting (i.e., no bifurcation stenting) has been performed.

After bypass graft surgery, CT can be of use to exclude graft obstruction. As subclinical occlusion may exist for years, because of competitive antegrade or collateral flow, assessment of the significance of an occluded graft late after revascularization requires some kind of functional imaging. Occasionally, the exact anatomy of the bypass graft procedure is unknown, or grafts cannot be located or engaged by catheter for other reasons, in which case CT can be very useful.

5.7   CT-Assisted Cardiac Interventions

Cardiac CT can provide unique three-dimensional information of the heart, which can benefit complex cardiac procedures such as electrophysiological ablation and coronary revascularization procedures.

Cardiac CT can provide potentially valuable information supplementing the angiographic projections obtained by invasive means. Information on the angulation of vessels or the presence and location of plaques at ostial or bifurcation sites is useful in complex coronary procedures. In chronic total occlusion, CT can provide information regarding the length and content of the occluded segment, proximal vessel tortuosity and stump morphology, and the presence of side branches (**Fig. 5.5** and **List 5.1**). Severe calcification and long occlusion predict a poorer outcome of revascularization procedures. These images may also be integrated in advanced catheter registration and navigation systems.

In patients undergoing electrophysiological procedures, three-dimensional imaging of the cardiac chambers is performed to assess (abnormal) anatomy, select the most optimal technique and equipment, avoid complications (by localization of the esophagus), guide catheters, and record proceedings.

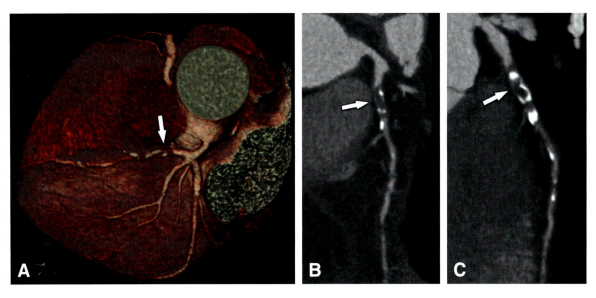

□ Fig. 5.5 Chronic total occlusion in the left anterior descending coronary artery of a 55-year-old woman with anginal symptoms. Short occlusion (*arrow*) with moderate amounts of calcium in the left anterior descending coronary artery. **Panel A** is a volume-rendered reconstruction, **Panels B** and **C** are curved multiplanar reformations and maximum-intensity projections

---

List 5.1. Predictors of revascularization failure in chronic total occlusion

1. Longer duration of the occlusion
2. Absence of antegrade collateral filling
3. Blunt rather than a tapered proximal stump
4. Occlusion length >15 mm[a]
5. Severe calcification[a]
6. Side branch at the occlusion site
7. Vessel tortuosity proximal to the occlusion

---

[a] Predictive value confirmed by CT

Prior to percutaneous implantation of aortic valves, cardiac CT can provide information concerning the size, shape, and angulation of the aortic root. This information is important for planning the procedure and selecting the size of the valve prosthesis.

5.8 Ventricular Function, Myocardial Infarction, and Valvular Heart Disease

The clinical mainstay of cardiovascular imaging is echocardiography. The technique is quick, inexpensive and can be performed at the bedside. When an acceptable echocardiographic window is available, echocardiography is the first choice for functional imaging of the heart. For more accurate or reproducible assessment of left ventricular function, MRI or nuclear imaging are generally performed (**Table 5.3**). While assessment of global left ventricular function by ECG-gated CT is possible, with good correlation to echocardiography, MRI, and nuclear imaging, it is not solely performed for this purpose unless other modalities are unavailable (Chap. 15). Dynamic display of cardiac CT can be used for assessment of segmental wall motion or valvular mobility, although CT has poorer temporal resolution than echocardiography and MRI and does not provide all functional parameters that can be determined with the latter two techniques. It should also be mentioned that full-cycle data is often unavailable with current dose-saving CT protocols (prospective acquisition, Chap. 8). CT provides detailed information on valve morphology during end-systole or mid-diastole but lacks the functional information afforded by Doppler measurement, often crucial in decision making. Aortic valve planimetry can be helpful in patients with poor acoustic windows (Chap. 16).

Myocardial infarction may be recognized as low myocardial attenuation on (coronary) CT angiograms. Chronic myocardial infarction may be differentiated from acute perfusion defects based on the lower myocardial attenuation resulting from the presence of fat tissue within the scar tissue. However, acute infarction within an area of subendocardial scarring will be difficult to

5

◼ **Table 5.3** Left ventricular function

Modality	Advantages	Disadvantages
Echocardiography	Easy, real-time, portable, low cost, safe and repeatable Velocity measurement	Acoustic accessibility Operator dependence Geometric assumptions[a]
Nuclear imaging	Accurate and reproducible No geometric assumptions	Radiation exposure Limited anatomy Arrhythmia No wall thickening[b] Hypoperfused myocardium delineation[c]
Magnetic resonance imaging	No ionizing radiation Flexible and reproducible	Limited availability and relatively time-consuming Pacemaker devices, claustrophobia, etc. Patient motion
Computed tomography	Available as part of conventional ECG-gated spiral CT High spatial resolution High contrast-to-noise ratio No geometric assumptions Reproducible	Unavailable with prospectively ECG-triggered acquisition protocols Contrast agent and radiation exposure Limited temporal resolution (wall motion)

[a] Largely overcome by three-dimensional echocardiography

[b] Radionuclide ventriculography

[c] Gated single-photon emission computed tomography

recognize based on these attenuation values. The area of early hypoenhancement may underestimate the total volume of infarcted myocardium, and late imaging after contrast injection ("delayed enhancement") is more accurate in quantifying myocardial infarction. Late-enhancement imaging by CT, like MRI, allows transmural infarction sizing, which is an advantage over nuclear techniques. However, current delayed-imaging CT techniques require more contrast agent to compensate for the generally lower contrast-to-noise levels and additional X-ray exposure, making it a second choice to MRI for myocardial viability assessment.

Recommended Reading

1   Arad Y, Goodman KJ, Roth M, Newstein D, Guerci AD (2005) Coronary calcification, coronary disease risk factors, C-reactive protein, and atherosclerotic cardiovascular disease events: the St. Francis heart study. J Am Coll Cardiol 46:158–165

2   Budoff MJ, Achenbach S, Blumenthal RS et al (2006) AHA Committee on Cardiovascular Imaging and Intervention; AHA Council on Cardiovascular Radiology and Intervention; AHA Committee on Cardiac Imaging, Council on Clinical Cardiology. Assessment of coronary artery disease by cardiac computed tomography: a scientific statement from the AHA Committee on Cardiovascular Imaging and Intervention, Council on Cardiovascular Radiology and Intervention, and Committee on Cardiac Imaging, Council on Clinical Cardiology. Circulation 114:1761–1791

3   Fox K, Garcia MA, Ardissino D et al (2006) Task force on the management of stable angina pectoris of the european society of cardiology; ESC Committee for Practice Guidelines (CPG). Guidelines on the management of stable angina pectoris: executive summary: The task force on the management of stable angina pectoris of the european society of cardiology. Eur Heart J 27:1341–1381

4   García-García HM, van Mieghem CA, Gonzalo N et al (2009) Computed tomography in total coronary occlusions (CTTO registry): radiation exposure and predictors of successful percutaneous intervention. EuroIntervention 4:607–616

5   Graham I, Atar D, Borch-Johnsen K et al (2007) European guidelines on cardiovascular disease prevention in clinical practice: full text. Fourth joint task force of the European society of cardiology and other societies on cardiovascular disease prevention in clinical practice. Eur J Cardiovasc Prev Rehabil 14(Suppl 2):S1–S113

6   Greenland P, Bonow RO, Brundage BH et al (2007) Society of Atherosclerosis Imaging and Prevention; Society of Cardiovascular Computed Tomography. ACCF/AHA 2007 clinical expert consensus document on coronary artery calcium scoring by computed tomography in global cardiovascular risk assessment and in evaluation of patients with chest pain: a report of the American College of Cardiology Foundation Clinical Expert Consensus Task Force (ACCF/AHA Writing Committee to Update the 2000 Expert Consensus Document on Electron Beam Computed Tomography) developed in collaboration with the Society of Atherosclerosis

Imaging and Prevention and the Society of Cardiovascular Computed Tomography. J Am Coll Cardiol 49:378–402

7 Hendel RC, Patel MR, Kramer CM et al (2006) ACCF/ACR/SCCT/SCMR/ASNC/NASCI/SCAI/SIR 2006 appropriateness criteria for cardiac computed tomography and cardiac magnetic resonance imaging. A report of the American College of Cardiology Foundation Quality Strategic Directions Committee Appropriateness Criteria Working Group. J Am Coll Cardiol 48:1475–1497

8 Jongbloed MR, Lamb H, Bax JJ et al (2005) Noninvasive visualization of the cardiac venous system using multislice computed tomography. J Am Coll Cardiol 45:749–753

9 Knez A, Becker A, Leber A et al (2004) Relation of coronary calcium scores by electron beam tomography to obstructive disease in 2, 115 symptomatic patients. Am J Cardiol 93:1150–1152

10 Lacomis JM, Goitein O, Deible C, Schwartzman D (2007) CT of the pulmonary veins. J Thorac Imaging 22:63–76

11 Lardo AC, Cordeiro MA, Silva C et al (2006) Contrast-enhanced multidetector computed tomography viability imaging after myocardial infarction: characterization of myocyte death, microvascular obstruction, and chronic scar. Circulation 113:394–404

12 Maintz D, Seifarth H, Raupach R et al (2006) 64-slice multidetector coronary CT angiography: in vitro evaluation of 68 different stents. Eur Radiol 16:818–826

13 McClelland RL, Chung H, Detrano R, Post W, Kronmal RA (2006) Distribution of coronary artery calcium by race, gender, and age: results from the Multi-Ethnic Study of Atherosclerosis (MESA). Circulation 113:30–37

14 Meijboom WB, van Mieghem CA, Mollet NR et al (2007) 64-slice computed tomography coronary angiography in patients with high, intermediate, or low pretest probability of significant coronary artery disease. J Am Coll Cardiol 50:1469–1475

15 Mollet NR, Hoye A, Lemos PA et al (2005) Value of preprocedure multislice computed tomographic coronary angiography to predict the outcome of percutaneous recanalization of chronic total occlusions. Am J Cardiol 95:240–243

16 Mowatt G, Cook JA, Hillis GS, Walker S, Fraser C, Jia X, Waugh N (2008) 64-Slice computed tomography angiography in the diagnosis and assessment of coronary artery disease: systematic review and meta-analysis. Heart 94:1386–1393

17 Nandalur KR, Dwamena BA, Choudhri AF, Nandalur MR, Carlos RC (2007) Diagnostic performance of stress cardiac magnetic resonance imaging in the detection of coronary artery disease: a meta-analysis. J Am Coll Cardiol 50:1343–1353

18 Schroeder S, Achenbach S, Bengel F et al (2008) Cardiac computed tomography: indications, applications, limitations, and training requirements: report of a Writing Group Deployed By The Working Group Nuclear Cardiology And Cardiac CT of the European Society of Cardiology and the European Council of Nuclear Cardiology. Working Group Nuclear Cardiology and Cardiac CT; European Society of Cardiology; European Council of Nuclear Cardiology. Eur Heart J 29:531–556

19 Schuetz GM, Zacharopoulou NM, Schlattmann P, Dewey M (2010) Meta-analysis: noninvasive coronary angiography using computed tomography versus magnetic resonance imaging. Ann Intern Med 152:167–177

20 Soon KH, Cox N, Wong A et al (2007) CT coronary angiography predicts the outcome of percutaneous coronary intervention of chronic total occlusion. J Interv Cardiol 20:359–366

21 Vanhoenacker PK, Decramer I, Bladt O et al (2008) Multidetector computed tomography angiography for assessment of in-stent restenosis: meta-analysis of diagnostic performance. BMC Med Imaging 8:14

Clinical Indications

M. Dewey

Abstract

The clinically most relevant indications for cardiac CT are presented.

6.1 Suspected Coronary Artery Disease

The most obvious indication for cardiac CT is to exclude coronary artery disease (CAD) in symptomatic patients with a low-to-intermediate pretest likelihood of disease, which is defined as a likelihood of approximately 20–70% (**Fig. 6.1**). This group includes patients with inconclusive findings in previous stress tests and those presenting with atypical angina. On the one hand, patients with a higher pretest likelihood of CAD (>70%; e.g., with typical angina, risk factors, and a positive stress test) should not undergo cardiac CT as the first-line modality, because more patients in this subgroup will require subsequent conventional coronary angiography as the negative predictive value of CT is reduced (making a negative CT result less reliable). On the other hand, the positive predictive value is rather low in patients with a very low pretest likelihood of CAD (<20%; e.g., with nonanginal chest pain and a negative stress test), and the CT findings would lead to many unnecessary conventional coronary angiographies.

Thus, the preferred patient population for CT coronary angiography has a pretest likelihood of CAD of 20–70%. In **Tables 6.1–6.3**, patients with a pretest likelihood in this range are highlighted in blue. The markings in the tables make it easy to identify those patients who are most likely to benefit from coronary CT angiography and to simultaneously exclude others who should not undergo this test. These tables may also be helpful in increasing the cost-effectiveness of coronary CT

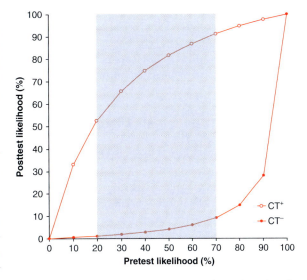

Fig. 6.1 The patient population with suspected CAD that is clinically most suitable for undergoing coronary CT angiography is highlighted in *blue* and has a pretest likelihood of disease of 20–70%. CT coronary angiography is very accurate in ruling out disease over a wide range of clinical presentations, as can be seen in the very low posttest likelihood after a negative CT (below 10% for pretest likelihoods of up to 70%). Thus, coronary CT angiography allows reliable exclusion of disease. However, patients with a likelihood of less than 20% may not benefit from noninvasive testing because of the very low positive predictive value in this group, which may lead to a rather high rate of unnecessary conventional coronary angiographies. This calculation, made according to the Bayes theorem, is based on the overall sensitivity and specificity of coronary CT angiography in patients with suspected CAD, as specified in Chap. 20 and modified from Schuetz GM et al., Ann Intern Med 2010

M. Dewey, *Cardiac CT*,
DOI: 10.1007/978-3-642-14022-8_6, © Springer-Verlag Berlin Heidelberg 2011

Table 6.1 Likelihood (in %) of CAD according to sex, age, and symptoms[a]

Women				Men			
Age (years)	Nonanginal chest pain[b]	Atypical angina[c]	Typical angina[d]	Age (years)	Nonanginal chest pain[b]	Atypical angina[c]	Typical angina[d]
30–39	0.8	4	26	30–39	5	22	70
40–49	3	13	55	40–49	14	46	87
50–59	8	32	79	50–59	22	59	92
60–69	19	54	91	60–69	28	67	94

[a] The range of patients who are most likely to benefit from coronary CT angiography is highlighted in blue (those with a likelihood of 20–70%). In the 30–69-year age range, all men with atypical symptoms would be expected to benefit from CT, whereas women with atypical angina pectoris would be suitable candidates for coronary CT angiography only if they were older than 50 years of age. Modified from Diamond and Forrester, New Engl J Med 1979

[b] Only one of the three characteristics of angina pectoris is present (either retrosternal localization of pain, pain precipitated by exercise or decreased at rest, or on nitrate medication)

[c] Only two of the three characteristics of angina pectoris are present

[d] All of the three characteristics of angina pectoris are present

angiography, as costly and unnecessary secondary examinations, which are more likely in very low (<20%) and high-likelihood patients (>70%), can potentially increase societal costs related to the diagnosis of CAD.

6.2   Other Appropriate Clinical Indications

Other justified indications for cardiac CT in addition to suspected CAD are summarized in **Table 6.4**. The most common of these indications is in patients presenting with acute chest pain (with normal enzymes and without ECG changes); a subgroup of patiens for whom results from single-center studies and the multicenter CT-STAT trial are now available. These studies suggest that management of low-risk patients with acute chest pain might be streamlined using CT (greater cost-effectiveness and a significant reduction in the length of hospital stay of 50%) in comparison to standard of care (single-photon emission computed tomography perfusion imaging). In contrast, the so-called "triple rule-out" CT (to exclude coronary stenosis, pulmonary embolism, and aortic dissection) in acute patients is still limited by the fact that no generally accepted scanning protocols are available, and the patient population that might benefit from such a comprehensive examination remains to be clearly defined (**Table 6.6**). Further larger studies investigating the benefit of CT in this respect are necessary before its general use can be considered and we regard this indication as inappropriate at this point in time. Another important argument against routine triple rule-out CT is that, according to Stillman et al., only two of the three diseases are actually suspected and need to be ruled out in most of the acute chest pain patients. Thus, the technical approach may better individually focus on two of the vascular beds ("double-rule out"), which will increase practicality and image quality.

Imaging and follow-up of symptomatic patients with coronary artery bypass grafts (e.g., recurrent chest pain; Chaps. 12 and 20) is an important appropriate indication. There is good evidence that CT allows highly accurate assessment of both the native coronaries and the bypass grafts in a single examination. However, the native coronary arteries in patients after bypass grafting are not as easily assessed as are the bypasses themselves (Chap. 12), and only a few studies have addressed the combined reading of coronaries and bypasses. Thus, scientific evidence most strongly supports the use of CT for exclusion of CAD in patients with low-to-intermediate pretest likelihood (e.g., patients with suspected CAD and inconclusive findings and complaints).

The presence of coronary artery anomalies (Chap. 17) is also readily ruled out with CT, which is superior to magnetic resonance imaging (MRI) in depicting the distal parts of the coronaries and visualizing the entire course of anomalous vessels. Moreover, CT is well suited for follow-up of coronary aneurysms; however, in young patients, such as those with Kawasaki syndrome, MRI should be the first-line imaging tool because it does not involve radiation exposure, and there is no need for contrast agent administration.

◨ **Table 6.2** Posttest likelihood (in %) of CAD in women after an electrocardiographic stress test (ST depression), according to age and symptoms[a]

ST depression (mm)	Age (years)	Women			
		Asymptomatic	Nonanginal chest pain[b]	Atypical angina[c]	Typical angina[d]
0–0.5	30–39	0.1	0.2	1	7
	40–49	0.2	0.7	3	22
	50–59	0.8	2	10	47
	60–69	2	5	21	69
0.5–1.0	30–39	0.3	0.7	4	24
	40–49	0.9	3	12	53
	50–59	3	8	31	78
	60–69	7	17	52	90
1.0–1.5	30–39	0.6	2	9	42
	40–49	2	6	25	72
	50–59	7	16	50	89
	60–69	15	33	72	95
1.5–2.0	30–39	1	3	16	59
	40–49	4	11	39	84
	50–59	12	28	67	94
	60–69	25	49	83	98
2–2.5	30–39	3	8	33	79
	40–49	10	24	63	93
	50–59	27	50	84	98
	60–69	47	72	93	99.1
>2.5	30–39	11	24	63	93
	40–49	28	53	86	98
	50–59	56	78	95	99.3
	60–69	76	90	98	99.7

[a] The range of women who are most likely to benefit from coronary CT angiography is highlighted in blue (20–70%). Modified from Diamond and Forrester, New Engl J Med 1979

[b] Only one of the three characteristics of angina pectoris is present (either retrosternal localization of pain, pain precipitated by exercise or decreased at rest, or on nitrate medication)

[c] Only two of the three characteristics of angina pectoris are present

[d] All of the three characteristics of angina pectoris are present

Please note that 1.0 mm is equal to 0.1 mV

■ **Table 6.3** Posttest likelihood (in %) of CAD in men after an electrocardiographic stress test (ST depression), according to age and symptoms[a]

ST depression (mm)	Age (years)	Men			
		Asymptomatic	Nonanginal chest pain[b]	Atypical angina[c]	Typical angina[d]
0–0.5	30–39	0.4	1	6	25
	40–49	1	4	16	61
	50–59	2	6	25	73
	60–69	3	8	32	79
0.5–1.0	30–39	2	5	21	68
	40–49	5	13	44	86
	50–59	9	20	57	91
	60–69	11	26	65	94
1.0–1.5	30–39	4	1	38	83
	40–49	11	26	64	94
	50–59	19	37	75	96
	60–69	23	45	81	97
1.5–2.0	30–39	8	19	55	91
	40–49	20	41	78	97
	50–59	31	53	86	98
	60–69	37	62	90	99
2.0–2.5	30–39	18	38	76	96
	40–49	39	65	91	99
	50–59	54	75	94	99.2
	60–69	61	81	96	99.5
> 2.5	30–39	43	68	92	99
	40–49	69	87	97	99.6
	50–59	81	91	98	99.8
	60–69	85	94	99	99.8

[a] The range of men who are most likely to benefit from coronary CT angiography is highlighted in blue (20–70%). Modified from Diamond and Forrester, New Engl J Med 1979

[b] Only one of the three characteristics of angina pectoris is present (either retrosternal localization of pain, pain precipitated by exercise or decreased at rest, or on nitrate medication)

[c] Only two of the three characteristics of angina pectoris are present

[d] All of the three characteristics of angina pectoris are present

Please note that 1.0 mm is equal to 0.1 mV

□ Table 6.4 Appropriate clinical indications for cardiac CT

	Pros	Cons
Exclusion of CAD in symptomatic patients with low to intermediate pretest likelihood	High negative predictive value of CT Noninvasive CT is highly accepted by patients	Only little data available on possible advantages of CT over other modalities such as stress ECG, and on possible advantages for patient management
Patients with suspected CAD and equivocal stress-test results	High negative predictive value of CT Noninvasive CT is highly accepted by patients	Only little data available on possible advantages for patient management
Acute chest pain with negative ECG and positive enzymes	Reliable exclusion of CAD in these patients is possible Patients can be discharged earlier	An outcome benefit over the standard of care has not been shown. However, very large and long-term studies may be needed to show this.
Follow-up of symptomatic patients with coronary artery bypasses	Reliable visualization of the entire bypass, including the proximal and distal anastomoses Noninvasive CT is highly accepted by patients	Only little data available on possible advantages for patient management Numerous studies, but in small patient populations
Exclusion of or delineation of the course of coronary artery anomalies	Excellent evaluation of the course of anomalous coronaries (malignant vs. benign) Unlike MRI, CT allows reliable visualization of the entire course of the vessel	Its competitor, MRI, is to be preferred, especially in younger patients, because it does not involve radiation exposure Unreliable in visualizing coronary collaterals
Assessment of pulmonary vein anatomy prior to and after electrophysiology procedures (e.g., in patients with atrial fibrillation)	CT has high spatial resolution Data can be acquired without ECG gating and thus with lower radiation exposure	MRI does not require radiation exposure and is able to visualize scar tissue after ablation using delayed-enhancement techniques
Analysis of global and regional cardiac function and valvular function[a]	CT has high spatial resolution[b] All data needed for functional analysis can be derived from CT coronary angiography without the need for an additional scan	Temporal resolution of CT is limited MRI and echocardiography are the established scientific and clinical gold standards

[a] Analysis of cardiac function is very fast and easy to perform using recent software tools, and because of its clinical importance, it should be performed and reported in every patient undergoing cardiac CT with retrospective gating. In only rare cases there is a clinical indication for cardiac function analysis alone. Functional analysis is nearly always done as part of coronary CT angiography performed for other clinical indications

[b] CT performs better than echocardiography and cineventriculography

CT is also highly accurate in analyzing global and regional cardiac function (Chap. 15). Coronary CT angiography has the crucial advantage that the images necessary for cardiac function analysis are inherently part of a standard retrospectively acquired dataset, and no additional injection of contrast agent or radiation exposure is required. Therefore, because of the importance of global as well as regional cardiac function for the patient's prognosis and further management (Chap. 11), we strongly encourage the inclusion of cardiac function analysis in the reports of all patients undergoing retrospectively gated coronary CT angiography. Nevertheless, because of the radiation exposure and the need for a contrast medium, CT is rarely indicated for analysis of cardiac function alone, but rather for use in combination with other clinical questions to be answered.

6.3   Potential Clinical Indications

CT coronary stent imaging is one of the potential clinical indications (**Table 6.5**). However, the available evidence (Chaps. 13 and 20) clearly indicates a reduced diagnostic accuracy in stents with a diameter of less than 3.5 mm. Also, because such stents represent 70–80% of all implanted coronary stents, in patients with more than two coronary stents the diagnostic accuracy will very likely be limited. Thus, there is no general indication for follow-up using currently available CT technology in patients after stent placement (**Table 6.5**). Also, the positive predictive value of CT is limited in coronary stent imaging (Chap. 23). The decision for or against CT should be made individually on the basis of the stent material and diameter; however, selected patients with low and stable heart rates and proximal large stents can successfully be analyzed using CT angiography.

□ Table 6.5 Potential clinical indications for cardiac CT

	Pros	Cons
Ruling out CAD prior to noncoronary cardiac surgery	Reliable exclusion of CAD in these patients may be possible Conventional coronary angiography may be avoided	There ar e as yet no results from studies in larger patient populations Unclear outcome benefit over established tests
Follow-up of patients with coronary artery stents	High negative predictive value for some stents Can be used for non-invasive follow-up	Evaluation of stents with an internal diameter <3.5 mm is still limited Current CT technology does not provide functional information on blood flow direction
Prior to reoperative cardiac surgery	Important pathology (such as sternal wire near bypasses) and dimensions (e.g., distance of sternum to bypass) can be detected prior to operation	There are as yet no results from studies in larger patient populations
Assessment of cardiac tumors	CT has high spatial resolution and best allows assessment of calcifications	MRI does not require radiation exposure and due to better soft tissue contrast enables better differentiation of certain tumor types
Suspected pericardial disease	Excellent depiction of calcified pericarditis ("armored heart") and pericardial effusion	CT provides only limited functional information MRI and echocardiography yield good results without radiation exposure

6.4 Currently No Clinical Indications

Besides triple rule-out CT, screening is another application that we currently do not consider an established clinical indication for coronary CT angiography (**Table 6.6**) because its predictive value for the presence of significant stenoses is too low in this patient population (**Fig. 6.1**). In contrast, the negative predictive value is very low in patients with typical symptoms and/or positive results of noninvasive tests (high pretest likelihood), so that CT is also not reliable enough to exclude coronary stenoses in this group.

Visualization and analysis of myocardial viability and perfusion is likewise not an accepted clinical indication for CT (**Table 6.6**). The main drawback of myocardial viability and perfusion imaging by CT is that extra scans with additional radiation exposure are necessary, whereas MRI yields excellent results without radiation exposure (Chap. 21).

◘ Table 6.6 Currently no clinical indications for cardiac CT

	Pros	Cons
Screening of asymptomatic individuals	May conceivably be more accurate than other noninvasive modalities in reliably excluding disease	The positive predictive value is unacceptably low in screening patients with a very low pretest likelihood of CAD (**Fig. 6.1**) Study results are not yet available
High pretest likelihood of CAD based on typical symptoms or positive results of other noninvasive tests	High negative predictive value	The negative predictive value is unacceptably low in patients with high pretest likelihood of CAD (**Fig. 6.1**) Intervention is likely required
Triple rule-out (to exclude coronary stenoses, pulmonary embolism, and aortic dissection)	Comprehensive examination	Generally accepted scanning protocols, and the target population remain to be defined No outcome studies
Assessment (including characterization and quantification) of coronary plaques	CT has reasonable accuracy in detection and characterization of plaques	Interobserver variability of CT is considerable and exact analysis of plaque dimension is limited Analysis is rather time-consuming Clinical implications have not been fully explored
Analysis of myocardial viability and perfusion	CT has higher spatial resolution than MRI	Stress echocardiography and MRI have good clinical accuracy without involving radiation exposure Analysis of myocardial vitality and perfusion by CT requires an additional scan after coronary angiography

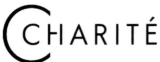

Referred by

Name: ....

Phone: ....

Address: ....

Referral for Coronary CT Angiography

Charité Campus Mitte   ○ **FAX:**

Dept. of Radiology   +49 (0)30/450 527 911

Charité platz 1

10117 Berlin, Germany

I request a **CT coronary angiography** for the following patient:

Last name: .... First name: .... D.O.B.:   .   .   .

Address: ....Phone: ....

Reason for exam: ○ Suspected CAD   ○ Follow-up bypass   ○ Follow-up stent   ○ Other: ....
Indication/Question/Risk factors:

....

....

If the patient has undergone previous tests: Which? **(please attach reports)**
○ ECG   ○ Stress ECG   ○ Echo   ○ Stress echo   ○ Cardiac scintigraphy   ○ MRI   ○ CT

In patients with bypasses: No. of bypassess: .... Date of operation: ....
○ LIMA to ......   ○ RIMA to ......   No. of veins to: ○ LAD: ......   ○ LCX: ......   ○ RCA: ......○ Other: ....

Provision of the following information is **mandatory** in patients with stents to decide whether CT is reasonable:
No. of stents: ...... Stent diameter (mm): ..../......../......../........
Stent length (mm): ..../......../......../........ Stent site: ..../......../......../........

Did the patient have a conventional coronary angiography? Date :   .   .   .
Findings: ....

We ask for the following information so that we can exclude contraindications to CT:
Creatinine: .... ○ Hyperthyroidism (TSH: ....)   ○ Allergic reaction to iodinated contrast agent
○ Irregular heart rate (e.g. atrial fibrillation): ....   ○ Severe asthma (if high heart rate)
Please contact us by phone (+49 (0)30 450 527 133) if your patient has a contraindication or if you have
further questions.

▪ **Fig. 6.2** Example of a referral form that can be used for coronary CT angiography

6.5   Patient Referral

We recommend using a special referral form, to be completed by physicians referring a patient for cardiac CT (**Fig. 6.2**). The information provided in the form makes it easier to decide whether the patient will benefit most from CT or another test. It also helps standardize and facilitate communication with referring physicians. Moreover, possible contraindications (Chap. 7) can be identified before an appointment is made, and the radiologist can choose in advance the most appropriate kind of coronary CT angiography (Chaps. 8 and 9) to be performed in the patient (**Fig. 6.2**).

In summary, the decision as to whether there is a clinical indication for coronary CT angiography should always be made on an individual basis and should take into account the patient's pretest likelihood and possible contraindications.

Recommended Reading

1   Achenbach S (2006) Computed tomography coronary angiography. J Am Coll Cardiol 48:1919–1928

2   Bluemke DA, Achenbach S, Budoff M et al (2008) Noninvasive coronary artery imaging: magnetic resonance angiography and multidetector computed tomography angiography: a scientific statement from the american heart association committee on cardiovascular imaging and intervention of the council on cardiovascular radiology and intervention, and the councils on clinical cardiology and cardiovascular disease in the young. Circulation 118:586–606

3   Cademartiri F, Schuijf JD, Pugliese F et al (2007) Usefulness of 64-slice multislice computed tomography coronary angiography to assess in-stent restenosis. J Am Coll Cardiol 49:2204–2210

4   Cordeiro MA, Lima JA (2006) Atherosclerotic plaque characterization by multidetector row computed tomography angiography. J Am Coll Cardiol 47:C40–C47

5   de Roos A, Kroft LJ, Bax JJ, Geleijns J (2007) Applications of multislice computed tomography in coronary artery disease. J Magn Reson Imaging 26:14–22

6   Dewey M, Hamm B (2007) CT coronary angiography: examination technique, clinical results, and outlook on future developments. Fortschr Röntgenstr 179:246–260

7   Dewey M, Müller M, Eddicks S et al (2006) Evaluation of global and regional left ventricular function with 16-slice computed tomography, biplane cineventriculography, and two-dimensional transthoracic echocardiography: comparison with magnetic resonance imaging. J Am Coll Cardiol 48:2034–2044

8   Dewey M, Teige F, Schnapauff D et al (2006) Noninvasive detection of coronary artery stenoses with multislice computed tomography or magnetic resonance imaging. Ann Intern Med 145:407–415

9   Diamond GA, Forrester JS (1979) Analysis of probability as an aid in the clinical diagnosis of coronary-artery disease. N Engl J Med 300:1350–1358

10   Ehara M, Kawai M, Surmely JF et al (2007) Diagnostic accuracy of coronary in-stent restenosis using 64-slice computed tomography: comparison with invasive coronary angiography. J Am Coll Cardiol 49:951–959

11   Feuchtner GM, Dichtl W, Friedrich GJ et al (2006) Multislice computed tomography for detection of patients with aortic valve stenosis and quantification of severity. J Am Coll Cardiol 47:1410–1417

12   Feuchtner GM, Dichtl W, Schachner T et al (2006) Diagnostic performance of MDCT for detecting aortic valve regurgitation. AJR Am J Roentgenol 186:1676–1681

13   Garcia MJ, Lessick J, Hoffmann MH (2006) Accuracy of 16-row multidetector computed tomography for the assessment of coronary artery stenosis. JAMA 296:403–411

14   Gaspar T, Halon DA, Lewis BS et al (2005) Diagnosis of coronary in-stent restenosis with multidetector row spiral computed tomography. J Am Coll Cardiol 46:1573–1579

15   Gasparovic H, Rybicki FJ, Millstine J et al (2005) Three dimensional computed tomographic imaging in planning the surgical approach for redo cardiac surgery after coronary revascularization. Eur J Cardiothorac Surg 28:244–249

16   Gilard M, Cornily JC, Pennec PY et al (2006) Assessment of coronary artery stents by 16 slice computed tomography. Heart 92:58–61

17   Hamon M, Biondi-Zoccai GG, Malagutti P, Agostoni P, Morello R, Valgimigli M (2006) Diagnostic performance of multislice spiral computed tomography of coronary arteries as compared with conventional invasive coronary angiography: a meta-analysis. J Am Coll Cardiol 48:1896–1910

18   Hamon M, Champ-Rigot L, Morello R, Riddell JW (2008) Diagnostic accuracy of in-stent coronary restenosis detection with multislice spiral computed tomography: a meta-analysis. Eur Radiol; 18:217–225

19   Hendel RC, Patel MR, Kramer CM et al (2006) ACCF/ACR/SCCT/SCMR/ASNC/NASCI/SCAI/SIR 2006 appropriateness criteria for cardiac computed tomography and cardiac magnetic resonance imaging. J Am Coll Cardiol 48:1475–1497

20   Hoffmann MH, Shi H, Schmitz BL et al (2005) Noninvasive coronary angiography with multislice computed tomography. JAMA 293:2471–2478

21   Hoffmann U, Pena AJ, Cury RC et al (2006) Cardiac CT in emergency department patients with acute chest pain. Radiographics 26:963–978, discussion 79–80

22   Jones CM, Athanasiou T, Dunne N et al (2007) Multi-detector computed tomography in coronary artery bypass graft assessment: a meta-analysis. Ann Thorac Surg 83:341–348

23   Leber AW, Johnson T, Becker A et al (2007) Diagnostic accuracy of dual-source multi-slice CT-coronary angiography in patients with an intermediate pretest likelihood for coronary artery disease. Eur Heart J; 28:2354–2360

24   Mahnken AH, Muhlenbruch G, Gunther RW, Cardiac WJE (2007) Cardiac CT: coronary arteries and beyond. Eur Radiol 17:994–1008

25   Malagutti P, Nieman K, Meijboom WB et al (2006) Use of 64-slice CT in symptomatic patients after coronary bypass surgery: evaluation of grafts and coronary arteries. Eur Heart J 28:1879–1885

26   Martuscelli E, Romagnoli A, D'Eliseo A et al (2004) Evaluation of venous and arterial conduit patency by 16-slice spiral computed tomography. Circulation 110:3234–3238

27   Meijboom WB, Mollet NR, Van Mieghem CA et al (2006) Preoperative computed tomography coronary angiography to detect significant coronary artery disease in patients referred for cardiac valve surgery. J Am Coll Cardiol 48:1658–1665

28   Meijboom WB, van Mieghem CA, Mollet NR et al (2007) 64-slice computed tomography coronary angiography in patients with high, intermediate, or low pretest probability of significant coronary artery disease. J Am Coll Cardiol 50:1469–1475

29   Meyer TS, Martinoff S, Hadamitzky M et al (2007) Improved non-invasive assessment of coronary artery bypass grafts with 64-slice computed tomographic angiography in an unselected patient population. J Am Coll Cardiol 49:946–950

30   Mollet NR, Cademartiri F, Nieman K et al (2004) Multislice spiral computed tomography coronary angiography in patients with stable angina pectoris. J Am Coll Cardiol 43:2265–2270

31   Poon M, Rubin GD, Achenbach S et al (2007) Consensus update on the appropriate usage of cardiac computed tomographic angiography. J Invasive Cardiol 19:484–490

32   Raff GL, Chinnaiyan KM, Berman DS et al (2009) Coronary Computed Tomography for Systematic Triage of Acute Chest Pain Patients to Treatment – (The CT-STAT Trial). Circulation 120:2160

33   Rixe J, Achenbach S, Ropers D et al (2006) Assessment of coronary artery stent restenosis by 64-slice multi-detector computed tomography. Eur Heart J 27:2567–2572

34   Ropers U, Ropers D, Pflederer T et al (2007) Influence of heart rate on the diagnostic accuracy of dual-source computed tomography coronary angiography. J Am Coll Cardiol 50:2393–2398

35   Schoepf UJ, Zwerner PL, Savino G, Herzog C, Kerl JM, Costello P (2007) Coronary CT angiography. Radiology 244:48–63

36   Schuetz GM, Zacharopoulou NM, Schlattmann P, Dewey M (2010) Meta-analysis: noninvasive coronary angiography using computed tomography versus magnetic resonance imaging. Ann Intern Med 152:167–177

37   Stillman AE, Oudkerk M, Ackerman M et al (2007) Use of multidetector computed tomography for the assessment of acute chest pain: a consensus statement of the North American Society of Cardiac Imaging and the European Society of Cardiac Radiology. Eur Radiol 17:2196–2207

38   van der Vleuten PA, Willems TP, Gotte MJ et al (2006) Quantification of global left ventricular function: comparison of multidetector computed tomography and magnetic resonance imaging. a meta-analysis and review of the current literature. Acta Radiol 47:1049–1057

39   Van Mieghem CA, Cademartiri F, Mollet NR et al (2006) Multislice spiral computed tomography for the evaluation of stent patency after left main coronary artery stenting: a comparison with conventional coronary angiography and intravascular ultrasound. Circulation 114:645–653

40   Weustink AC, Meijboom WB, Mollet NR et al (2007) Reliable high-speed coronary computed tomography in symptomatic patients. J Am Coll Cardiol 50:786–794

Patient Preparation

M. Dewey

Abstract

Patient preparation is the key to success in cardiac CT, and the relevant aspects of this step are discussed in detail in this chapter.

7.1   Patient Information Sheets

As patient preparation is the cornerstone of a successful cardiac CT, a well-trained nurse, physician assistant, technician, or a physician (according to state and/or federal legal regulations) should discuss the entire procedure with the patient and obtain written informed consent. Patient education can be facilitated by sending the patient an information sheet and questionnaire before the appointment (**Figs. 7.1** and **7.2**). The information asked in the questionnaire also serves to verify the patient's clinical indication for cardiac CT (Chap. 6) and exclude possible clinical contraindications to the examination.

7.2   General Information

The patient should be assured that CT is a noninvasive diagnostic procedure and that it does not take long to perform the examination. The short duration of the CT examination (about 15 min in the scanner room) and the comfortably wide and short gantry (in contrast to the narrow, claustrophobia-inducing bore in MRI) are major advantages of CT over MRI and should be stressed while talking to the patient. On the one hand, clearly explaining these aspects before the patient enters the scanner room reduces psychological stress and may relax the patient as well as reduce heart rate in some cases. On the other hand, the patient must also be given explicit information about the radiation exposure, which is the most important disadvantage of cardiac CT. As it does not mean much to a layperson that the effective exposure of a typical retrospectively gated exam is approximately 10–20 mSv, meaningful comparisons should be used, such as "the radiation exposure of cardiac CT angiography is five to ten times the annual background radiation" or "the effective radiation dose is the same as that of 100–200 chest X-rays." Using prospective gating ("step-and-shoot") will dramatically reduce the effective dose of cardiac CT to below 5 mSv in nearly all patients with low and stable heart rates (Chap. 8). Such effective doses are lower than necessary for nuclear myocardial perfusion imaging (about 8–12 mSv) and conventional coronary angiography (about 8 mSv). Thus, in patients with low and stable heart rates, the radiation exposure of CT is lower than that of alternative diagnostic tests. Nevertheless, especially in younger patients with a higher lifetime risk of cancer induced by CT, it is essential to carefully consider alternative imaging tests that might yield the same clinical information without radiation exposure.

Patients should know that lower heart rates (<60 beats per min) are associated with longer cardiac rest periods and thus improve image quality and diagnostic accuracy while they also help to reduce radiation dose. Informing them about the entire procedure prevents inadvertent reactions to unexpected events that might increase their heart rate. Hence, patients should be informed that they might experience a sensation of warmth when the contrast medium is injected and should also be told beforehand about the expected duration and number of breath-hold periods.

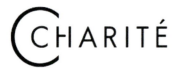

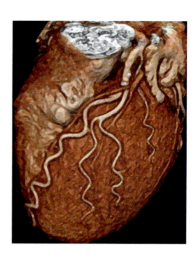

Patient Information
CT Coronary Angiography

7

Dear Ms./Mr. ....,

Your doctor has referred you for an examination of your heart vessels (coronary arteries) to look for narrowings (stenoses) and deposits (plaques). The examination is performed on a computed tomography (CT) scanner. CT identifies stenoses and plaques in the coronary arteries with a reliability of over 90% and we expect that the information gained by the examination will help improve your further treatment.

You should fast for four hours before the examination (most importantly, you should not drink coffee or tea) and should continue to take your usual medications. If you take the antidiabetic drug called metformin, you must stop taking this medication for 48 hours after the test.

Please carefully complete the questionnaire provided with this information sheet (see **Figure 7.2**). The details about your symptoms and other tests that you have had in the past will help us make the correct diagnosis by CT. A written report of the CT findings will be sent to your doctor after the examination.

Please send the completed form to the address or fax number given below or bring it along when you come in for your examination on day: .... at: ....

Address:

Charité

Institut für Radiologie, CT

Luisenstr. 68 (Hochhaus)

10117 Berlin

FAX No.:

+49 (0)30/450 527 911

Phone:

+49 (0)30/450 527 133

Most patients with one of the following conditions cannot undergo a CT scan of the heart:

1. Irregular heart beat (e.g., atrial fibrillation)
2. Severe bronchial asthma (if high heart rate is present)
3. Intake of certain erectile dysfunction pills (e.g., Viagra)
4. Reduced kidney function (creatinine level > 1.5 – 2.0 mg/dl)
5. Allergic reactions to X-ray contrast media
6. Manifest overactivity of the thyroid (hyperthyroidism)

If one of these conditions applies in your case, please contact us before the examination

🔲 **Fig. 7.1** Example of an information sheet that is sent out to the patient prior to the examination. Patients are asked to inform us in case contraindications to coronary CT angiography might be present that have been overlooked during the prior referral procedure (Chap. 6)

Patient Questionnaire

Name: .... Address: .... Phone No.: ....

FAX: ....Email: ....@...

1. **D.O.B.**:   .   .   . **Height**:   .   m/inches **Weight**: .... kg/pounds **male** ○ **female** ○

2. Do you have **pain** in the chest? yes ○ no ○, If yes, please describe the location and type of pain:

....

   Does the pain increase when you **exercise**? yes ○ no ○ How long does the pain last? ....

   Does the pain decrease **at rest or after nitro spray**? yes ○ no ○

3. Do you **smoke**? yes ○ no ○ If yes, for how long? .... years, how many cigarettes per day? ......

4. **Did you smoke**? yes ○ no ○ If yes, for how long? .... years, how many cigarettes per day? ......

5. Do you have **high blood lipid levels** (hyperlipidemia)? yes ○ no ○

   Total cholesterol: ....(p≥200 mg/dl) **LDL**: ...... (p≥120 mg/dl) **TG**: ......(p≥200mg/dl)

6. Do you take **statins** or other drugs to lower cholesterol? yes ○ no ○ - for how long? .... years

7. Do you have **high blood sugar** (diabetes mellitus)? yes ○ no ○

8. Do you have **high blood pressure** (hypertension)? yes ○ no ○

9. Do you take **beta blockers** to lower blood pressure? yes ○ no ○ - for how long? .... years

10. Have you had a **heart attack** (myocardial infarction)? yes ○ no ○, If yes, please bring the report with you.

11. Do you have **stents** that keep the heart vessels open? yes ○ no ○, If yes, please bring the report with you.

12. Have you had **widening of a vessel** with a catheter? yes ○ no ○, If yes, please bring the report with you.

13. Do you have any cardiac **bypasses**? yes ○ no ○, If yes, please bring the report with you.

14. Have you had an **electrocardiogram** (ECG)? yes ○ no ○, If yes, please bring the report with you.

15. Have you had an **exercise (treadmill) ECG**? yes ○ no ○, If yes, please bring the report with you.

16. Have you had an **echocardiogram**? yes ○ no ○, If yes, please bring the report with you.

17. Have you had a **stress echocardiogram**? yes ○ no ○, If yes, please bring the report with you.

18. Have you had **myocardial scintigraphy**? yes ○ no ○, If yes, please bring the report with you.

19. Have you had a **cardiac catheter examination**? yes ○ no ○, If yes, please bring the report(s) with you.

20. Have you had a **CT scan/MRI** of the heart? yes ○ no ○, If yes, please bring the reports with you.

21. Which **medications** are you taking? Please list, **with doses**:

   - ....   - ....

   - ....   - ....

   - ....   - ....

▢ **Fig. 7.2** Example of a medical history questionnaire that is also sent out to the patient prior to the examination. This questionnaire elicits information about the patient's entire cardiovascular medical history and is very valuable for diagnostic procedures in the outpatient setting

Patients who are aware that the target structures are just a few millimeters in size will better understand that any motion during the breath-hold periods may severely degrade the images and may even result in a nondiagnostic scan. They also need to be informed that they should hold their breath after submaximal inspiration (ca. 75% of maximum inspiration), a maneuver that should be taught either prior to the examination or during scanning as part of the training related to the breath-hold commands (Chap. 9). The submaximum depth of inspiration is important, because maximal inspiration may increase intrathoracic pressure (Valsava maneuver) and reduce inflow of the contrast medium.

The length of the breath-hold periods varies between 3 and 30 s, depending on the scanner used and the examination performed (Chap. 2). Breath-hold training on the scanner table is therefore also important to determine whether a patient is able to hold his or her breath for the required duration, or whether oxygen administration is needed to improve compliance. Preoxygenation is rarely required when the examination is performed on a 64-row CT scanner, with scan times of only 8–12 s. Using wide-volume scanning (320-rows) or fast prospective spiral acquisitions with second-generation dual-source CT, the scanning time is greatly reduced to just a single heart beat and breath-hold time is about 3–5 s (Chap. 2).

7.3   Contraindications

When informing the patient about cardiac CT, the examiner should make sure that the patient is in sinus rhythm. This assessment is most easily accomplished by feeling the radial pulse when meeting the patient. In the case of patients with atrial fibrillation or frequent extrasystoles (at least one or two within the expected scanning period), the per-patient diagnostic accuracy is still unsatisfactory; for this reason, it is advisable that the examination be performed at a later time, for example after medical or electrical cardioversion.

At the same time, the patient should also be questioned about general contraindications to contrast agents (**List 7.1**), as well as contraindications to nitroglycerin (**List 7.2**) and beta blockers (**List 7.3**). The considerable radiation exposure involved precludes coronary CT angiography in young and pregnant women. It is usually safe to administer nitroglycerin and/or beta blockers for the CT scan to patients who are taking these two medications on a regular basis without problems. Whether

CT can be performed without nitroglycerin and/or beta blocker administration in patients with contraindications must be decided on an individual basis and depends on the clinical question and the patient's heart rate. It is generally desirable to administer nitroglycerin because of the beneficial vasodilatory effect. The CT scan should be postponed by at least 24 h in patients who have taken phosphodiesterase inhibitors (**List 7.2**).

List 7.1. Contraindications to iodinated contrast agents

1. Renal insufficiency (creatinine level >1.5–2.0 mg/dl, absolute contraindication unless evidence-based measures to prevent contrast-induced nephropathy can be taken)
2. Intake of metformin-containing medications (metformin needs to be discontinued for 48 h after contrast injection)[a]
3. Prior allergic reactions to iodinated contrast agents (switching to a different contrast agent and antiallergic premedication may enable imaging in those patients)
4. Manifest hyperthyroidism

---

[a] In patients with abnormal renal function, metformin also needs to be discontinued for 48 h prior to elective examinations, according to the ESUR guideline.

List 7.2. Contraindications to nitroglycerin

1. Intake of phosphodiesterase inhibitors (such as sildenafil, tadalafil, and vardenafil)
2. Arterial hypotension (systolic blood pressure below 100 mmHg)
3. Severe aortic stenosis
4. Hypertrophic obstructive cardiomyopathy
5. Nitroglycerin intolerance (e.g., severe headache)

List 7.3. Contraindications to beta blockers

1. Severe asthma
2. Severe obstructive lung disease
3. Bradycardia (below 50 beats per min)
4. Second or third degree atrioventricular block
5. Beta blocker intolerance (e.g., psoriasis)

Recommended Reading

1 Achenbach S (2006) Computed tomography coronary angiography. J Am Coll Cardiol 48:1919–1928

2 Achenbach S, Rost C, Ropers D, Pflederer T, von Erffa J, Daniel WG (2007) Non-invasive coronary angiography: current status and perspectives. Dtsch Med Wochenschr 132:750–756

3 Dewey M, Hamm B (2007) CT coronary angiography: examination technique, clinical results, and outlook on future developments. Fortschr Röntgenstr 179:246–260

4 Dewey M, Hoffmann H, Hamm B (2006) Multislice CT coronary angiography: effect of sublingual nitroglycerine on the diameter of coronary arteries. Fortschr Röntgenstr 178:600–604

5 Einstein AJ, Henzlova MJ, Rajagopalan S (2007) Estimating risk of cancer associated with radiation exposure from 64-slice computed tomography coronary angiography. JAMA 298:317–323

6 Hoffmann U, Ferencik M, Cury RC, Pena AJ (2006) Coronary CT angiography. J Nucl Med 47:797–806

7 Pannu HK, Alvarez W Jr, Fishman EK (2006) Beta-blockers for cardiac CT: a primer for the radiologist. AJR Am J Roentgenol 186:S341–S345

8 Schoepf UJ, Zwerner PL, Savino G, Herzog C, Kerl JM, Costello P (2007) Coronary CT angiography. Radiology 244:48–63

9 Schönenberger E, Schnapauff D, Teige F, Laule M, Hamm B, Dewey M (2007) Patient acceptance of noninvasive and invasive coronary angiography. PLoS ONE 2:e246

10 Schuetz GM, Zacharopoulou NM, Schlattmann P, Dewey M (2010) Meta-analysis: noninvasive coronary angiography using computed tomography versus magnetic resonance imaging. Ann Intern Med 152:167–177

11 Weigold WG (2006) Coronary CT angiography: insights into patient preparation and scanning. Tech Vasc Interv Radiol 9:205–209

The ESUR guideline on contrast media can be accessed at: http://www.esur.org/Contrast-media.51.0.html.

Physics Background and Radiation Exposure

J. Geleijns and M. Dewey

Abstract

This chapter outlines the physical background of cardiac CT and different scanning approaches including aspects of radiation exposure.

8.1 Physics of CT

The mathematical principle underlying computed tomography (CT) was formulated by the Austrian mathematician Johann Radon in 1917. The inverse Radon transform can be used to calculate tomographic reconstructions from line integrals of the attenuation of X-rays. In CT, the Radon transform is often visualized as a sinogram. The sinogram represents the raw data space of a CT scan. It took until the early 1970s before Allan Cormack and Sir Godfrey Hounsfield were able to generate the first 2D reconstructions of a human brain in preclinical laboratory experiments. This lead to the clinical introduction of CT in 1974 with the installation of 60 head scanners. Allan Cormack and Sir Godfrey Hounsfield shared the Nobel Prize in Physiology or Medicine in 1979 for their pioneering work in the development of CT.

The first CT scanners were manufactured exclusively for CT examinations of the brain (**Fig. 8.1**) since the bore was too small to fit the trunk of an adult patient. An impressive milestone for the development of cardiac imaging of the heart was reported by Harrel and his research group as early as June 1976. They used a new whole-body CT scanner and a rotation time of 6 s to perform what they termed "stop-action computed tomography." Their total scan time of 18 s consisted of two 6-s

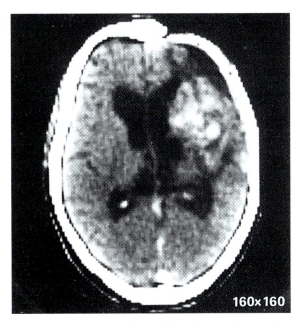

Fig 8.1 Early brain image from a CT head scanner. Reconstruction performed on a 160² matrix

M. Dewey, *Cardiac CT*,
DOI: 10.1007/978-3-642-14022-8_8, © Springer-Verlag Berlin Heidelberg 2011

rotations separated by 6 s, allowing imaging of the heart within one breath-hold. The resulting 12-s data acquisition included 13½ heartbeats. By simultaneously recording the raw data and the ECG, combined with a sophisticated reconstruction technique, they were able to reconstruct images corresponding to any phase of the cardiac cycle with a temporal resolution of 250 ms. However, a serious limitation of the technique developed by Harrel was that they could only reconstruct images of a single plane of the heart. The same research group presented their first results on coronary CT angiography in 1979 (**Fig. 8.2**). The basic principles of their reconstruction technique and particularly their method of obtaining a short snapshot of the heart are still applied today in what is now known as multisegment reconstruction.

It took about 25 years of research and development after Harell's initial experiment to develop CT scanners suitable for routine cardiac imaging. Good in-plane spatial resolution and good low-contrast resolution were already accomplished with the single detector row CT (step-and-shoot, axial) scanners available in 1976. Volume acquisitions became feasible with the introduction of helical single-row CT in 1989, and a small slice thickness of about 1 mm was available as early as 1981. However, it took the introduction of helical 4-row CT scanners with rotation times below 1 s in 1998 to combine small slice thickness and sufficient volume coverage within one breath-hold. With the 4-row CT scanners it became possible for the first time to assess cardiac function and coronary arteries in a clinical setting. Further developments leading to 16- and 64-row CT scanners provided considerable improvements in image quality (Chap. 2). Even more sophisticated performance in cardiac CT is offered by recent achievements, such as second-generation dual-source CT (Somatom Definition Flash, Siemens; Chap. 10b) and volumetric cone-beam CT (Aquilion ONE, Toshiba; Chap. 10a).

CT images are typically reconstructed using a 512 × 512 axial image matrix. The numerical value assigned to each pixel represents the average linear X-ray attenuation coefficient of the tissues within the associated voxel relative to the attenuation coefficient of water, and are given in Hounsfield units, see **Table 8.1**. The Hounsfield unit for a voxel that contains different tissues expresses the average attenuation within the voxel; this averaging is referred to as the partial volume effect.

The basic acquisition parameters for a CT scan are the number of active detector rows, slice thickness (mm), X-ray tube rotation time (s), tube current (mA), and tube voltage (kV). In axial step-and-shoot CT, the

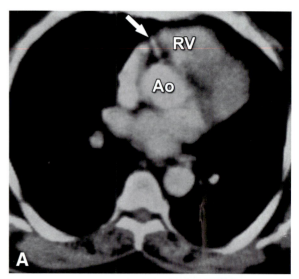

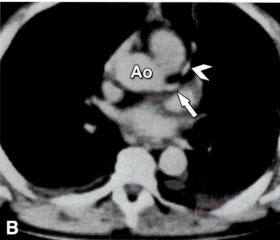

◘ **Fig. 8.2** First images of coronary CT angiography. **Panel A** shows the proximal right coronary artery (*arrow*) and **Panel B** the left main (*arrow*) and left anterior descending coronary artery in another patient (*arrowhead*). *Ao* aorta; *RV* right ventricle. With permission from Guthaner et al., AJR 1979 (American Roentgen Ray Society)

table translation between axial acquisitions is referred to as the table increment, in helical CT the pitch factor defines the table increment per rotation. These parameters must be optimized to achieve contradictory goals such as minimal motion artifacts, coverage within one breath-hold, good spatial resolution, good contrast resolution, and minimal radiation exposure. The parameters relevant for high-quality reconstruction in CT are the reconstruction field of view, the reconstructed slice thickness, the reconstructed slice increment, and the reconstruction filter.

Table 8.1 Attenuation values of different tissues and materials		
Substance	**Hounsfield unit (HU)**	**Range of HUs**
Compact bone	+1,000	(+300 to +2,500)
Contrast-enhanced blood[a]	+400	(+200 to +600)
Calcified plaque	+400	(+130 to +1,000)
Noncalcified fibrotic plaque	+80	(+30 to +130)
Noncalcified lipid plaque	+10	(−40 to +40)
Liver	+ 60	(+50 to +70)
Blood	+ 55	(+50 to +60)
Kidneys	+ 30	(+20 to +40)
Muscle	+ 25	(+10 to +40)
Brain, gray matter	+ 35	(+30 to +40)
Brain, white matter	+ 25	(+20 to +30)
Water	0	
Fat	− 90	(−100 to −80)
Lung	− 750	(−950 to −600)
Air	− 1,000	

[a] Enhanced aorta, ventricle or coronary artery

8.2   Physics of Cardiac CT

Users of CT scanners aim at producing images of good diagnostic quality whilst maintaining the radiation exposure of the patient as low as reasonably achievable. In cardiac CT it is crucial to achieve excellent spatial resolution (to be able to visualize the small coronaries), excellent temporal resolution (to avoid motion-induced blurring), and short scan time (to avoid breathing artifacts). In addition, image noise should be low enough and the contrast-to-noise ratio high enough for visualization of the coronary arteries. What distinguishes cardiac CT from most other CT applications is the need for appropriate synchronization of the image reconstruction with the simultaneously recorded ECG.

8.2.1   Spatial Resolution

Spatial resolution plays an important role in coronary CT angiography, particularly in the visualization of distal segments with diameters down to less than 1 mm. A voxel size of about $0.5 \times 0.5 \times 0.5$ mm or smaller in combination with an intrinsic spatial resolution (expressed as FWHM[1]) of about 0.5–0.7 mm is sufficient for coronary imaging. However, for accurate visualization of very small structures, such as early atherosclerotic lesions within the coronary wall, even better spatial resolution is required but not possible with current CT scanners. Spatial resolution in the reconstructed images also depends on the reconstruction filter used; in cardiac CT for example a dedicated stent or coronary reconstruction filter. Small objects such as stents and calcifications may also be visualized inappropriately due to artifacts related to motion, partial volume effect, and beam hardening.

8.2.2   Temporal Resolution

Good temporal resolution is required in cardiac CT to guarantee that the motion of the fast moving coronary arteries does not lead to substantial artifacts. This can be achieved by hardware that allows fast data acquisition, e.g., a fast rotating gantry and/or a gantry equipped with two X-ray tubes. The rotation time of the X-ray tube should be as short as possible, but is limited by engineering since short rotation times lead to very high g-forces, up to 20–30 g, on all components mounted on the rotating gantry. Rotation times of current CT scanners are in the range of 0.27–0.35 s. Optimal temporal resolution can also be enhanced by dedicated reconstruction algorithms. CT images are generally reconstructed from one full (360°) rotation. In cardiac CT, images are reconstructed from half (180°) rotations because, according to the mathematics of CT, this yields the minimum required amount of information.

---

[1]Physicists measure spatial resolution as the point spread function (PSF) and express the performance of CT scanners with regard to spatial resolution as the full width half maximum (FWHM) of the PSF. The FWHM defines whether or not two adjacent structures will be represented separately in the images; two structures separated by at least one FWHM can in general be distinguished from each other, two structures separated by less than one FWHM are bound to merge together in the reconstructed image.

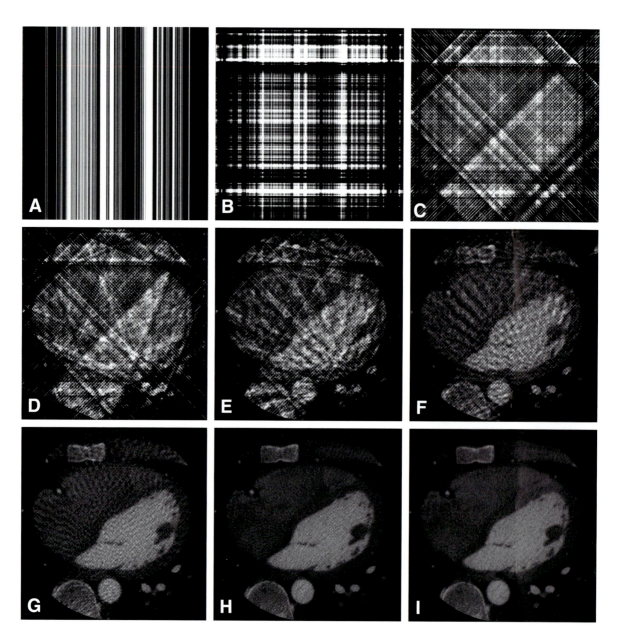

🔳 **Fig. 8.3** Simulation of the effect of the number of backprojections on image quality. Reconstructed axial cardiac CT images are shown using 1, 2, 4, 8, 16, 32, 64, 128, and 1024 backprojections in **Panels A–I**, respectively

Fig. 8.3 illustrates that hundreds of views are required to reconstruct artifact-free images. Temporal resolution can be further improved by a factor of two with the incorporation of two X-ray tubes (dual-source CT). Improved temporal resolution can also be achieved by including attenuation profiles acquired during two or more heartbeats in the reconstruction. In this latter case, raw data from multiple heartbeats are combined during the reconstruction. This is referred to as a multisegment reconstruction, i.e., more than one RR interval is used for image reconstruction.

8.2.3   Image Noise and Radiation Exposure

Low image noise provides better image quality. Image noise may be decreased by raising the tube current (mA), but this comes at the cost of increased patient exposure. Currently, the choice of tube current in cardiac CT acquisitions is based on clinical experience and provides a balance between low patient dose and sufficient image quality (Chap. 10). Computer simulations of the image quality of cardiac CT resulting from a lower tube current can be performed and may provide an evidence base for selection of the most appropriate tube current (**Fig. 9.11**). In addition, image quality, and the contrast-to-noise ratio, in cardiac CT may be enhanced by selecting a lower tube voltage (e.g., 100 or 80 kV), which improves the visualization of iodine. Particularly in patients with a normal or low body mass index, a lower tube voltage can be used to achieve better image quality at the same radiation exposure or to reduce the dose whilst maintaining image quality.

8.2.4   Retrospective ECG Gating and Prospective ECG Triggering

Essential in cardiac CT is synchronization of the image reconstruction with the patient's ECG and selection of the best cardiac phase. Current cardiac CT scanners only provide good image quality, without motion artifacts, when the reconstructed images correspond to the optimal rest phase of the coronary arteries. The principles of retrospective ECG-gated reconstruction and prospective ECG-triggered reconstruction are illustrated in **Fig. 8.4**.

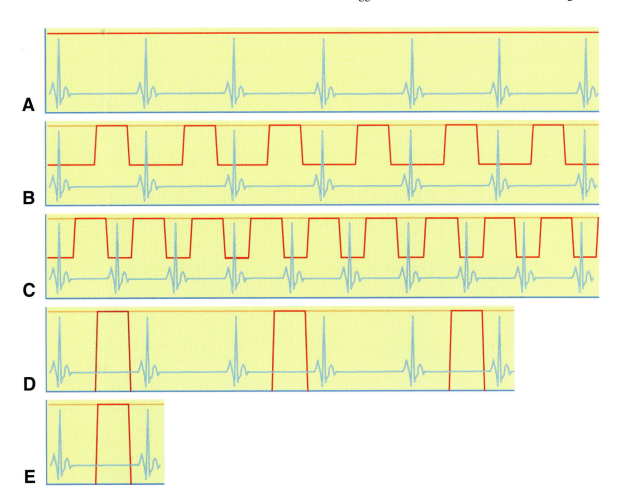

◻ **Fig. 8.4** ECG (blue lines) and tube current during different acquisitions (*red lines*). **Panel A** shows that during a retrospective helical acquisition with a 64-row CT scanner, the tube current remains constant during six RR intervals. **Panel B** shows how the tube current can be modulated during a helical acquisition based on the recorded ECG to achieve good image quality for assessment of the coronary arteries (where the tube current remains high, peaks of the *red line*) and at the same time sufficient image quality for assessment of cardiac function (where the tube current is reduced). **Panel C** shows that at a higher heart rate, there is less opportunity to reduce tube current during the helical acquisition and less opportunity to reduce patient exposure. All helical acquisitions depicted in **Panels A–C** allow assessment of cardiac function. **Panel D** shows how an acquisition on a 64-row CT scanner is done in five heartbeats with "step-and-shoot" covering the entire heart with lower dose at the assumed coronary rest phase. Different axial steps are separated by at least one heartbeat to allow for translation of the patient. **Panel E** shows that some CT scanners allow prospective scanning of the entire heart within a single heartbeat: a fast dual-source CT scanner is capable of performing a helical acquisition of the entire heart within one heartbeat (Siemens Definition Flash), and a wide cone beam CT scanner performs an axial acquisition of the entire heart (Toshiba Aquilion ONE) within one heartbeat. Such novel "single heartbeat" techniques carry the promise of further dose reduction and image quality improvement

Reconstruction based on retrospective cardiac phase selection requires helical registration of the raw data and the ECG during several complete cardiac cycles. **Fig. 8.4A** shows that retrospective ECG gating allows reconstruction of the scanned volume at any cardiac phase. Effective dose can be reduced using ECG-triggered tube current modulation (**Fig. 8.4B**). **Fig. 8.4C** shows that at higher heart rates, there is less opportunity to reduce the tube current during helical acquisitions.

An alternative to retrospective helical ECG-gated reconstruction is prospective "step-and-shoot" acquisition (**Fig. 8.4D**). Step-and-shoot techniques have the advantage of reducing patient dose, but the required stitching of several images is prone to artifacts at the borders of the prospectively acquired slabs, especially in arrhythmic patients. Of course, prospectively acquired step-and-shoot scans do not allow assessment of cardiac function since they only cover the (assumed) best cardiac phase. Also, prospective ECG gating is preferred in patients with low and stable heart rates, in whom the center of the acquisition window is located at approximately 70–80% of the RR interval. Some CT scanners allow prospective scanning of the entire heart within a single heartbeat: a fast dual-source CT scanner is capable of performing a helical acquisition of the entire heart (Siemens Definition Flash), and a wide cone beam CT scanner performs an axial acquisition of the entire heart (Toshiba Aquilion ONE) within one heartbeat (**Fig. 8.4E**). Such novel "single heartbeat" techniques carry the promise of further dose reduction. The appearance of helical and axial scans on film that is exposed on the CT table is shown in **Fig. 8.5**.

Scans that require image acquisition during more than one cardiac cycle are inherently sensitive to arrhythmia, this is true for both retrospective and prospective acquisitions. But even CT angiography scans acquired within a single heartbeat are prone to artifacts caused by arrhythmia, since it is not possible to predict if the subsequent heartbeat will be stable or irregular. A volume CT scanner covering the entire heart in an axial snapshot (Aquilion ONE, Toshiba) may be more robust with regard to arrhythmia due to the lack of table movement (**Fig. 8.6**).

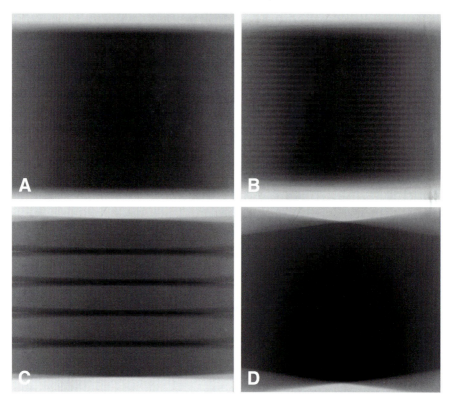

■ **Fig. 8.5** Appearance of coronary scans covering 16 cm in the Z-axis with different collimations on films exposed on the CT table. **Panel A** shows a retrospectively ECG-gated helical scan performed using 16-row CT whereas **Panel B** shows retrospectively ECG-gated scanning using 64-row CT. There is significant overscanning visible on the films exposed using these approaches. Triggered (prospectively ECG-gated) scanning using 5 axial acquisitions in the step-and-shoot mode is shown in **Panel C** with the overlapping areas of the prospectively acquired slabs clearly visible. Nevertheless, there is relevant reduction of overscanning. **Panel D** is a representation of a single shot with volume CT using 320 simultaneous detectors. We are thankful to R. Juran Ph.D. and J. Mews RT for their assistance with this figure

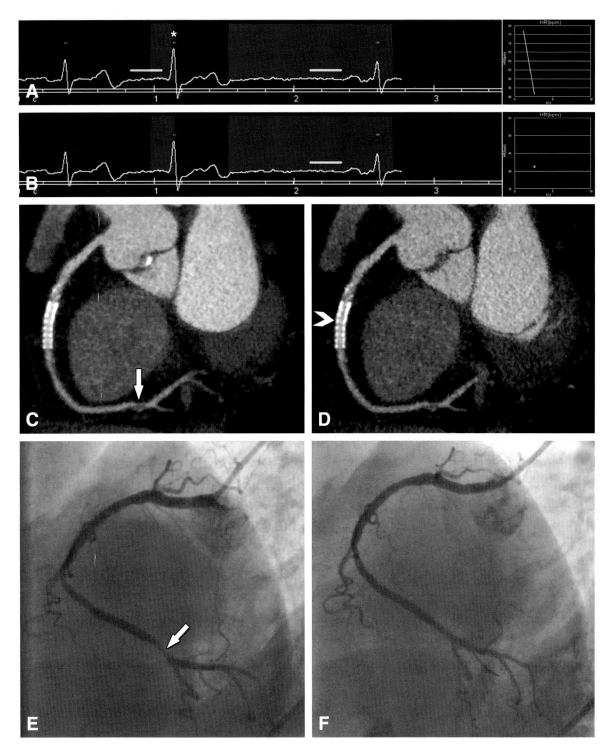

◘ Fig. 8.6 Advantage of volume coronary CT angiography in arrhythmia. Example of a 66-year-old woman who had a premature atrial contraction during the heartbeat intended for volumetric scanning (*asterisk* in **Panel A**). Scanning was immediately stopped when the arrhythmia occurred and was continued during the subsequent beat with a safety window (**Panel A**). These two beats had a rate of 77 and 41 beats per min (**Panels A** and **B**). Only the second, nonarrhythmic beat was used for reconstruction of images (**Panel B**). Reconstructions with a soft filter showed a significant (70% diameter) stenosis of segment 3 of the right coronary artery (RCA, *arrow* in **Panel C**), whereas significant in-stent restenosis of the 3.0-mm mid-RCA stent was excluded in reconstructions with a stent filter (**Panel D**). Conventional coronary angiography confirmed the significant distal RCA stenosis (*arrow* in **Panel E**), which was treated during the same interventional session (**Panel F**)

8.3   Patient Dosimetry and Radiation Exposure

8.3.1   Dosimetry

Dosimetry is used to measure the energy imparted by ionizing radiation to matter. Physicists provide the basis for radiation dosimetry with the definition of the fundamental physical quantity for radiation dosimetry, being the quantity absorbed dose (D). Absorbed dose is the quotient of the energy imparted by ionizing radiation (energy (E); unit Joule (J)) and the mass of the exposed matter (mass (m); unit kilogram (kg)). The unit of absorbed energy is Joule per kilogram (J/kg), but in radiation dosimetry absorbed dose is expressed as gray (Gy). Dose levels that occur in CT are generally much lower than 1 Gy, therefore doses are usually expressed in milligray (1 mGy = 0.001 Gy).

Dose measurements must be performed during installation, acceptance testing, and constancy testing of CT scanners. During such tests the normalized output of the scanner is generally established as the CT dose index per unit of tube charge (CTDI/Q; unit mGy/mAs). The radiation exposure of specific CT acquisition protocols is expressed either as CTDI (mGy) or as dose length product (DLP, Gy.cm). The CTDI represents the radiation output of the CT scanner during one full rotation of the X-ray tube; and the DLP represents the radiation exposure during a complete helical or axial acquisition and takes into account the total number of tube rotations during the CT scan. Both CTDI and DLP are very useful for comparing the radiation exposure of different CT acquisition protocols.

Dosimetric quantities that are most often used in the context of biomedical dose assessment are the equivalent organ dose[2] (H_T, mSv) and the effective dose (E, mSv). The effective dose is the pragmatic weighted sum of equivalent organ doses, where the tissue weighting factors (w_T) are used to take into account the relative sensitivity of organs to carcinogenic and hereditary effects.

---

[2]The equivalent dose is the product of absorbed dose (D, mGy) and a radiation weighting factor (wR, mSv/mGy). The radiation weighting factor for X-rays is 1, so absorbed dose and the equivalent dose are numerically equal.

■ **Table 8.2** Tissue weighting factors published by the ICRP in 1972 (ICRP publication 26), 1991 (ICRP publication 60), and 2007 (ICRP publication 103)

Organ	ICRP 26, 1972	ICRP 60, 1991	ICRP 103, 2007
Breast	0.15	0.05	0.12
Bone marrow	0.12	0.12	0.12
Lung	0.12	0.12	0.12
Colon	–	0.12	0.12
Stomach	–	0.12	0.12
Thyroid	0.03	0.05	0.04
Bone surface	0.03	0.01	0.01
Gonads	0.25	0.20	0.08
Other	0.30	0.05	0.12

Tissue weighting factors are regularly revised on the basis of new scientific insights (**Table 8.2**). Particularly relevant for cardiac CT are the changes in the tissue weighting factor for breast tissue. It was 0.15 in 1972 and was decreased to 0.05 in 1991. Since 2007, the tissue factor breast has been 0.12 according to the most recent ICRP recommendation. As a result of this latest change, effective doses for cardiac CT calculated according to the most recent ICRP publication are generally higher compared to effective doses calculated according to the previous ICRP publication.

8.3.2   Computed Tomography Dose Index (CTDI) and Dose Length Product (DLP)

The computed tomography dose index (CTDI, mGy) applies to one 360° rotation of the X-ray tube and is defined as the integral of the dose profile along the Z-axis divided by the nominal beam width. Measurements are performed with a 100 mm long pencil ionization chamber (**Fig. 8.7**). A derivative of the CTDI has been defined that is based on weighting of the five CTDIs measured at

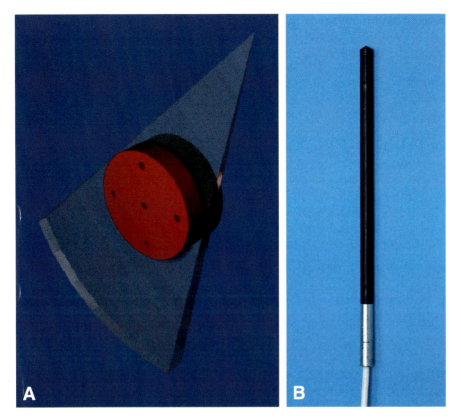

Fig. 8.7 Measurement of CTDI. **Panel A** shows in red the CT dose body phantom with five positions for inserting a CT ionization chamber (one in the center, four at the periphery of the phantom). **Panel B** shows a pencil CT ionization chamber, which was specifically developed for CT dosimetry. The length of the ionization chamber is 100 mm

central and peripheral positions of the phantoms, yielding the weighted CTDI (CTDIw, mGy). The CTDIw can be conveniently applied to axial step-and-shoot CCTA scans. For helical CCTA acquisitions it is common practice to correct the CTDIw by dividing it by the pitch factor, yielding the volume CTDI (CTDIvol, mGy). Both the CTDIw and the CTDIvol are approximations of the average dose in a cross section of the cylindrical CT dose phantom. The dose length product (DLP, mGy.cm) is calculated by multiplying the CTDIw (axial step-and-shoot acquisition) or CTDIvol (helical acquisition) by the actual scan range. Modern CT scanners give the weighted CTDI or volume CTDI and DLP on the scanner console for each acquisition. Generally these dose values are also stored in, and can be retrieved from, the DICOM header of the CT examination.

8.3.3   Organ and Tissue Doses

Organ doses cannot be measured directly during clinical CT examinations. An exception is the entrance skin dose, which can be measured with small dosimeters that can be attached safely to the skin. Particularly relevant in cardiac CT is the assessment of the exposure of organs such as breast, lung, liver, esophagus, and stomach. There is software available for calculating organ doses incurred during a CT scan. An example is the generic ImPACT CT Patient Dosimetry Calculator (ImPACT, http://www.impactscan.org/ctdosimetry.htm). These software applications do not require special user skills, it is sufficient to specify the scanned range, the type of CT scanner, and some basic acquisition parameters such as tube voltage, tube current, rotation time, pitch (helical) or table increment (axial), slice thickness, and number of active

detector rows. These generic computer applications are suitable for solving most clinical dosimetric questions in CT (**Fig. 8.8**). A disadvantage is that they may not be updated for new types of scanners, only provide dose estimations for standard sized patients (adults), and do not integrate tube current modulation schemes in their dose calculation.

Fig. 8.9 shows the contours of a virtual patient model (MIRD phantom) represented as a voxel phantom that can be used for Monte Carlo computer simulations, which are more accurate than generic software calculations. Accurate organ doses can easily be estimated from the calculated dose distribution of these more sophisticated models. Rough estimates of organ doses resulting from cardiac CT in average-sized patients are presented in **Table 8.3**. Clearly, female breast tissue and lung tissue receive the highest doses. Organs in the

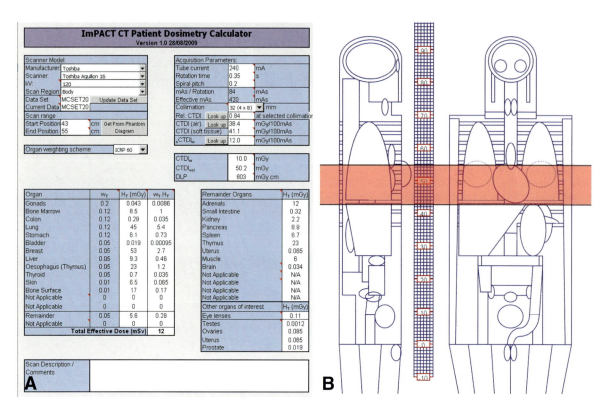

◘ **Fig. 8.8** Two screenshots of the ImPACT CT Patient Dosimetry Calculator (http://www.impactscan.org/ctdosimetry.htm). **Panel A** shows the worksheet for entering the scan details, in this example a retrospectively gated helical cardiac CT, and the dosimetric results, equivalent organ dose, and effective dose. **Panel B** shows a drawing of the patient model with the scan range in *red*

◘ Fig. 8.9 Organ doses and effective dose are often derived from computer simulations. **Panel A** shows the contours of some organs of a virtual, average-sized patient (phantom). **Panel B** shows the dose distribution (colors) in this virtual patient; the dose distribution is calculated for a single-shot cardiac acquisition using a 320-row CT scanner. Note the lighter the color, the higher the absorbed dose; the contours of the skeleton are shown in gray in **Panel B**

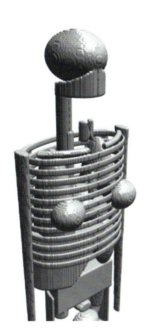

A

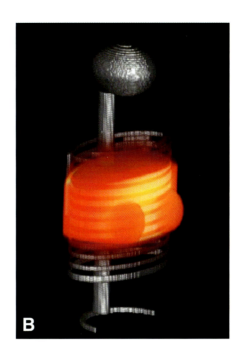

B

◘ Table 8.3 Typical equivalent organ doses (mGy) for different acquisition techniques

	Equivalent organ dose, mGy			
	Retrospectively ECG-gated reconstruction, no tube current modulation[a]	Retrospectively ECG-gated reconstruction with tube current modulation[a]	Prospectively triggered axial acquisition	Ultra-low-dose technique (volumetric CT, dual source CT)
Breast	40	32	10	5
Lung	35	28	9	5
Liver	30	24	8	4
Esophagus	25	20	7	3
Stomach	25	20	7	3
Bone surface	20	16	5	3
Red bone marrow	15	12	4	2
Skin	5	4	1	0.7
Colon	1.5	1	0.4	0.2
Bladder	0.1	0.1	0.03	0.01
Ovaries	0.1	0.08	0.03	0.01
Testes	0.01	0.008	0.003	0.001

[a] Note that only retrospectively gated acquisition allows assessment of cardiac function in addition to CCTA

upper abdomen are also exposed to substantial levels of radiation, and exposure is usually highest for retrospective helical acquisitions. A modest dose reduction in helical CT can be achieved using tube current modulation. Substantial dose reduction can be achieved with prospectively triggered axial acquisitions; these can be performed either in one single acquisition if the X-ray beam width covers the entire heart (volumetric or fast dual-source CT) or in two to five shots for scanners that cover part of the heart. Clinical studies are necessary to identify the clinical indications for which ultra-low-dose protocols are best used.

8.3.4 Effective Dose

The most pragmatic approach for calculating effective dose is to record the DLP and to multiply this value with a conversion factor. This conversion factor expresses the effective dose (mSv) per unit of dose length product (mGy.cm). Such conversion factors have been published for CT scans of different parts of the body. For general chest CT (120 kV, entire chest CT scan) conversion factors in the range of 0.014–0.017 mSv/mGy.cm have been published (effective dose according to ICRP 60). These conversion factors are also frequently used for calculating effective dose for cardiac CT but may not be the most accurate choice here. More appropriate for typical cardiac CT scans (120 kV, 120–140 mm range) are conversion factors of about 0.020 mSv/mGy.cm (according to ICRP 60) and 0.030 mSv/mGy.cm (according to ICRP 103). Even more accurate estimates of the effective dose for patients undergoing CCTA can be derived from the generic software applications, which take into account the actually exposed range (see Sect. 8.3.3).

Table 8.4 provides typical effective dose values for chest and cardiac imaging. The effective dose values clearly show that radiation exposure from chest radiography is negligible compared to nuclear medicine, conventional coronary angiography, and CT. There is also a trend towards lower effective doses in cardiac CT, from up to 20 mSv for retrospective acquisitions to less than 2 mSv for ultra-low-dose protocols. The order of magnitude of the effective dose for established cardiac imaging tests such as SPECT, PET, and conventional coronary angiography is about 8 mSv.

▫ Table 8.4 Typical exposure values according to ICRP 60

Chest radiography	
PA chest radiograph	0.02 (0.01–0.04) mSv
LAT chest radiograph	0.04 (0.02–0.08) mSv
SPECT, myocardial perfusion	
Rest; technetium Tc-99 m tetrofosmin, 500 MBq	3.8 mSv
Stress; technetium Tc-99 m tetrofosmin, 500 MBq	3.5 mSv
PET, myocardial viability	
18F-Fluorodeoxyglucose (FDG), 400 MBq	7.6 mSv
Conventional coronary angiography	
Diagnostic catheterization	8.0 (4.0–16) mSv
Percutaneous coronary intervention	12.0 (8.0–20) mSv
Cardiac CT	
CT radiography, planscan	0.05 (0.02–0.10) mSv
Bolus tracking	0.15 (0.10–0.20) mSv
Calcium scoring	2.0 (1.0–2.0) mSv
Coronary CT angiography	
Retrospectively gated reconstruction, no tube current modulation	15.0 (10.0–20.0) mSv
Retrospectively gated reconstruction, ECG-triggered tube current modulation	12.0 (5.0–15.0) mSv
Prospectively triggered axial acquisition	4.0 (2.0–8.0) mSv
Ultra-low-dose (volumetric CT, fast dual-source CT)	< 2.0 mSv

SPECT single photon emission computed tomography; *PET* positron emission tomography

Recommended Reading

1   Achenbach S, Marwan M, Ropers D et al (2010) Coronary computed tomography angiography with a consistent dose below 1 mSv using prospectively electrocardiogram-triggered high-pitch spiral acquisition. Eur Heart J 31:340–346

2   Buzug TM (2008) Computed tomography: from photon statistics to modern cone-beam CT. Spinger, Berlin

3   Cody DD, Mahesh M (2007) AAPM/RSNA physics tutorial for residents: technologic advances in multidetector CT with a focus on cardiac imaging. Radiographics 27:1829–1837

4   Dewey M, Zimmermann E, Deissenrieder F et al (2009) Noninvasive coronary angiography by 320-row CT with lower radiation exposure and maintained diagnostic accuracy: comparison of results with cardiac catheterization in a head-to-head pilot investigation. Circulation 120:867–875

5   Dirksen MS, Bax JJ, de Roos A et al (2002) Usefulness of dynamic multislice computed tomography of left ventricular function in unstable angina pectoris and comparison with echocardiography. Am J Cardiol 90:1157–1160

6   Earls JP, Berman EL, Urban BA et al (2008) Prospectively gated transverse coronary CT angiography versus retrospectively gated helical technique: improved image quality and reduced radiation dose. Radiology 246:742–753

7   Guthaner DF, Wexler L, Harell G (1979) CT demonstration of cardiac structures. AJR Am J Roentgenol 133:75–81

8   Harell GS, Guthaner DF, Breiman RS et al (1977) Stop-action cardiac computed tomography. Radiology 123:515–517

9   Hsieh J (2002) Computed tomography: principles, design, artifacts, and recent advances, vol PM114. SPIE Press Monograph, Bellingham

10   Valentin J (ed) (2007) Annals of the ICRP, PUBLICATION 102. Managing Patient Dose in Multi-Detector Computed Tomography (MDCT). Elsevier

11   Valentin J (ed) (2007) Annals of the ICRP, PUBLICATION 103. The 2007 recommendations of the international commission on radiological protection. Elsevier

12   Kak AC, Slaney M (1988) Principles of computerized tomographic imaging. IEEE Press, New York (free PDF at http://www.slaney.org/pct/)

13   Kalender W (2005) Computed tomography: fundamentals, system technology, image quality, applications. Publicis Corporate Publishing, Erlangen

14   Kobayashi Y, Lardo AC, Nakajima Y, Lima JA, George RT (2009) Left ventricular function, myocardial perfusion and viability. Cardiol Clin 27:645–654

15   Kroft LJ, de Roos A, Geleijns J (2007) Artifacts in ECG-synchronized MDCT coronary angiography. AJR Am J Roentgenol 189:581–591

16   Lell M, Marwan M, Schepis T et al (2009) Prospectively ECG-triggered high-pitch spiral acquisition for coronary CT angiography using dual source CT: technique and initial experience. Eur Radiol 19:2576–2583

17   McNitt-Gray MF (2002) AAPM/RSNA physics tutorial for residents: topics in CT. Radiation dose in CT. Radiographics 22(6):1541–1553

18   Nieman K, Oudkerk M, Rensing BJ et al (2001) Coronary angiography with multi-slice computed tomography. Lancet 357:599–603

19   Rybicki FJ, Otero HJ, Steigner ML et al (2008) Initial evaluation of coronary images from 320-detector row computed tomography. Int J Cardiovasc Imaging 24:535–546

Examination and Reconstruction

M. Dewey

Abstract

In this chapter, the examination-related procedures are described.

9.1 Examination

The CT examination should be performed in a calm and comfortable atmosphere (e.g., lights should be dimmed, and the staff should speak quietly), avoiding anything that might affect the patient's heart rate, because a constant rate is crucial for image quality and diagnostic accuracy in coronary CT angiography. Patients should likewise avoid anything that can increase their heart rate, such as talking during the scan or moving too much. The steps involved in cardiac CT are summarized in **List 9.1**. The entire examination procedure takes approximately 15–20 min.

List 9.1. Steps in performing cardiac CT

1. Reassure the patient that the examination will be short and uncomplicated – consider oral beta blockers
2. Place the patient in a comfortable supine position
3. Place ECG electrodes to obtain good R-wave signals
4. Check heart rate and rhythm – consider injecting beta blockers
5. Plan scan range, and adjust scan and contrast agent parameters individually
6. Administer nitroglycerin sublingually
7. Provide breath-hold training
8. Repeat beta blocker injection if necessary
9. Inject the contrast agent – adjust scan delay individually
10. Perform the scan, and make sure that the patient is feeling fine afterward

---

9.1.1 Calcium Scoring

Unlike coronary CT angiography, coronary calcium scoring is always performed with prospective triggering and without contrast administration, typically using 3-mm slice collimation, and can help reduce radiation exposure by allowing exact determination of the scan range required for subsequent cardiac CT (from about 1 cm above to 1 cm below the coronaries). The clinical benefit of calcium scoring is not in detecting or ruling out coronary artery disease, but in risk stratification of individual patients (Chap. 5). Combined coronary calcium scoring and angiography can be easily performed, and it prolongs the examination by only 3–5 min.

However, in symptomatic patients, especially young ones, with low-to-intermediate pretest likelihood of coronary artery disease, calcium scoring should not be performed alone, since angiography will demonstrate significant coronary stenoses in a considerable number of patients without coronary calcium or a low coronary calcium score. Very high calcium scores (above 600 or 1000) are considered by some groups to preclude reliable reading of coronary CT angiography and may be used as a gatekeeper prior to noninvasive angiography. This approach, however, requires calculating or estimating the score during the examination and may reduce workflow. In our experience, neither image quality nor diagnostic accuracy is significantly reduced in patients with somewhat higher calcium scores, and patients with atypical angina pectoris and a 20–70% pretest likelihood of coronary disease only rarely have very high calcium scores. Therefore, on our 64-row scanner, we did not routinely perform calcium scoring in our patients with low-to-intermediate pretest likelihood of coronary artery disease. For single heart beat imaging with the 320-row

CT scanner or fast prospective spiral acquisition using dual-source CT, we now always perform coronary calcium scoring to adjust the scan range to individual heart size (Chaps. 10a and 10b). To sum up, the decision whether to perform coronary CT angiography alone or in combination with calcium scoring largely depends on the local situation and the individual patient's needs.

9.1.2 Positioning and ECG

Once the patient has been placed on the table in the supine position with the arms above the head (**Fig. 9.1**), he or she should not move, in order to ensure that the planned scan region matches the region actually scanned and that the entire coronary tree is imaged (**Fig. 9.2**). Spatial resolution is highest in the center of the scan field, which is why the patient should be shifted slightly to the right side of the table, so that the heart is as close to the center as possible (**Fig. 9.1**). The ECG electrodes should be placed so that they do not disturb the patient (**Fig. 9.1**), while ensuring optimal identification of R-wave signals (**Fig. 9.3**). The optimal electrode position is as close as possible to the heart but outside the anatomic scan field (**Fig. 9.4**), in order to avoid artifacts.

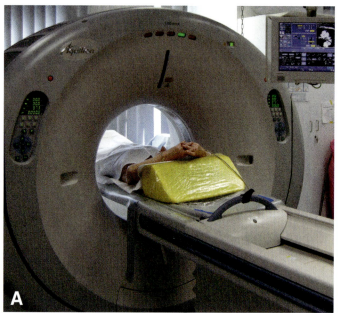 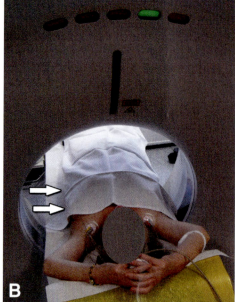

🔲 **Fig. 9.1** Patient positioning for cardiac CT. Examining the patient feet-first (**Panel A**) has the advantage of providing better access to the patient than with head-first positioning. The arms are comfortably placed above the head to improve penetration of the chest by the X-rays, thereby reducing artifacts and radiation exposure. The patient is placed in an offset position, slightly to the right side of the table (*arrows*, **Panel B**), to ensure that the heart is as close as possible to the center of the scan field. ECG electrodes are attached in the area of the supraclavicular fossa after the patient has elevated his or her arms. The ECG electrodes should not be attached near the biceps or deltoid muscles, in order to minimize the effects of muscle tremor on the ECG (**Fig. 9.5**)

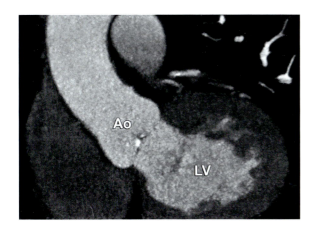

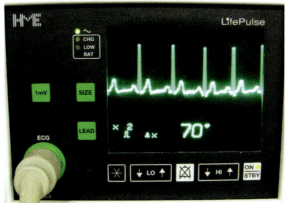

▫ **Fig. 9.2** Motion of the patient between planning of the scan and the actual scan resulted in a scan range that extended too far cranially, and therefore the caudal portions of the heart were missed. Oblique coronal maximum-intensity projection in the left ventricular outflow tract view. *Ao* aorta; *LV* left ventricle

▫ **Fig. 9.3** ECG monitor with regular ECG and sufficiently high R waves for gating of the examination. However, heart rate reduction using beta blockade should be considered

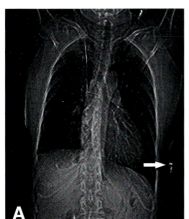

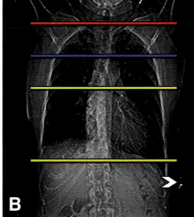

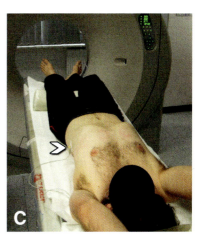

▫ **Fig. 9.4** Positioning of ECG leads and planning of the scan. A typical anterior scanogram (**Panel A**) with a too-high electrode (*arrow*) on the left side of the chest, which can lead to artifacts over the cardiac structures. Such artifacts can be easily avoided by lower placement of the electrode (*arrowhead* in **Panels B** and **C**). The typical anatomic scan range for patients with suspected or known coronary artery disease is indicated by the *yellow lines* and extends from above the left atrium to immediately below the heart (**Panel B**). Because of the high effective dose, the scan range should be as short as reasonably achievable. For imaging of venous (*blue line*) or internal mammary artery bypass grafts (*red line*), the beginning of the scan range needs to be extended (**Panel B**)

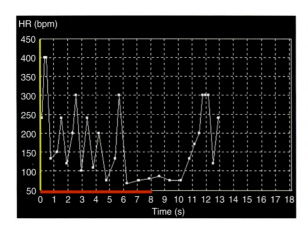

Fig. 9.5 Unconscious muscle shivering led to a highly variable (between 60 and 400 beats per min) and unreliable heart rate recording. Covering the patient with a blanket will reduce shivering, and the ECG will very likely become normal

If the electrodes are too far away from the chest (e.g., near the biceps or deltoid muscles), involuntary muscle shivering may be superimposed on the cardiac electrical activity (**Fig. 9.5**).

9.1.3   Nitroglycerin

Sublingual nitroglycerin administration increases the diameter of the coronary arteries (**Fig. 9.6**) and therefore facilitates image interpretation and comparability of the results (percent diameter stenosis) with those of cardiac catheter examination (which is often performed with intracoronary nitroglycerin administration). The onset of action of sublingual nitroglycerin spray (**Fig. 9.7A**) is about 10–20 s after administration, and its effect lasts for about 10 min. Patients should be given two to three sprays of sublingual nitroglycerin (corresponding to a dose of about 0.8–1.2 mg). Complications of nitroglycerin administration include tachycardia and hypotension (which may cause headaches). Relevant reflex tachycardia is rare, and this unlikely event should not prevent physicians from taking advantage of the beneficial vasodilatory effect of nitroglycerin (**Fig. 9.6**).

9.1.4   Beta Blockade and I$_f$ Channel Blockade

The heart rate can be reduced (**Fig. 9.8**) by oral administration of a beta blocker about 1 h before CT scanning (e.g., 50–150 mg atenolol, **Fig. 9.7B**), or intravenous administration of an agent with rapid onset of action and

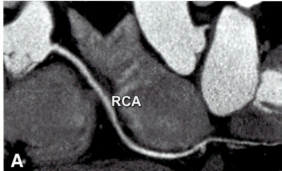

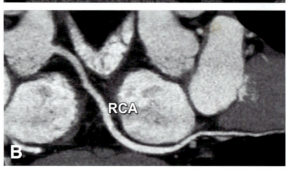

Fig. 9.6 Effect of sublingual nitroglycerin on the coronary vessel diameters. Curved multiplanar reformation of the right coronary artery (RCA) in a patient who underwent coronary CT angiography without (**Panel A**) and after sublingual nitroglycerin (**Panel B**). Nitroglycerin administration leads to a relevant increase in the coronary diameter (on average 12–21%), which also improves visibility of the distal vessel segments

shorter duration of action (e.g., esmolol at a dose of 25–50 mg min^{-1} [0.5 mg kg^{-1} bodyweight per min], **Fig. 9.7C**; or metoprolol at 2.5–5 mg min^{-1}, **Fig. 9.7D**) with the patient on the table. All intravenous beta blockers should be injected slowly, and the examiner must wait and see how the patient reacts to the initial dose (e.g., 20–30 mg of esmolol) before determining the further injection protocol. The onset of action of esmolol is approximately 2–5 min, and the half-life is only 9–10 min. Therefore, a lower risk of complications such as bradycardia can be expected with intravenous beta blockade, while oral beta blockers tend to lower heart rate more effectively. Thus, beginning with oral beta blockade and adding intravenous beta blockers if needed is the most common approach to lowering the heart rate. Another important effect of beta blockers is the reduction of heart rate variability, which significantly improves image quality.

In our experience, a resting heart rate of 60 beats per min is a good threshold above which to give oral beta blockers. Up to a threshold of about 65 beats per min, good image quality can almost always be achieved and

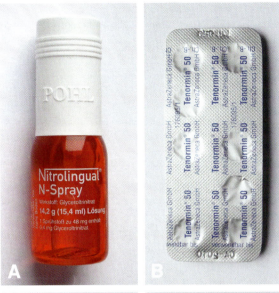

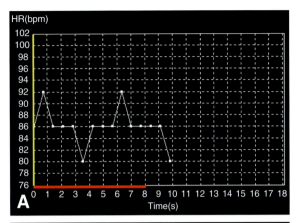

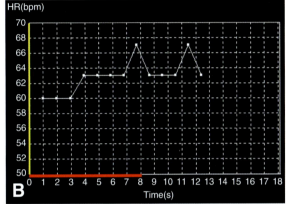

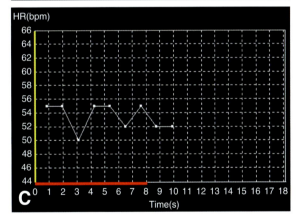

Fig. 9.7 Drugs for premedication in patients undergoing coronary CT. Sublingual nitroglycerin (**Panel A**) increases coronary vessel diameters and facilitate comparison of the findings to conventional coronary angiography. Oral (**Panel B**, metoprolol or atenolol) and/or intravenous beta blockade (**Panels C** and **D**, esmolol or metoprolol) is important to reduce heart rate in order to improve image quality and increase diagnostic accuracy as much as possible

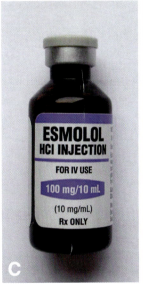

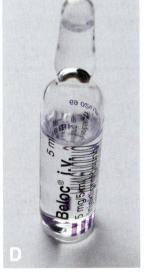

prospective acquisitions protocols ("step-and-shoot") with reduced effective dose can be applied. In patients with heart rates of more than 80 beats per min, a combination of oral and intravenous beta blockers is very likely needed to reduce the heart rate sufficiently. A potent alternative that avoids the contraindications of beta blockers (Chap. 7) is the oral administration of ivabradine

Fig. 9.8 Heart rate reduction using intravenous beta blockade. The patient (90 kg) had an initial heart rate of 80–92 beats per min during breath-hold training (**Panel A**). An initial dose of 10 mg metoprolol (equivalent to approximately 100 mg esmolol) reduced the heart rate to 60–67 beats per min (**Panel B**). After a second injection of 10 mg metoprolol, the patient's heart rate was adequately reduced to 50–55 beats per min during the final breath-hold training period (**Panel C**). Following contrast injection, the heart rate remained stable at 55 beats per min. In this case, the dose of intravenous beta blockers might have been reduced if oral beta blockers had been administered before the patient entered the scanner room (e.g., 5 mg 1 h before CT). This drug is a selective I_f channel blocker and has the largest heart rate reducing effect in patients with high heart rates.

In general, beta blockers should be administered in accordance with local practice and guidelines where applicable. Note that atropine must be available as an antidote whenever beta blockers are given. Complications of beta blockers are bradycardia, hypotension, and acute asthmatic episodes. The foremost measure to alleviate the initial symptoms of bradyicardia and hypotension is to elevate the patient's legs and administer saline intravenously. In case of severe hypotension, 0.5–1.0 mg atropine should be given intravenously. Nevertheless, serious complications of beta blockers are very rare and, in patients with high heart rates, should not prevent us from making use of the positive effects of beta blockers in terms of improved image quassssssslity and diagnostic accuracy at a markedly decreased effective dose. In case of an insufficient effect of beta blockade, intravenous conscious sedation (e.g., 1 mg of midazolam or lorazepam) is a very effective alternative to slow the patient's heart rate.

9.1.5   Planning the Scan

When a CT scan is performed for suspected coronary disease or follow-up of coronary artery stents, the scan range extends from above the left atrium to immediately below the heart (**Figs. 9.4** and **9.9**). As 1 cm of a retrospective helical scan is equal to an effective dose of 1–2 mSv, every effort should be made to limit the scan range as much as possible. For imaging of the ascending aorta or the aortic and/or pulmonic valve, the start of the scan range needs to be extended above the aortic arch (**Fig. 9.4**). This scan range is also sufficient for patients who have undergone sole venous coronary bypass grafting, whereas in patients with left or right internal mammary artery grafts, the scan should start approximately in the middle of the clavicle (**Fig. 9.4**) to include the full length of these grafts. These different scan lengths highlight the importance of taking into account clinical information about previous treatments and diagnostic tests to tailor the examination to the individual patient's needs.

The scan field of view (axial extension of the radiated area) should be as small as possible to reduce the radiation exposure and, most important, to increase the spatial resolution (since small focus spots are used). We use, for instance, 320-mm scan fields of view (medium size) for coronary imaging, which reduces radiation exposure by 20–25% when compared with large scan fields of view (**Fig. 9.9**). The scan field of view needs to be differentiated from the smaller reconstruction field of view, which determines the size of the images to which the standard 512×512 CT matrix is applied. If the scanner allows the determination of this reconstruction field of view during the scanning procedure, it is clearly advisable to do so (**Fig. 9.9**), as this precaution will avoid potential mistakes, such as forgetting to reduce the reconstruction field of view afterward and reconstructing the coronary images on large fields of view.

9.1.6   Breath-Hold Training

Temporal resolution can be improved by testing the patient's heart rate before the examination using the same breathing

Fig. 9.9 Planning and conducting the scan. The scan range for a typical coronary CT extends from above the left atrium to immediately below the heart (*dotted lines* in **Panel A**). We then perform a single axial scan at the level of the largest diameter of the heart (**Panel B**), which is indicated by a *yellow line* in **Panel A**. We use this axial image to determine the 180–200 mm reconstruction field of view (*yellow circular region* in **Panel C**) to make optimal use of the maximum resolution provided by CT scanners (10 line pairs per cm). Breath-hold training not only familiarizes the patient with the breathing instructions for the actual coronary scans but also allows monitoring of heart rate and variability during this period (**Panel D**). If the heart rate variability is above 10% (43–60 beats per min), as shown in **Panel D**, either further relaxation of the patient or beta blockade is necessary to reduce the RR interval variability to less than 10%, as shown in **Panel E** (55–57 beats per min). By obtaining another axial scan at the level of the planned beginning of the helical coronary acquisition (**Panel F**), we can make sure that no coronary vessels are visible on this axial image (**Panel G**) that might not be included in the planned scan region. Alternatively, the unenhanced calcium scan can be used to define the start and end of the coronary scan. This axial image (**Panel G**) is also used to define a circular region of interest (*arrowhead*) in the descending aorta. This region of interest is subsequently used to track the arrival of the contrast agent bolus (**Panel H**) and to start the helical scan at a threshold of 180 Hounsfield units. Once the threshold has been reached, a simple, 5-s breathing instruction is given ("Please breathe in and then hold your breath"). The helical scan is then started with a delay of 3 s, to allow the heart to return to normal after inspiration. During the subsequent helical acquisition, the moving position of the online images is indicated by a *yellow line* on the scanogram (**Panel I**). These online images (**Panel J**, in this case showing an example at the level of the largest diameter of the heart) can be used to stop the acquisition once the caudal border of the heart has been reached, in order to reduce radiation as much as possible. The results of this coronary CT angiography are shown in **Panel K**

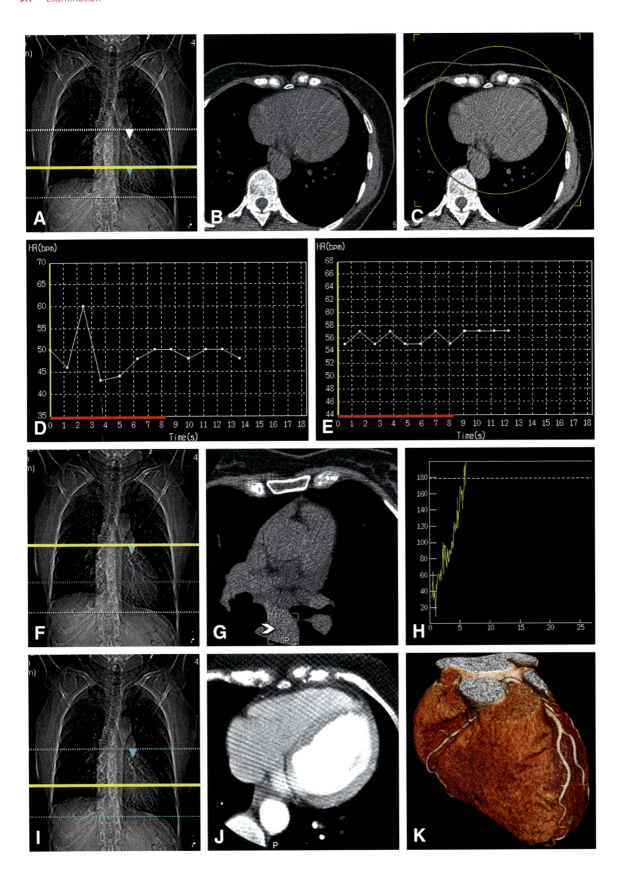

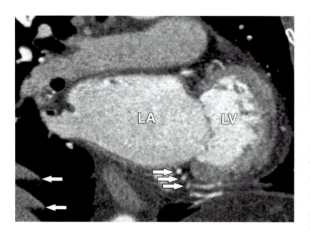

Fig. 9.10 Breathing-related motion artifacts leading to multiple visualizations of the right coronary artery and diaphragm and degraded images of the caudal portions of the heart (*arrows*). Such artifacts can be avoided in most patients by breath-hold training to ensure that the patient can hold his or her breath as long as is required for scanning. If the patient is unable to do so, breath-hold capacity can be improved by preoxygenation. *LA* left atrium; *LV* left ventricle

instructions ("Please breathe in and then hold your breath") as during the actual scan (**Fig. 9.9**). The information on the individual patient's heart rate range during the trial breath-hold can be used on some scanners to automatically adjust scan parameters such as pitch and gantry rotation time to the individual heart rate and heart rate variability. Even more importantly, breath-hold training ensures that a patient can actually hold his or her breath as long as necessary for the scan (**Fig. 9.10**). Heart rate variability during breath-hold training should be less than 10% (**Fig. 9.9**),

because greater variability will degrade image quality. Breath-hold training is also a good opportunity to remind the patient that scanning is not performed at full inspiration but at about 75% of maximum inspiration, because the increased intrathoracic pressure at full inspiration (Valsalva maneuver) might reduce inflow of the contrast agent.

9.1.7   Scanning Parameters

Tube current should be adjusted to the patient's body weight to ensure a constant high image quality regardless of body mass, while keeping the effective radiation dose to a minimum (**Table 9.1** and **Fig. 9.11**). The effective dose can be reduced most effectively by choosing the smallest possible scan, since a range of about 1 cm of a retrospective scan corresponds to the effective radiation dose of 5–10 mammographies (each an effective dose of approximately 0.2 mSv). A further significant reduction of 10–40% and 60–90% can be achieved by ECG-gated tube current modulation and prospective ECG triggering ("step-and-shoot"), respectively. Nevertheless, these techniques should only be used in patients with slow heart rates (≤65 beats per min) and low heart rate variability to maintain adequate image quality. In patients with low body mass index, use of a lower tube voltage of 80 or 100 kV is another useful approach to reduce effective dose without a loss of image quality.

9.1.8   Contrast Agent

The flow of contrast agent, and thus its amount, should also be adjusted to the patient's body weight (**Table 9.2**) in order to compensate for the greater attenuation of X-rays in heavier patients and to achieve comparable contrast between the contrast-filled coronary lumen and the surrounding tissue over a wide range of body weights (**Table 9.2**). When coronary artery stents are being imaged, a higher density in the vessel lumen is beneficial (Chap. 13), whereas for coronary plaque imaging, the density should not be too high (to avoid influencing of plaque density values, and potentially also plaque volumes, Chap. 14). Thus, contrast agent flow may also have to be adapted to reflect the clinical question to be answered by cardiac CT.

Injection of the contrast agent followed by a saline flush (using a dual-head injector) results in a more compact contrast bolus in the heart and ensures that only little contrast medium is left in the right ventricle and atrium when the coronary scan is started with an adequate delay. Ensuring this washout of the right ventricle and atrium

Table 9.1 Scanner settings for CT coronary angiography

Body weight	kV	mA	
		Pitch of 0.2 to <0.225[a]	Pitch of ≥ 0.225
<60 kg (<132 lb)	120	300	300
60–80 kg (132–176 lb)	120	340	360
>80 kg (>176 lb)	120	360	400

[a] The pitch can be adjusted according to the heart rate and heart rate variability during breath-hold training (see Chap. 9.1.6). The mA settings above are valid for Toshiba's Aquilion 64 scanner only. Optimal mA settings may be different on other scanners (Chap. 10). As a general rule, the mA should always be reduced in patients with lower body weight or body mass index and increased in heavier patients. An increase in kV (e.g., to 140) may be considered in very heavy patients (above 100 or 120 kg)

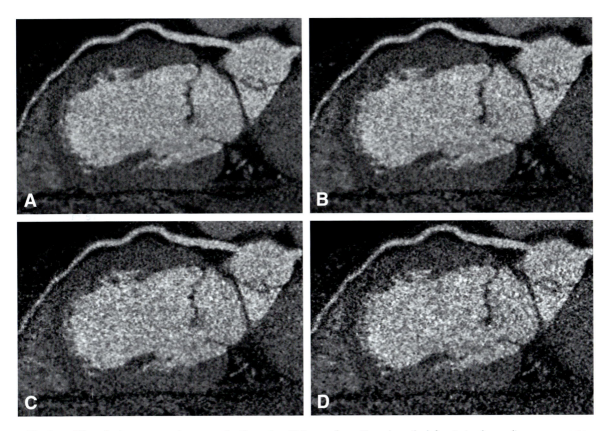

⬛ **Fig. 9.11** Effect of tube current on image quality. Curved multiplanar reformations along the left anterior descending coronary artery in a patient with a body weight of 110 kg and a body-mass index of 32. The scan was acquired with a mA of 360 and is shown in **Panel A**. Using the raw data for this patient, we simulated (**Panels B–D**) what the images would look like with lower mA settings (performed in cooperation with Toshiba; Okumura-san and Noshi-san). These panels represent mA settings of 300 (**Panel B**), 250 (**Panel C**), and 200 (**Panel D**). Already at 300 mA (**Panel B**), the curved multiplanar image looks much grainier (salt-and-pepper appearance). At the lowest mA settings (**Panel D**), it becomes impossible to rule out significant stenoses and plaques in the mid-segment of this vessel. This situation illustrates the importance of adjusting the tube current to the size of each patient. It is important to note that these images represent simulations, and the differences would be even larger in actual repeated scanning (which would be unethical)

⬛ **Table 9.2** Contrast agent injection rates

Body weight	Rate (ml/s)[a]
<60 kg (<132 lb)	3.5
60–80 kg (132–176 lb)	4.0
>80 kg (>176 lb)	5.0

[a] The amount of iodine injected should be about 1.3–2.0 g s^{-1} to ensure adequate opacification of the coronary arteries. The flow rates given in the table are thus valid for contrast agents with an iodine concentration of 350–400 mg ml^{-1}. For contrast agents with a lower iodine concentration (e.g., 320), the flow needs to be increased to achieve the same iodine influx of 1.3–2.0 g s^{-1}. Higher flow rates can also be used with 350–400 mg ml^{-1} contrast agents to make the bolus more compact and increase vessel lumen density (e.g., for stent assessment), but this will also increase the risk of adverse reactions. We feel that the suggestions above are a reasonable compromise between image quality and patient safety

significantly reduces the likelihood of streak artifacts arising from the right cardiac chambers, which can otherwise severely degrade the capacity to assess the right coronary artery. This simple bolus of contrast agent followed by saline is sufficient for coronary artery imaging. Because of the very low density in the right cardiac chambers, however, the septal wall might not be easily discernible, making it difficult to evaluate both regional and global left and right ventricular function. Thus, whenever cardiac function assessment is pivotal, two injection protocols can be used to improve the images: (1) dual-phase contrast agent injection (e.g., 5 ml s^{-1} for 80% of the contrast agent, and 2 ml s^{-1} for the rest) followed by saline, or (2) after the first contrast agent injection phase, injection of a mixture of contrast agent and saline (second phase), again followed by saline (third phase). In most "rule out coronary disease" patients, however, such sophisticated contrast agent injection techniques are not a must, and simple contrast agent administration followed by a saline flush is sufficient.

What is clearly more important than these issues is that at least a 20-gauge intravenous line is used for contrast agent injection. The right cubital veins are clearly preferable over the left side or hand veins, because the distance to the cardiac chambers is shortest this way and the contrast bolus is the least diluted. Moreover, using the right cubital vein is preferable because this approach avoids problems with streak artifacts from contrast agent in the left subclavian vein that might obscure the most common arterial bypass graft (left internal mammary artery).

Another area of concern is how to estimate and standardize the contrast agent amount that is injected for cardiac CT. The following formula can be used to calculate the amount of contrast agent for CT angiography on a 64-row scanner according to the individual helical scan duration:

Contrast agent amount [ml] $= (10 \text{ s} + \text{scan duration in seconds}) \times \text{contrast agent flow in ml/s}^a$

First example: 70 kg patient undergoing a 10-s coronary helical scan

$$(10s + 10s) \times 4 mls^{-1} = 80 ml$$

Second example: 105 kg patient undergoing a 15-s coronary bypass scan

$$(10s + 15s) \times 5 mls^{-1} = 125 ml$$

^{a}See **Table 9.2** for calculating contrast agent injection rates. The 10 s is a constant.

9.1.9   Starting the Scan

Properly connecting the contrast agent line to the patient's intravenous access and making sure that there is no air in the injection system are essential to preventing air from being injected into the cardiac chambers or pulmonary arteries (**Fig. 9.12**). Before starting the contrast agent injection, it is important to reassure the patient that the next breath-hold is the last one and that it takes as long as the one during breath-hold training. Again, mentioning that the patient might feel some warmth can be important for those who are nervous. It is always a good idea to have someone on site to monitor the injection of the contrast agent for at least a few seconds to avoid extravasation.

Immediately prior to injecting the contrast agent, make a "final check" to ensure that the heart rate is still

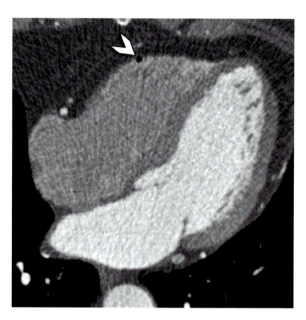

Fig. 9.12 Four-chamber view showing a very small air bubble at the ventral wall of the right ventricle (*arrowhead*). The bubble was most likely introduced when the contrast agent line was connected to the patient's intravenous line. Such small amounts are unlikely to harm the patient. Care must be taken not to inject relevant amounts of air into the cardiac chambers or pulmonary arteries, by properly connecting the contrast agent line and excluding any air that is in the injection system

in an acceptable range and the ECG is detected by the system. There are two options for timing the start of the helical scan after intravenous contrast administration: (1) monitoring the arrival of the contrast agent during the injection of the main bolus and starting the helical scan once a threshold has been reached ("bolus tracking"), and (2) injecting a test bolus to determine the individual patient's circulation time and adjusting the scanning parameters accordingly ("test bolus"). The second approach has the disadvantage that any changes between the test bolus and the actual bolus used for coronary opacification (such as relevant heart rate changes) can alter the patient's circulation time. We think that the test bolus approach more commonly leads to mistiming of the coronary helical scan (**Fig. 9.13**), and it has also been shown that the coronary enhancement is less homogenous when this approach is used. We therefore strongly recommend the bolus tracking approach (for 64-row CT), which also reduces the total amount of contrast agent injected, as no test bolus is needed.

We perform bolus tracking (which should be initiated 10–15 s after the start of contrast injection) by analyzing Hounsfield unit density in a region of interest in the descending aorta (**Fig. 9.9**). The spiral scan at a threshold

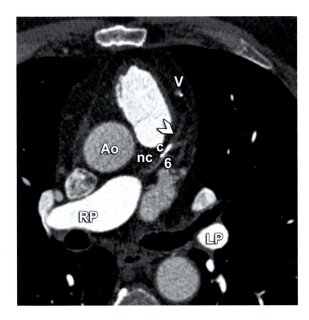

☐ **Fig. 9.13** Too-early initiation of the coronary acquisition, with most of the contrast agent still in the pulmonary arteries (LP and RP). As a result, there is very little contrast in the aorta (Ao) and the coronary arteries (*arrowhead*) in this patient with a history of venous coronary bypass grafting (V). Because of the poor opacification, it is very difficult to identify the stenosis in segment 6 of the left anterior descending coronary artery caused by noncalcified (nc) and calcified (c) plaques. In this patient, a test bolus was used to calculate the appropriate delay time for initiation of the coronary scan, but a heart-rate change after contrast agent administration led to incorrect timing of the coronary helical scan. *LP* left pulmonary artery; *RP* right pulmonary artery

initiation of the scan has been reached, a simple 5-s breathing instruction is given ("Please breathe in and then hold your breath"). Since there is often a brief increase in heart rate after inspiration, there is an additional gap of 3 s before the scan is started, so that the heart rate can normalize after submaximal inspiration.

9.1.10 After the Scan

As soon as the prospectively or retrospectively gated coronary scan is completed, we return to the scanning room to make sure that the patient has tolerated the contrast agent well. Because of the nitroglyerin and possible beta blockade, it is advisable that the patient gets up slowly to avoid orthostatic reactions. Most patients are eager to know the results of the examination immediately, which is difficult because a single cardiac CT can easily produce as many as 4,000–5,000 images.

The patient can be offered the opportunity to wait in the seating area after the scan is completed and to meet with the interpreting physician to discuss the results as soon as he or she has finished reading and interpreting the images. This offer is highly appreciated by some patients and many of our referring physicians. In addition, sending reconstructions of the coronary arteries to the referring physician together with the report not only improves further management of the patient but is also a strong marketing tool.

of 180 Hounsfield units is then initiated. We use the descending aorta, as opposed to the ascending aorta, for example, for bolus tracking because it is less likely for early-enhancing vessels such as the superior vena cava to affect this region of interest. As soon as the threshold for

9.2 Reconstruction

Image reconstruction is an integral component of the examination. The parameters for coronary and lung reconstructions are compiled in **Table 9.3**, and typical results of

☐ **Table 9.3** Reconstruction settings

	FOV (mm)	Slice thickness (mm)	Reconstruction increment (mm)	Kernel	RR intervals
Coronary images	180–200	0.5–0.75	0.3–0.5	Coronary, possibly stent kernel	0–90% at 10% increments[a] and/or minimal cardiac motion phases
Lung and mediastinal images	Scan field of view[b]	3–5	3–5	Lung and mediastinum	80%[c]

[a] Alternatively, one can reconstruct images at 5% increments around 70–80% of the RR interval

[b] Adapted to include the entire chest in the *xy*-plane

[c] This percentage refers to the center of the reconstruction window (as on Toshiba, Philips, and General Electric scanners). On other scanners (Siemens), the percentage phase given denotes the beginning of the reconstruction phase (which would be equal to approximately 65% or 70% instead)

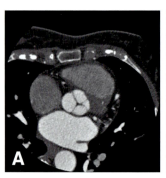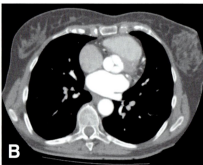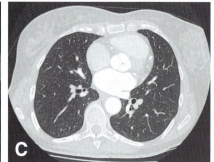

■ **Fig. 9.14** Typical axial images of coronary (**Panel A**), mediastinal (**Panel B**, soft tissue), and lung reconstructions (**Panel C**) at the level of the aortic valve. Please note that the coronary reconstructions here (**Panel A**) were performed on smaller fields of view in order to maximize spatial resolution. The mediastinal (**Panel B**) and lung (**Panel C**) reconstructions are less noisy because of the greater slice thickness (3–5 mm)

these reconstructions are shown in **Fig. 9.14**. The reconstruction of cardiac CT is summarized in **List 9.2**.

List 9.2. Steps in the reconstruction of cardiac CT images

1. Check whether the heart rate was regular throughout scanning
2. Perform ECG editing if necessary – consider automatic identification of minimal cardiac motion phases
3. Reconstruct coronary axial slices using specific kernels on small fields of view (180–200 mm) – consider stent kernels
4. Reconstruct lung and mediastinal axial slices using specific kernels on large fields of view to cover the entire chest width
5. Archive all reconstructed coronary images or only those indicated by the reading physician
6. Archive all lung and mediastinal images

9.2.1   Slice Thickness and Fields of View

For analysis of the small and tortuous coronary arteries, it is of utmost importance to keep the reconstructed slice thickness for the axial slices as thin as possible. A slice thickness of 3 or 2 mm is clearly inadequate for coronary imaging, but there is also a remarkable difference between 0.5 and 1.0-mm reconstructions (**Fig. 9.15**). The reconstructed slice thickness is different from the reconstruction increment. This increment between the centers of adjacent slices can be thinner (e.g., 0.4 mm) than the slice thickness (e.g., 0.5 mm) to improve the three-dimensional reconstructions by spatial interpolation. However, the true spatial resolution is defined by the actual slice thickness, and a reduction in the slice increment may impose too large a burden on the local picture archiving and communication system. Thus, it clearly depends on the local situation whether it is advisable to use this spatial interpolation approach or not.

What is much more important than slice interpolation is the use of a minimally small reconstruction field

■ **Fig. 9.15** Importance of slice collimation for image quality, as shown in curved multiplanar reformations along the right coronary artery (*first column*), left anterior descending coronary artery (*middle column*), and left circumflex coronary artery (*third column*). Slice thicknesses of 3 mm (**Panels A–C**) and 2 mm (**Panels D–F**) are clearly inadequate for coronary imaging, as can be seen in the step-like appearance of the vessel on curved multiplanar reformations. These slice thicknesses were commonly used with electron-beam CT and 4-row CT. But there is also an image-quality difference (step-like appearance) between 0.5 and 1.0-mm slice thickness reconstructions available on different 16 and 64-row CT scanners (**Panels G–I** and **Panels J–L**). All reconstructions were performed using raw data that were acquired with 64 × 0.5-mm detector collimation in a single patient

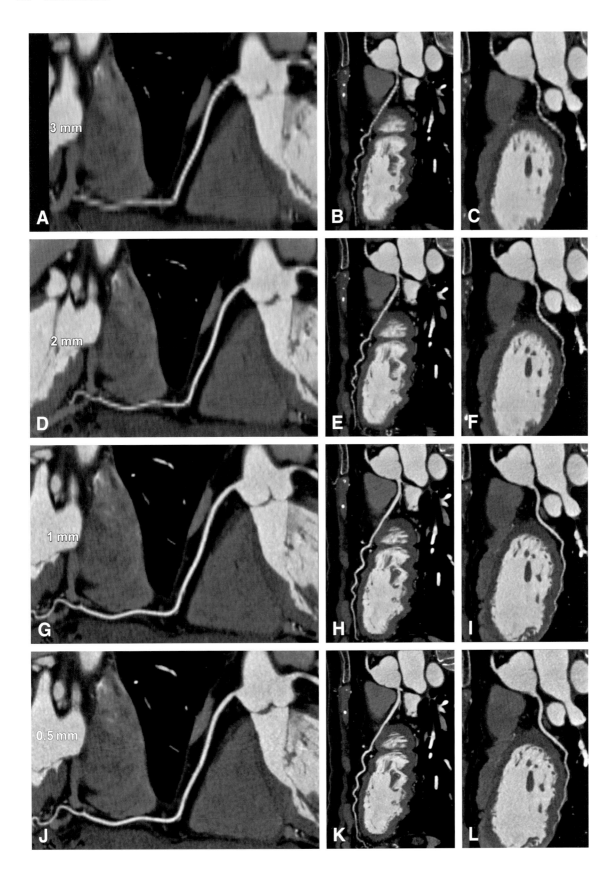

9

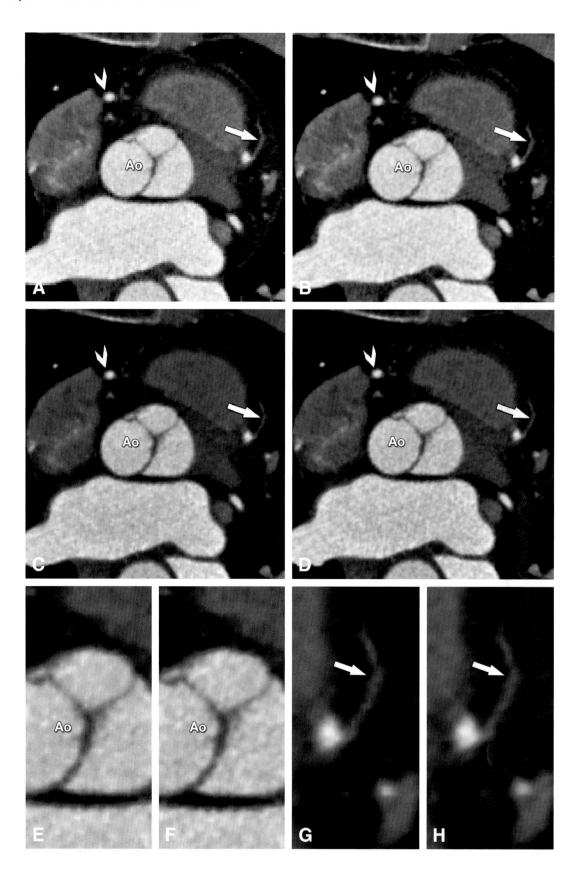

Fig. 9.16 Effect of the reconstruction field of view (320 vs. 180 mm) on the image quality of coronary artery reconstructions. The original axial images of the 320-mm reconstruction field of view (**Panel A**) are compared with the 180-mm reconstruction fields of view (**Panel B**). The 320-mm reconstructions (**Panel A**) have markedly poorer spatial resolution with coarser pixels (ca. 0.625×0.625 mm² vs. 0.35×0.35 mm²), as illustrated by the right coronary artery (*arrowhead*) and a rather small side branch of the LAD (*arrow*). On workstations this difference appears to be somewhat blurred but is still present, as can be seen in the images at exactly the same anatomic level (**Panel C** vs. **D**). Magnified views of the aortic valve cusps (**Panel E** vs. **F**) and the small side branch of the LAD (**Panel G** vs. **H**) clearly show the considerable advantage of using small 180-mm reconstruction fields of view (**Panels F** and **H**). *Ao* aorta

of view (ca. 180–200 mm) to make optimal use of the maximal spatial resolution of the scanner (10 line pairs per cm) using a 512×512 image matrix (**Table 9.3**). With this image matrix, a 180-mm field of view results in a pixel size of 0.35×0.35 mm² (0.12 mm²). If one inadvertently uses a 320-mm field of view for reconstruction, the resulting pixel size is about 0.625×0.625 mm²

(0.4 mm²), which is almost four times larger. The effect on image quality is significant and is illustrated in **Figs. 9.16** and **9.17**. In contrast to the situation for coronary axial slices, it is ethically desirable to use the entire scanned field for reconstruction of the lung, the mediastinum, and the chest wall (**Fig. 9.14** and **Table 9.3**) to avoid overlooking any pathology in this area.

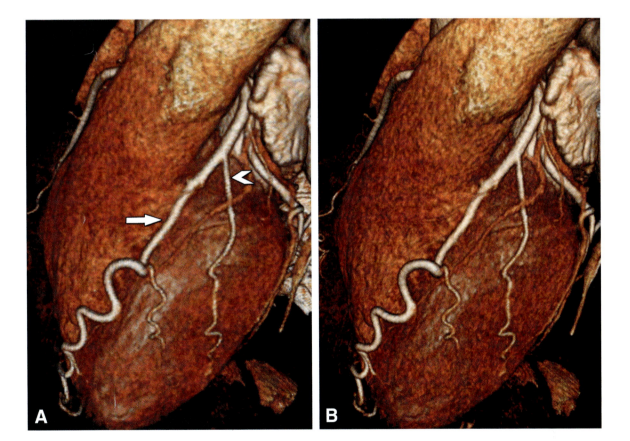

Fig. 9.17 Effect of the reconstruction field of view (320 vs. 180 mm) on the image quality of coronary artery reconstructions. Three-dimensional reconstructions of the LAD (of the same patient as in **Fig. 9.16**) show the relevantly lower spatial resolution obtained using the 320-mm reconstruction field of view (**Panel A**), when compared with the smaller 180-mm reconstruction field of view (**Panel B**), as illustrated by the mid-LAD (*arrow*) and the first diagonal branch (*arrowhead*)

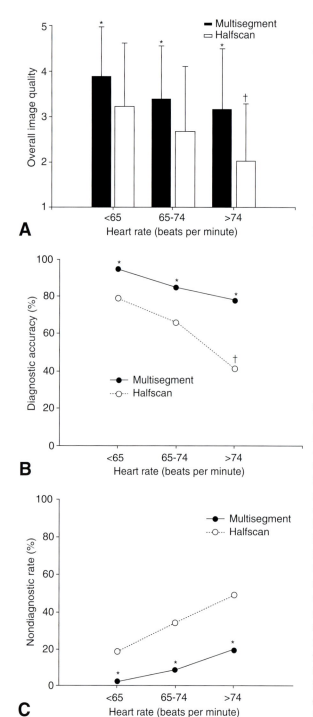

A

B

C

9.2.2 Temporal Resolution and the Cardiac Reconstruction Phase

Temporal resolution is still the major limitation of coronary CT and the main cause of nondiagnostic images, and therefore all possible measures must be taken to improve this parameter. One such measure is adaptive multisegment reconstruction, which should be used whenever available for patients with heart rates greater than about 60 beats per min (**Figs. 9.18** and **9.19**). An alternative approach that markedly improves temporal resolution is dual-source CT, which allows a 50% reduction in the length of the reconstruction window, regardless of the heart rate (**Fig. 9.20**). In this way, dual-source CT markedly reduces heart-rate dependence.

◻ **Fig. 9.18** Comparison of overall image quality (**Panel A**), per-patient diagnostic accuracy (**Panel B**), and per-patient nondiagnostic rate (**Panel C**) of CT coronary angiography obtained using adaptive multisegment and standard halfscan reconstructions in three heart rate groups. There is a trend toward reduced overall image quality and accuracy at higher heart rates, which was significant in the case of the halfscan reconstructions when the 65–74 and above 74 beats-per-min groups were compared (*dagger*). Nevertheless, regardless of whether multisegment reconstruction is available or not, the heart rate should be reduced to below 65 beats per min by beta blocker administration whenever possible. For all three heart rate groups, overall image quality, diagnostic accuracy, and nondiagnostic rate are significantly superior for multisegment reconstruction than for standard halfscan reconstruction (*asterisk*). Therefore, whenever available, adaptive multisegment reconstruction should be used instead of halfscan reconstruction. A very recent important alternative to improve temporal resolution is DSCT (**Fig. 9.20**). Note that the image quality and accuracy obtained with multisegment reconstruction at high heart rates (>74 beats per min) are comparable with the results obtained using standard halfscan reconstruction at low heart rates (<65 beats per min). From Dewey et al., Eur Radiol 2007

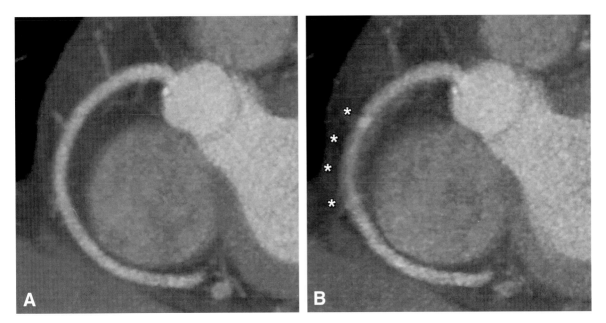

Fig. 9.19 Advantages of multisegment reconstruction (**Panel A**) over halfscan reconstruction (**Panel B**), as illustrated by a cath view along the right coronary artery in a patient with a heart rate of 66–68 beats per min during 320-row CT scanning. There are multiple motion artifacts resulting from insufficient temporal resolution with halfscan reconstruction, which cause blurring of the vessel wall (*asterisks*, **Panel B**)

Fig. 9.20 Technical realization of second-generation dual-source computed tomography (DSCT). One detector (A) covers the entire scan field of view with a diameter of 50 cm, while the other detector (B) is restricted to a slightly smaller field (33 cm). With first-generation DSCT the second field of view was restricted to 26 cm and the two gantries were mounted at a 90° angle. With second-generation DSCT this space limitation was reduced by having a 95° off-set between the gantries. Using DSCT, the length of the image reconstruction window can be reduced by a factor of 2 when compared with standard halfscan reconstruction using a single X-ray source, to one-fourth of the gantry rotation time. Thus, temporal resolution is significantly improved. Image courtesy of Thomas Flohr

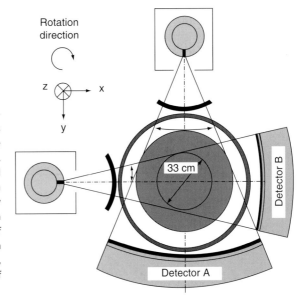

Reconstruction can be done throughout the cardiac cycle at 10% intervals, resulting in 10 phases, or around a mid-diastolic interval at 5% increments (about 70–80% of the RR interval) (**Table 9.3**). Most of the suitable reconstruction phases (intervals) within the cardiac cycles are mid-diastolic phases (e.g., 75%) and end-systolic phases (e.g., 40%). The latter are especially suitable for analysis in patients with higher heart rates. Reconstruction of several phases throughout the RR interval has the advantage that the resulting data can be used for high-resolution analysis of regional and global cardiac function without having to perform any additional reconstructions. It is important to note that the designations of the phases are not defined consistently by the different vendors. The percentage of the RR interval refers either to the center of the reconstruction phase (Toshiba, Philips, and General Electric) or the beginning of the reconstruction phase (Siemens). As a result, there are different recommendations regarding minimal cardiac motion phases, but these can be matched (thus, the start of the reconstruction phase at about 65–70% of the RR interval corresponds to a center of the phase at about 75–80%). In patients with severe arrhythmias (e.g., atrial fibrillation)

an absolute temporal reconstruction approach (in ms) might be superior to relative reconstruction intervals (% of the RR interval).

In discussing the number of phases to be reconstructed and the distance between phases, one must bear in mind that the reconstruction window in coronary CT angiography is about 50–175 ms long, corresponding to about 8–20% of the RR interval. Therefore, there will not be great differences between reconstructions at intervals ≤2%.

Heart rate is crucial in determining the position of the minimal cardiac motion phase that is most suitable for reconstruction. In patients with higher heart rates, end-systolic phases (e.g., 30–40%) are often superior to diastolic phases in terms of image quality. Selection of the reconstruction phase has considerable influence on the diagnostic accuracy of coronary CT angiography. It has been shown, for example, that a single reconstruction phase (typically with the center of the reconstruction window at 80%) results in optimal quality and diagnostic accuracy in only half of the patients. Two reconstruction phases are necessary in 40% of patients, and at least three phases in 10%, to optimally evaluate

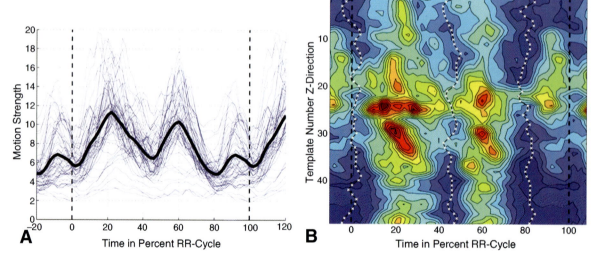

◻ **Fig. 9.21** Motion strength curve and motion map samples. **Panel A** shows a representative mean curve of the motion strength function for all voxels within a single axial plane. Motion strength (corresponding to inverse similarity) is plotted against phase point propagation of one cardiac cycle. The *curve* shows low motion troughs for the end-systolic phase (~46%) and the mid-diastolic or diastasis phase (~80%). **Panel B** shows the corresponding motion map, with color-coded (*blue*, low motion; *red*, high motion) motion strength curves plotted against the cardiac phase (*x*-axis) and against *z*-axis propagation of the helical scan (*y*-axis truncated at a value of 50 to confine the coverage to aortic root position, *y*-axis value = 0, down to the diaphragmatic surface of the heart, *y*-axis value = 49). A low-motion phase becomes apparent as a *blue valley* between *red-colored* systolic contraction (0–40% longitudinally) and rapid diastolic filling (50–70% longitudinally). Atrial contraction is apparent as a hump around 90%. *Lines with crosses* track the valleys of lowest motion; *dashed vertical lines* mark the beginning and the end of the cardiac cycle (R to R peak). Used with permission from Hoffmann et al., Eur Radiol 2006

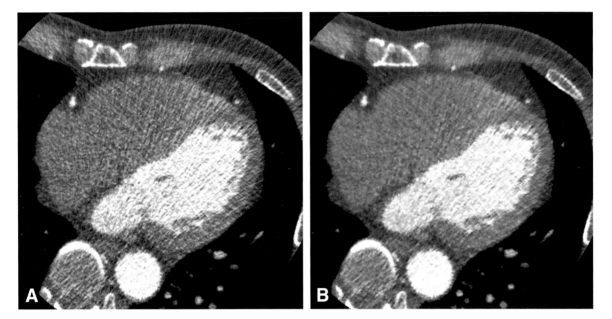

Fig. 9.22 Example of cardiac CT reconstructed with standard filtered back projection (**Panel A**) and iterative reconstruction (**Panel B**). Imaging was performed on a 320-row CT using 120 kV and 60 mA translating into an effective dose of about 0.6 mSv. There is significant reduction in image noise using adaptive iterative dose reduction reconstruction (**Panel B**) in comparison to standard filtered back projection (**Panel A**) on these axial images. Images courtesy of Kazuhiro Katada, Fujity University

the entire coronary artery tree by CT angiography. Automatic determination of minimal cardiac motion using software approaches based on the raw data (e.g., "Best Phase") using motion maps (**Fig. 9.21**) is likely to considerably simplify identification of the optimal cardiac phase for coronary artery analysis (Chap.11).

9.2.3   Iterative Reconstruction

Recently, several vendors have introduced iterative reconstruction for routine clinical use. This reconstruction takes slightly longer than standard filtered back projection but also reduces image noise significantly. Thus the mA during scanning may be lowered while image quality is maintained and effective dose relevantly reduced (**Fig. 9.22**).

Recommended Reading

1   Achenbach S (2006) Computed tomography coronary angiography. J Am Coll Cardiol 48:1919–1928

2   Cademartiri F, Luccichenti G, Marano R, Runza G, Midiri M (2004) Use of saline chaser in the intravenous administration of contrast material in non-invasive coronary angiography with 16-row multislice computed tomography. Radiol Med (Torino) 107:497–505

3   Cademartiri F, Maffei E, Palumbo AA et al Influence of intra-coronary enhancement on diagnostic accuracy with 64-slice CT coronary angiography. Eur Radiol 18:576–83

4   Cademartiri F, Mollet NR, Runza G et al (2006) Improving diagnostic accuracy of MDCT coronary angiography in patients with mild heart rhythm irregularities using ECG editing. AJR Am J Roentgenol 186:634–638

5   Cademartiri F, Mollet NR, Runza G et al (2005) Influence of intracoronary attenuation on coronary plaque measurements using multislice computed tomography: observations in an ex vivo model of coronary computed tomography angiography. Eur Radiol 15:1426–1431

6   Cademartiri F, Nieman K, van der Lugt A et al (2004) Intravenous contrast material administration at 16-detector row helical CT coronary angiography: test bolus versus bolus-tracking technique. Radiology 233:817–823

7   Cademartiri F, Runza G, Mollet NR et al (2005) Impact of intravascular enhancement, heart rate, and calcium score on diagnostic accuracy in multislice computed tomography coronary angiography. Radiol Med (Torino) 110:42–51

8   Chun EJ, Lee W, Choi YH et al (2008) Effects of nitroglycerin on the diagnostic accuracy of electrocardiogram-gated coronary computed tomography angiography. J Comput Assist Tomogr 32:86–92

9   Dewey M, Hamm B (2007) CT coronary angiography: examination technique, clinical results, and outlook on future developments. Fortschr Röntgenstr 179:246–260

10   Dewey M, Hoffmann H, Hamm B (2006) Multislice CT coronary angiography: effect of sublingual nitroglycerine on the diameter of coronary arteries. Fortschr Röntgenstr 178:600–604

11   Dewey M, Laule M, Krug L et al (2004) Multisegment and halfscan reconstruction of 16-slice computed tomography for detection of coronary artery stenoses. Invest Radiol 39:223–229

12   Dewey M, Teige F, Laule M, Hamm B (2007) Influence of heart rate on diagnostic accuracy and image quality of 16-slice CT coronary angiography: comparison of multisegment and halfscan reconstruction approaches. Eur Radiol 17:2829–2837

13   Dewey M, Teige F, Rutsch W, Schink T, Hamm B (2007) CT coronary angiography: influence of different cardiac reconstruction intervals on image quality and diagnostic accuracy. Eur J Radiol

14   Earls JP, Berman EL, Urban BA et al (2008) Prospectively gated transverse coronary CT angiography versus retrospectively gated helical technique: improved image quality and reduced radiation dose. Radiology 246:742–753

15   Einstein AJ, Moser KW, Thompson RC, Cerqueira MD, Henzlova MJ (2007) Radiation dose to patients from cardiac diagnostic imaging. Circulation 116:1290–1305

16   Engelken F, Lembcke A, Hamm B, Dewey M (2009) Determining optimal acquisition parameters for computed tomography coronary angiography: evaluation of a software-assisted, breathhold exam simulation. Acad Radiol 16:239–243

17   Flohr TG, McCollough CH, Bruder H et al (2006) First performance evaluation of a dual-source CT (DSCT) system. Eur Radiol 16: 256–268

18   Hoffmann MH, Lessick J, Manzke R et al (2006) Automatic determination of minimal cardiac motion phases for computed tomography imaging: initial experience. Eur Radiol 16:365–373

19   Horiguchi J, Fujioka C, Kiguchi M et al (2007) Soft and intermediate plaques in coronary arteries: how accurately can we measure CT attenuation using 64-MDCT? AJR Am J Roentgenol 189:981–988

20   Horiguchi J, Shen Y, Hirai N et al (2006) Timing on 16-slice scanner and implications for 64-slice cardiac CT: do you start scanning immediately after breath hold? Acad Radiol 13:173–176

21   Hur G, Hong SW, Kim SY et al (2007) Uniform image quality achieved by tube current modulation using SD of attenuation in coronary CT angiography. AJR Am J Roentgenol 189:188–196

22   Husmann L, Valenta I, Gaemperli O et al (2008) Feasibility of low-dose coronary CT angiography: first experience with prospective ECG-gating. Eur Heart J 29:191–197

23   Kim DJ, Kim TH, Kim SJ et al (2008) Saline flush effect for enhancement of aorta and coronary arteries at multidetector CT coronary angiography. Radiology 246:110–115

24   Leber AW, Johnson T, Becker A et al (2007) Diagnostic accuracy of dual-source multi-slice CT-coronary angiography in patients with an intermediate pretest likelihood for coronary artery disease. Eur Heart J;28:2354–2360

25   Leschka S, Wildermuth S, Boehm T et al (2006) Noninvasive coronary angiography with 64-section CT: effect of average heart rate and heart rate variability on image quality. Radiology 241:378–385

26   Maffei E, Palumbo AA, Martini C et al (2009) "In-house" pharmacological management for computed tomography coronary angiography: heart rate reduction, timing and safety of different drugs used during patient preparation. Eur Radiol

27   Mahesh M, Cody DD (2007) Physics of cardiac imaging with multiple-row detector CT. Radiographics 27:1495–1509

28   Morin RL, Gerber TC, McCollough CH (2003) Radiation dose in computed tomography of the heart. Circulation 107:917–922

29   Paul JF, Abada HT (2007) Strategies for reduction of radiation dose in cardiac multislice CT. Eur Radiol 17:2028–2037

30   Ropers U, Ropers D, Pflederer T et al (2007) Influence of heart rate on the diagnostic accuracy of dual-source computed tomography coronary angiography. J Am Coll Cardiol 50:2393–2398

31   Schnapauff D, Zimmermann E, Dewey M (2008) Technical and clinical aspects of coronary computed tomography angiography. Semin Ultrasound CT MR 29:167–175

32   Schuetz GM, Zacharopoulou NM, Schlattmann P, Dewey M (2010) Meta-analysis: noninvasive coronary angiography using computed tomography versus magnetic resonance imaging. Ann Intern Med 152:167–177

33   Shapiro MD, Pena AJ, Nichols JH et al (2007) Efficacy of pre-scan beta-blockade and impact of heart rate on image quality in patients undergoing coronary multidetector computed tomography angiography. Eur J Radiol

34   Yoshimura N, Sabir A, Kubo T, Lin PJ, Clouse ME, Hatahu H (2006) Correlation between image noise and body weight in coronary CTA with 16-row MDCT. Acad Radiol 13:324–328

9

Toshiba Aquilion 64 and Aquilion ONE

E. Zimmermann

Abstract

This chapter outlines how the heart is examined and reconstructed on Toshiba CT scanners.

10a.1 Examination

10a.1.1 Preparation

The patient is positioned on the scanner table in a comfortable supine position with the arms raised above the head and feet first. To image the heart in the isocenter of the scanner, the patient should be positioned slightly to the right side of the table. It is recommended that the 20 or 18-gauge cannula be checked by means of a physiologic saline flush immediately before scanning to avoid contrast extravasation. Care must be taken to remove all foreign materials that can cause image artifacts (e.g., electrocardiography electrodes/cables and other metal-dense foreign bodies) from the scan field. It is also important to make sure that the ECG electrodes make good contact with the patient's skin and that a good R-wave is displayed on the monitor (**Fig. 10a.1**). Details of patient preparation for coronary CT angiography on all scanner types are presented in Chaps. 7 and 9.

10a.1.2 Defining the Scan Range

A low-dose planning scan (scanogram with 50 mA) is obtained on the Aquilion 64 to define the start and end of the spiral scan, identify the widest dimension of the heart, and place the SureStart (**Figs. 10a.2–10a.4**). The start position is placed just above the origins of the coronary arteries, using the left atrial appendage for orientation. The scan ends just below the heart, and can be stopped manually. The SureStart is placed at the start of the spiral scan, by positioning the active line exactly over the upper boundary of the scan as illustrated in **Fig. 10a.2**. The SureStart should not contain the coronary arteries or be placed too high (**Fig. 10a.4**). Careful planning of the scan is essential for achieving an optimal result while minimizing radiation exposure.

M. Dewey, *Cardiac CT*,
DOI: 10.1007/978-3-642-14022-8_10, © Springer-Verlag Berlin Heidelberg 2011

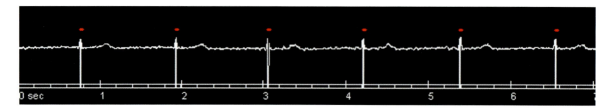

Fig. 10a.1 Illustration of optimal ECG recordings. A clear R-wave and sinus rhythm are essential for reconstruction of the image data. Here, the *red dot* indicates identification of the R-wave. An incorrect R-wave can be removed by clicking on the *red dot* (ECG editing). In patients with arrhythmia, it may be helpful to add "virtual R-waves" by clicking on additional *red dots* or to remove incorrectly identified R-waves. The goal is to obtain a highly regular ECG in order to minimize image artifacts

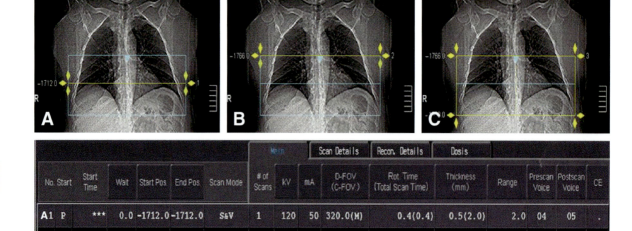

	No. Start	Start Time	Wait	Start Pos	End Pos	Scan Mode	# of Scans	KV	mA	D-FOV (C-FOV.)	Rot. Time (Total Scan Time)	Thickness (mm)	Range	Prescan Voice	Postscan Voice	CE
A1	P	***	0.0	-1712.0	-1712.0	S&V	1	120	50	320.0(M)	0.4(0.4)	0.5(2.0)	2.0	04	05	.
B2	P	***	0.0	-1766.0	-1766.0	S&V	1	120	50	320.0(M)	0.4(0.4)	0.5(2.0)	2.0	04	05	.
3	P	***	15.0	***	***	SureStart	***	120	50	320.0(M)	0.4(40.0)	0.5(2.0)	***	00	00	ON
C4	A		0.0	-1766.0	-1650.0	Helical	1	120	320	320.0(M)	0.4(8.876)	0.5(32.0)	116.0	04	05	ON

Fig. 10a.2 Planning the acquisition. A planning scan (scanogram) is acquired to identify the greatest circumference of the heart (**Panel A**), position the SureStart (**Panel B**), and define the scan length (**Panel C**) for the subsequent helical coronary examination. *Yellow* indicates the active area, while *blue* indicates inactive areas. As anatomical structures may be displaced as a result of respiratory motion, we recommend defining the start of the scan about 1 cm above the assumed coronary artery origins and the end of the scan about 1 cm below the heart base. **Panel A** shows a single slice (low-dose scan, 50 mA) that defines the greatest circumference of the heart. **Panel B** shows another low-dose single slice (50 mA) (**Fig. 10a.4**) that defines the SureStart, which serves to trigger the spiral scan once the desired density threshold has been reached. The scan is automatically started after 15 s. **Panel C** defines the scan length. The start of the spiral scan corresponds to the SureStart position. The tube current for the spiral scan is selected according to the patient's weight and is higher in obese patients to ensure an adequate image quality

10a.1.3   Surestart

Planning the individual scan delay on the Aquilion 64 using the SureStart bolus tracking tool is illustrated in **Fig. 10a.4**. The selected scan plane, just above the origin of the coronary arteries, is chosen to start the scan at the optimal time by monitoring the arrival of the contrast bolus in a region of interest (ROI) placed in the descending aorta (**Fig. 10a.5**). Important landmarks in this plane are the sternum anteriorly and the descending aorta

posteriorly. Also seen in this plane are a segment of the pulmonary trunk and a portion of the anterolateral chest wall. The ROI in the descending aorta is used to monitor the increase in Hounsfield units (HU) after initiation of contrast injection.

The scan delay after contrast injection can be determined in one of the two ways: (1) by injection of a test bolus to determine the patient's individual circulation time and optimize the spiral scan parameters accordingly, or (2) by bolus tracking, with automatic triggering of the

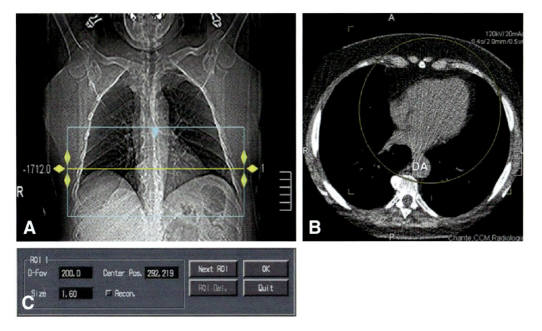

⬛ **Fig. 10a.3** Defining the FoV. The scan depicting the greatest circumference of the heart (**Panel A**) is used to define the FoV (**Panel B**) according to individual heart size, ensuring good image quality at the highest possible spatial resolution. In the majority of patients, if the FoV should be about 180–200 mm (**Panel C**), the FoV should comprise the descending aorta (DA) and part of the anterior chest wall. The descending aorta is more suitable for measuring contrast inflow than the ascending aorta because it is associated with fewer motion artifacts

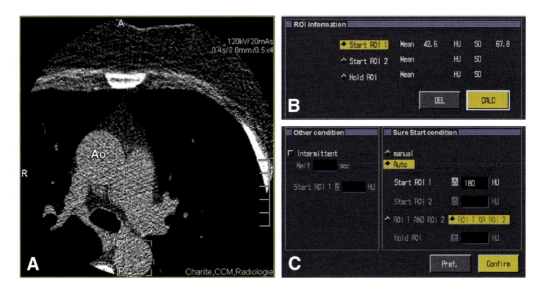

⬛ **Fig. 10a.4** Planning of the SureStart. Using the SureStart (**Fig. 10a.2**), a ROI is identified in the descending aorta (*circle* in **Panel A**); this region should be neither too large nor too small to avoid mistriggering the spiral scan. The ROI is placed in the descending aorta because there are fewer motion artifacts than in the ascending aorta (Ao). In this way, it is possible to avoid mistriggering of the scan as a result of effects of the superior vena cava, which is opacified very early. Another safeguard is checking attenuation in the ROI (**Panel A**) by clicking on "CALC" (calculation in **Panel B**). An attenuation of about 40 HU is optimal. Next, the threshold of 180 HU for starting the scan is defined (**Panel C**), and "Auto" is selected from the menu as the start position. The scan is then automatically started once the 180 HU threshold has been reached. Alternatively, the scan can be started manually by the examiner, on the basis of visual identification of the time of optimal contrast enhancement. Starting the scan manually results in considerable variation in coronary opacification, since the start is influenced by various factors such as individual reaction time and the examiner's level of experience

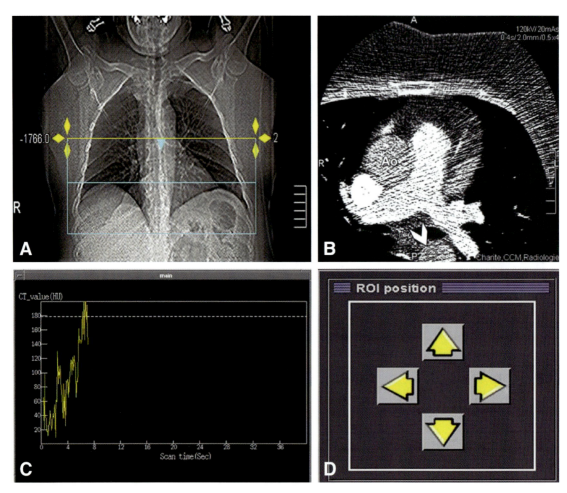

10a

□ **Fig. 10a.5** Start of the helical coronary examination. The position of the SureStart has been defined on the basis of the planning scan (**Panel A**). Next, a continuous low-dose scan (30–50 mA) is acquired at the level of the start of the spiral scan for triggering the spiral scan after IV contrast administration (**Panel B**). Contrast arrival can be tracked in real time. The continuous scan is started not earlier than 15 s after initiation of contrast administration for reasons of radiation protection and to ensure optimal opacification of the target vessels. Contrast arrival is measured in an ROI in the descending aorta (*arrowhead* and *small circle* in **Panel B**). The continuous increase in HU in the ROI over time is represented in **Panel C** in the form of a **graph**. The breathing command starts once the defined threshold of 180 HU has been reached. The scan then starts with a 3-s delay to allow the heart rate to normalize after inspiration. The *arrows* in **Panel D** represent cursor movements and can be clicked to correct the position of the ROI in the descending aorta if necessary. *Ao* ascending aorta

scan once a predefined Hounsfield threshold has been reached (**Figs. 10a.4** and **10a.5**). Use of the test bolus method increases the total amount of contrast injected and may be inaccurate because the circulation time may vary. Contrast agent injection is usually followed by an automatic 40-ml intravenous saline flush administered at a flow rate of 4 ml s^{-1}, which serves to wash out the right ventricle and improve coronary artery visualization.

Precontrast baseline attenuation is also measured in the descending aorta. In our experience, good results are achieved using a threshold of 180 HU when baseline attenuation is in the range of approximately 30–60 HU.

On the basis of our experience, we recommend the use of the SureStart bolus tracking option because it consistently yields good-quality images.

10a.1.4   Breath-Hold Training and Premedication

We recommend sublingual nitroglycerin administration (0.8–1.2 mg) before the breath-hold training. Nitroglycerin dilates the coronary arteries and improves the comparability of the CT findings with those of cardiac catheterization. The effect of nitroglycerin lasts for about 10–30 min.

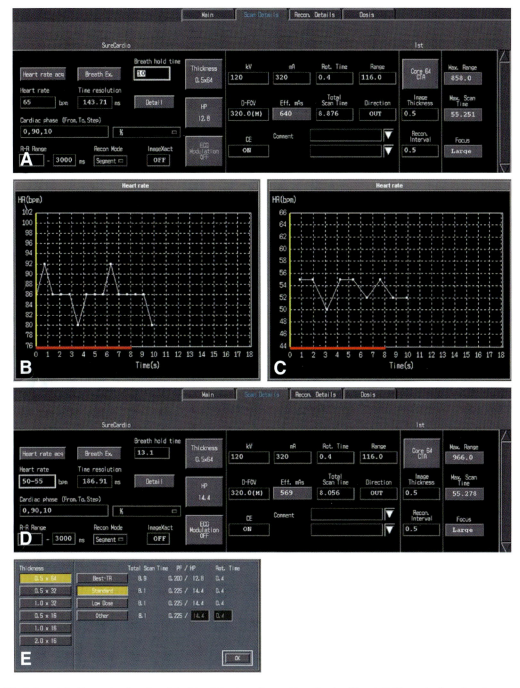

■ **Fig. 10a.6** Breath-hold examination. Breath-hold training is performed by selecting "Breath Ex." from the Scan Details menu. As can be seen in **Panel A**, the default breath-hold time should be 10 s for scanning of the coronary arteries. When bypasses are scanned, longer breath-hold periods are needed according to the scan length. The test is started by clicking on "Breath Ex."; the breathing commands that will also be used during the actual scan are then heard. The computer automatically calculates heart rate variability (which should be <10%), the optimal helical pitch (HP), and gantry rotation time. **Panel B** shows a case in which heart rate variability is in the upper normal range (80–92 beats per min). **Panel C** shows the results of a second test at a later time after intravenous beta blocker administration. The result is good, with a heart rate of 50–55 beats per min, and the examination can proceed. **Panel D** shows the results of the breath-hold test: a breath-hold time of 13.1 s, total scan time of 8.056 s, heart rate of 50–55 beats per min, and a recommended HP of 14.4. Other recommended scan parameters are shown in **Panel E**

Although nitroglycerin is usually well tolerated, patients should be monitored for the occurrence of possible hemodynamic side effects (e.g., hypotension).

In our department, we use an automatic speech system for the breathing commands ("Please breathe in and hold your breath"). The required breath-hold period is about 6–30 s, depending on the scanner used and the scan volume. Breath-hold training is done without radiation exposure, and the physician or technician should stand next to the patient to verify that the patient can hold his/her breath in submaximal inspiration for the required period and also to check for possible ECG alterations during inspiration. Toshiba scanners have a special function for breath-hold training. Heart rate variability should be less than 10% to achieve good results (**Fig. 10a.6**). Breath-hold training can be repeated if the ECG is suboptimal. If intravenous beta blocker injection is deemed necessary, it can be done at this stage. Heart rate variability is determined for individual adjustment of scan parameters such as pitch and gantry rotation time. A consistent image quality is achieved in all patients if the tube current is adjusted according to body weight (Chap. 9).

10a.2   Reconstruction

Following acquisition of the CT dataset, a few more steps are necessary to ensure good image quality as a basis for a reliable diagnosis. Motion of the individual coronary arteries, and even of their segments, varies during the different phases of the cardiac cycle. A number of reconstruction algorithms are available to depict the entire coronary arteries without motion. A basic prerequisite, as already mentioned, is sinus rhythm and low heart rate variability during data acquisition. Whether this has been the case during scanning should be verified by checking the ECG before proceeding to the next steps (**Fig. 10a.7**).

Image reconstruction starts automatically after completion of the examination, if this option has been selected in the scan protocol. In our department, we use adaptive multisegment reconstruction in increments of 10 from 0% to 90% of the RR interval if retrospective data have been acquired (**Fig. 10a.7**). Instead of percent-related or millisecond-related reconstructions, one can opt for so-called "BestPhase" and "Systole/Diastole" reconstructions. The "BestPhase" always corresponds to either "Systole" or "Diastole." For "Systole"

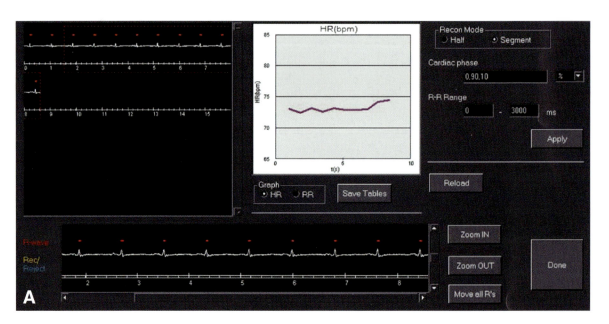

☐ **Fig. 10a.7** The reconstruction procedure. **Panel A** shows the ECG and heart rate variability [HR (bmp)] during scanning. The *red dots* indicate the R-waves identified

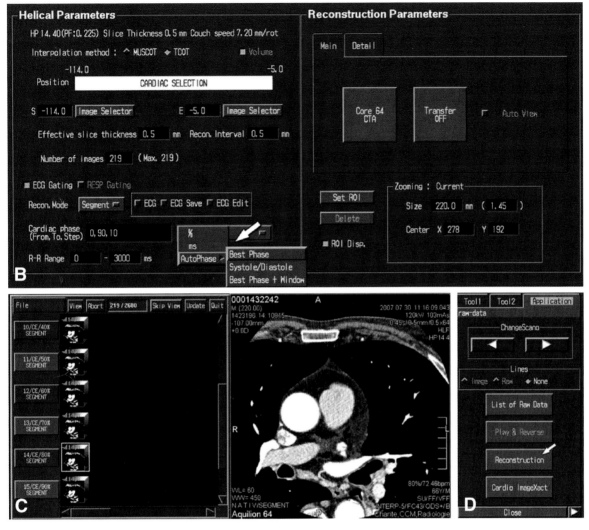

Fig. 10a.7 (continued) In **Panel B**, the reconstruction algorithm can be seen. In our example, we use adaptive multisegment reconstruction from 0–90% of the RR interval in increments of 10. These parameters are shown at the bottom of the dialogue window (0, 90, 10). The "Effective slice thickness" is 0.5 mm, and the reconstruction interval ("Recon. Interval") is 0.5 mm. In addition, "BestPhase" and "Systole/Diastole" reconstruction can be selected separately (*arrow*). The effective slice thickness and reconstruction interval are the same. The reconstruction FoV should be 180–220 mm for the coronary arteries and 320 mm for lung/soft tissue reconstruction (**Panel B,** *bottom right*). To send the images to the archive or a workstation, click on the "Transfer off" button to activate the transfer ("Transfer on") and select the target. The reconstructed segment is indicated in **Panel C** (*bottom right*), and any reconstructed image can be selected from a list (**Panel C,** *left part*). Finally, click on "Reconstruction" (*arrow*) to start the reconstruction (**Panel D**)

reconstruction, the systolic phase with the least coronary motion is reconstructed. The same holds true for "Diastole" reconstruction. To reduce storage requirements, one can select "Systole/Diastole" reconstruction alone as the standard option and then, after reviewing the images, retrospectively select individual phases for repeat reconstruction. On the basis of the scan field of view (FoV) selected before the examination, one should then reconstruct the so-called lung and soft tissue windows on large FoVs (**Fig. 10a.8**). It is quite common that accessory pulmonary, soft-tissue, or vascular changes are detected on the noninvasive coronary angiography scans. We use Vitrea workstations for the evaluation of noninvasive coronary angiography and generation of representative images for the patient and referring physician (**Fig. 10a.9**).

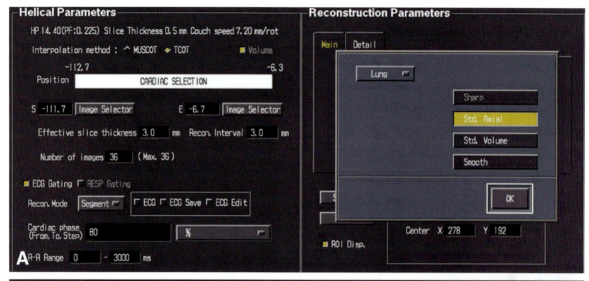

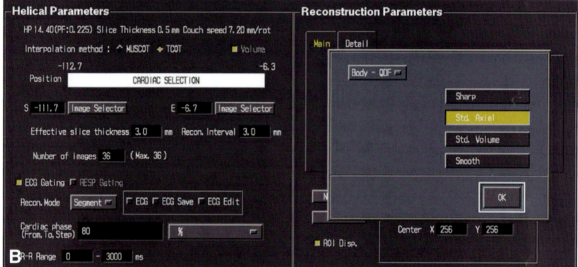

🔴 **Fig. 10a.8** Reconstruction of lung and soft tissue windows. The lung window (**Panel A**) and soft tissue window (**Panel B**) are reconstructed on large FoVs with an "Effective slice thickness" of 3 mm and a "Recon. Interval" of 3 mm at 80% of the RR interval and are selected by clicking on "Lung Std. axial" and "Body Std. Axial," respectively. Again, reconstruction is started by clicking on "Reconstruction"

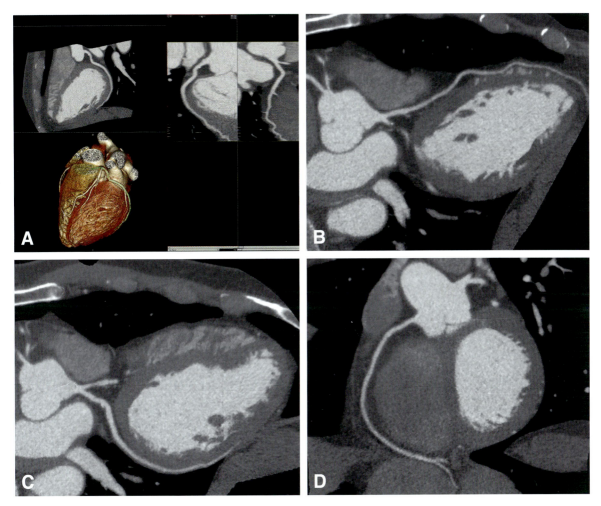

Fig. 10a.9 Reconstruction examples: Three-dimensional reconstructions of the heart are well suited for demonstrating the most important findings. The heart can be rotated to allow viewing from any direction (**Panel A**). An automatic tool identifies a vessel and traces a path along its course for generation of a curved multiplanar reformation (MPR, right upper corner in **Panel A**) or cath view (left upper corner in **Panel A**). On both the MPR and the cath view, the vessel is straightened and displayed in one plane. **Panel B** shows the curved MPR of the left anterior descending coronary artery (LAD). MPR is a fast and easy reconstruction method that provides good image quality and is very helpful in detecting and quantifying coronary stenosis. **Panel C** shows the curved MPR of the left circumflex coronary artery (LCX). **Panel D** shows the MPR of the right coronary artery (RCA)

10a.3 Aquilion ONE

With a gantry rotation time of 350 ms and 16-cm coverage along the Z-axis, the 320-row CT system is extremely well suited to perform CT examinations of the heart. Since nearly all hearts are smaller than 12 cm, the entire heart can be scanned with a single gantry rotation in the prospective acquisition mode (**Fig. 10a.10**), for the first time enabling scanning of the entire coronary tree with uniform enhancement along the Z-axis at one point in time.

10a.3.1 Preparation

Patient preparation is nearly the same as described above and is of crucial importance for obtaining a good scan with low effective dose with the new 320-row CT system as well. As with other CT scanners, a low heart rate is pivotal for good image quality. The 320-row system enables acquisition of a cardiac CT scan in a single heartbeat, which minimizes radiation exposure.

10a.3.2   The Role of the Cone Beam for Defining the Scan Range

The 15.2° cone angle of 320-row CT and the resulting cylindrical shape of the acquired volume makes it more difficult to plan the CT angiogram scan range from the scanogram alone (anteroposterior and lateral) compared with conventional CT scanners. The heart must lie in the center of the scan field (Chap. 9). The volume acquired with the 15.2° scan angle does not cover the cranial and caudal portions of the heart with a maximal axial field of view (**Fig. 10a.10**). The effects of the cone angle are best illustrated with the aid of coronal reconstructions (**Fig. 10a.11**). The resulting truncation of the volume was

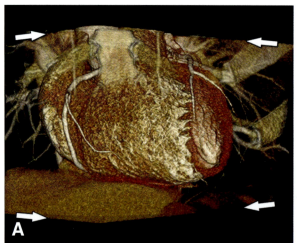

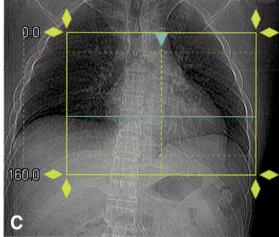

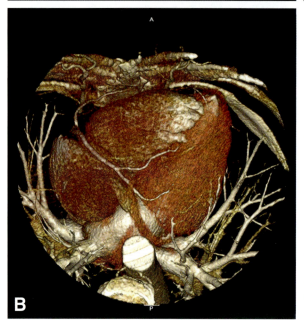

▪ **Fig. 10a.10** Imaging of the entire heart with a single gantry rotation using 320-row CT. Nearly all hearts are smaller than 12 cm and can be completely scanned with a single gantry roation using less than 320 simultaneous rows. The challenge of coronary CT angiography is to obtain good image quality with a minimum of radiation exposure. If the heart is not positioned in the center of the scan field (**Panel A**), there is the risk of "cutting off" cranial or caudal cardiac or coronary portions, and a stenosis of the left main coronary artery, for example, may be overlooked. **Panel A** is an anterior three-dimensional reconstruction of the heart, showing narrowing of the scan volume at the cranial and caudal ends (*arrows*) using 320-row CT; these portions cannot be reconstructed with the maximum axial FoV. **Panel B** shows a caudal three-dimensional reconstruction of the same heart. **Panel C** is the corresponding anteroposterior scanogram, illustrating the difficulty of exactly determining the heart size using only this image. The yellow rectangle indicates the scan range in the Z-axis. Note the two vertical broken yellow lines, which outline the scan length imaged with the maximum axial FoV

▪ **Fig. 10a.11** Effects of the 15.2° cone angle of 320-row CT. The 16-cm detector width of 320-row CT results in a cone angle of 15.2° (*arrows* in **Panel A**). It is important to correctly position the patient to preclude incomplete visualization of the target anatomy. **Panels A, C**, and **E** show coronal reconstructions of a properly positioned heart. The red horizontal lines in **Panels A, C,** and **E** indicate the positions of the corresponding axial slices (**Panels B, D**, and **F**). The left main coronary artery is depicted in the center in one of the cranial slices with a maximum axial FoV (**Panel B**). As a result, all four cardiac chambers are fully depicted at the level of the widest dimension of the heart in coronal (**Panel C**) and axial (**Panel D**) planes. The basal portions are also depicted in the center and with a maximum FoV (**Panels E** and **F**). *Ao* aorta; *DA* descending aorta; *LV* left ventricle; *RV* right ventricle

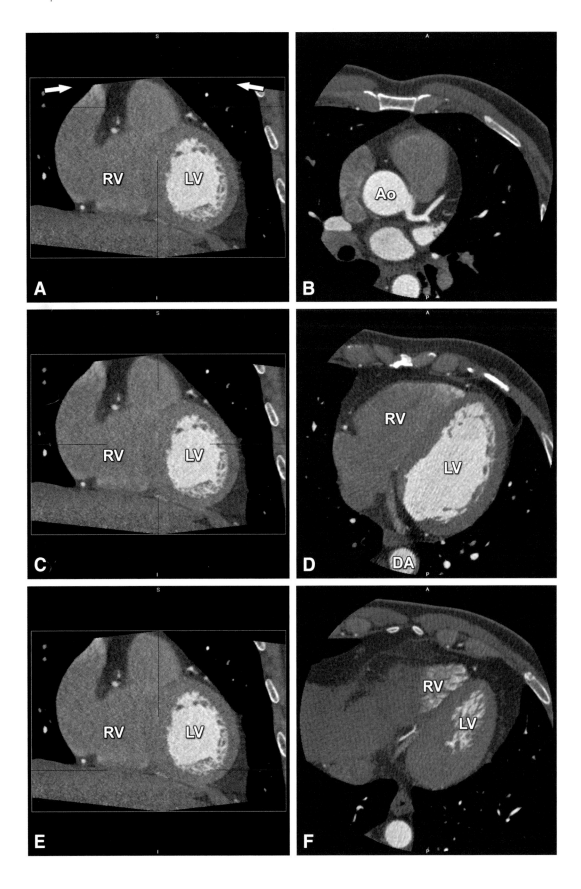

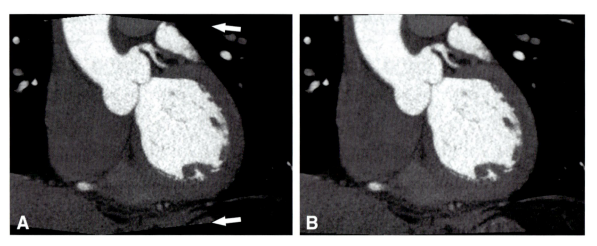

🔴 **Fig. 10a.12** Reduced truncation of the cylindrical volume obtained with 320-row CT shown on coronal reformations. Using VolumeXact + for reconstruction it is possible to reduce the truncation (**Panel A**) of the volume dataset (which occurs with the ConeXact reconsctruction based on the cone angle of 15.2° arrows, see **Fig. 10a.11**) by about 75% (**Panel B**). This greatly facilitates the planning process

reduced with recent software by 75% (**Fig. 10a.12**) which greatly facilitates planning of the coronary acquisition.

10a.3.3   Planning the Scan Range Using a Calcium Scan

A low-dose scanogram in two planes is acquired to define the proximal and distal ends of the low-dose calcium scan (**Fig. 10a.10**). The unenhanced axial slices of the calcium scan are used to individually plan the final length of the cardiac CT angiogram (**Fig. 10a.13**). Estimating individual heart size and planning the length of the CT scan in the Z-axis are much more difficult from the scanogram. Errors in planning may result in overestimation of the scan range required to cover the target anatomy, which may lead to unnecessary radiation exposure, or in underestimation with failure to capture the proximal or distal portions of the coronary arteries. **Fig. 10a.14** illustrates how the scan range is adjusted to the patient's heart size.

🔴 **Fig. 10a.13** Planning the 320-row CT angiogram from a low-dose calcium scan. Individual adjustment of the scan length of a cardiac CT angiogram to the patient's heart size can reduce the radiation exposure compared with the full 16-cm scan range in the z-direction. The heart size is determined from the axial slices of the calcium scan. The slice containing the most cranial segment of the coronary arteries, typically the left main coronary artery, is identified (**Panel A**). **Panel B** shows the slice with the anatomic landmark (aortic root with the left main coronary artery and the proximal segments of the left anterior descending and left circumflex coronary arteries) coded in green. The widest dimension of the heart is shown in **Panel C**. **Panel D** shows the four cardiac chambers, which are difficult to delineate on unenhanced scans, in green. The red dot is a cross-section of the RCA (**Panel D**). Next, the slice containing the most caudal portion of the heart is identified (**Panel E**), which is typically the apex of the heart (**Panel F**). To accommodate variations in the position of the heart with the phase of the respiratory cycle at which a patient holds his or her breath, an additional 10–15 mm are added at either end of the calculated scan length for the CT angiography. If the variation in inspiration depth is not taken into account, there is a risk of missing portions of the target anatomy despite accurate planning of the scan length. *Ao* aorta; *DA* descending aorta; *LV* left ventricle; *RV* right ventricle

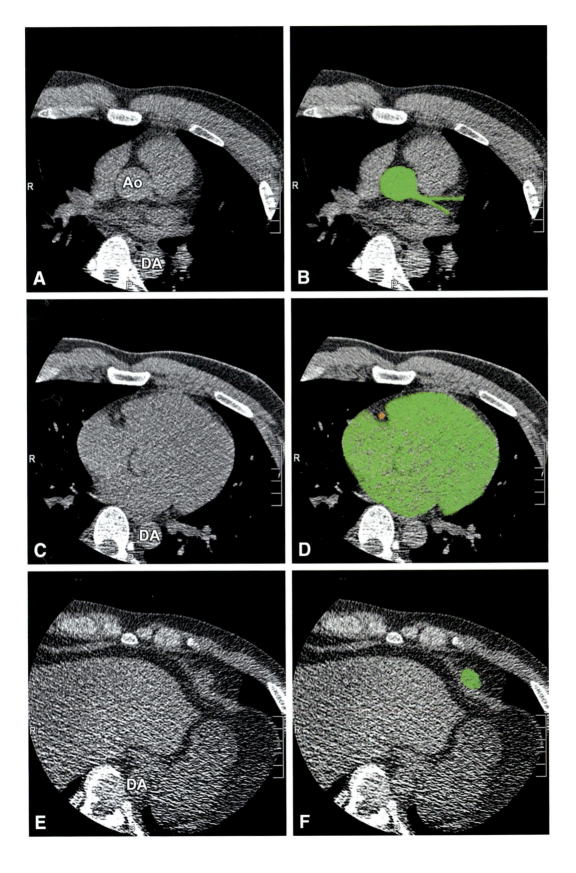

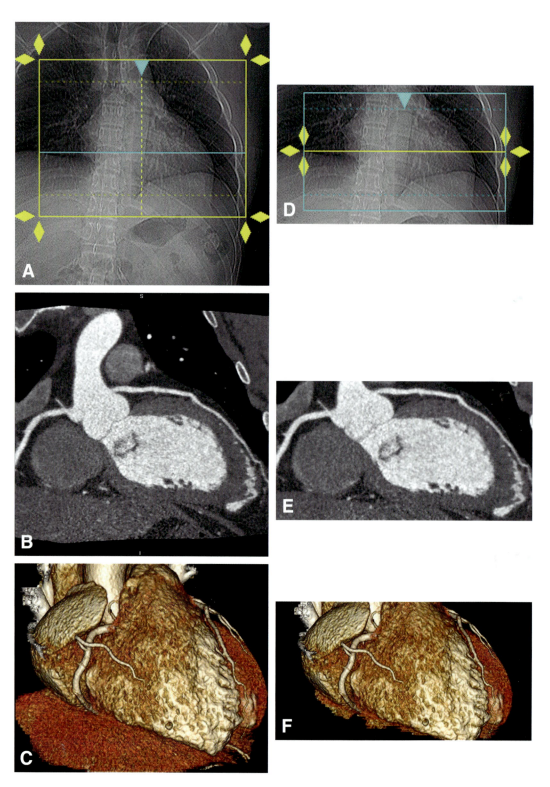

10a

■ **Fig. 10a.14** Comparison of the full 16-cm scan range of 320-row CT angiography with the scan range adjusted to individual heart size. **Panel A** shows how the 16-cm scan range is planned using a scanogram. In the same patient, the scan range was also planned on the basis of the actual heart size determined using a low-dose calcium scan (**Panel D**). The coronal (**Panels B and E**) and three-dimensional reconstructions (**Panels C and F**) nicely illustrate the effects of a meaningful limitation of the scan range, which allows a marked reduction of the radiation exposure

10a.3.4   Surestart

The 320-row CT system has the so-called Fast SureStart option (**Fig. 10a.15**) which allows initiation of the cardiac CT scan within one second after reaching the predefined threshold in the descending aorta. The SureStart protocol and contrast agent injection are started simultaneously, and acquisition of a low-dose monitoring scan starts after 10 s and is presented online. After another 4 s, the breathing command is given ("Please breathe in and hold your breath"), which lasts 4 s. The breathing command is followed by a 2-s delay, which is necessary to allow the heart

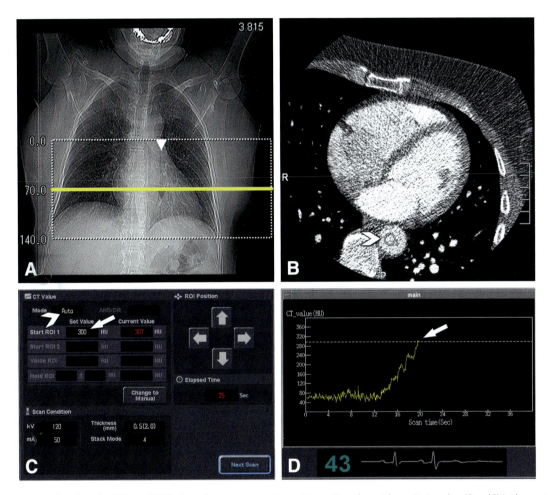

🔲 **Fig. 10a.15** SureStart for 320-row CT. The low-dose scanogram is used to position the axial monitoring slice (*Panel B*) in the center of the scan area (Z-axis) (**Panel A**). This slice (**Panel B**) is used for real-time monitoring of the inflowing contrast agent, which can be followed on its passage from the right atrium and ventricle to the left atrium and ventricle, and to the thoracic aorta. The CT angiogram can be started automatically or manually

(1) Automatically starting the CT angiogram after a predefined attenuation threshold (HU) has been reached. Arrival of the contrast agent is measured in a region of interest (ROI) in the descending aorta (*arrowhead*) (**Panel B**). The ROI can be displaced from the aorta by respiratory motion while the SureStart scan is running, which must be corrected in order not to miss the optimal time for starting the CT angiogram. The position of the ROI (**Panel B**, *arrowhead*) can be corrected with the cursor (**Panel C**, *right*). When the predefined threshold is exceeded (**Panel C**, *arrow*), the scan is started automatically. The increase in HU measured in the descending aorta is presented online in the form of a Hounsfield unit curve, which serves as a control of contrast administration (**Panel D**). If the threshold is not reached, the scan can be started manually by clicking on the "Next Scan" button (**Panel C**)

(2) Alternatively, the manual start option can be selected. When this option has been chosen, the user visually follows the inflow of the contrast agent on the monitor (**Panel B**) to start the scan. For this option, no threshold or ROI need to be defined. The scan mode is selected via the "Mode" button ("Auto" or "Manual," **Panel C**, *arrowhead*). In the manual mode, the CT angiogram is started by clicking on the "Next Scan" button (**Panel C**). The manual start option depends on the skills and experience of the operator but has a greater potential for reducing the amount of contrast agent administered. An optimal time point for starting the scan (automatically or manually) has been reached when there is good enhancement of the left ventricle and aorta and most of the contrast agent has been washed from the right ventricle (**Panel B**)

rate to normalize following the slight increase that may be induced by inspiration. This means that there is a delay of at least 20 s after the start of contrast injection before the cardiac CT scan can be started. In patients with a normal circulation time, optimal enhancement of the cardiac chambers will be seen after about 20–25 s. The amount of contrast agent is adjusted to the patient's body weight and ranges from 60 to 80 ml (administered at a flow rate of 3.5–5 ml/s), followed by a 40-ml saline chaser administered at the same flow rate, which serves to accelerate washout from the right ventricle.

The axial contrast agent monitoring slice for the SureStart protocol is defined on the basis of a scanogram. This axial slice provides an overview and is presented on the screen for real-time monitoring of the inflow of contrast agent into the right atrium and ventricle and its further passage into the left atrium and ventricle and the thoracic aorta. The optimal time for starting the CT angiogram is when most of the contrast agent has left the right ventricle and there is good enhancement of the left ventricle and aorta. Two options are available for starting the CT angiogram: (1) automatic start after a predefined Hounsfield threshold has been reached in the descending aorta (e.g., 300 HU) or (2) manual start based on visual assessment of enhancement in the cardiac chambers. **Fig. 10a.15** illustrates the individual steps of planning the CT scan and using the SureStart option.

10a.3.5   Scan Modes

The new scan mode, (**Fig. 10a.16**), so-called "Target CTA," allows the user to determine the radiation exposure before the scan by defining the number of beats to be used for data acquisition. However, this scan mode does not allow automatic arrhythmia control. The user also defines the center position of the exposure window in relation to the RR target phase in Target CTA (e.g., 75% of the RR interval) before the scan starts. The exposure window defines the duration of radiation exposure.

Unlike Target CTA, "Prospective CTA" allows arrhythmia control, which is why a maximum radiation exposure threshold cannot be defined beforehand. The individual heart rate registered during breath-hold training (SureCardio) serves to define the number of beats to be used for the prospective CTA scan, the exposure time, and the center position of the exposure window in relation to the RR interval.

Cardiac function analysis (CFA) can be done using one of two scan modes: (1) identical mA (CTA/CFA Cont.) for the entire scan, ensuring a constant image quality for both CTA and CFA or (2) modulated scan mode (CTA/CFA Mod.) with variable mA (high during diastole and 25% of this value during the other cardiac phases), resulting in a reduction of the effective dose (**Fig. 10.16**).

10a

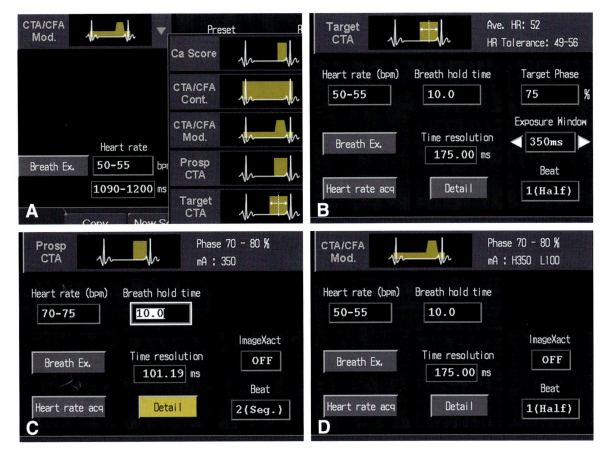

❑ **Fig. 10a.16** Scan modes available on the 320-row CT system. Select "Scan details" from the menu to make changes to the scan modes for each examination (**Panel A**). "Target CTA" (**Panel B**) is a scan mode allowing the user to define the number of beats and the target phase (position of the exposure window in relation to the RR interval) before the examination. Heart rate tolerance refers to the range of heart rates for which image reconstruction will be possible. Target CTA does not provide automatic arrhythmia control but sets an upper limit for radiation exposure. In contrast, "Prospective CTA" (**Panel C**) is a scan mode that automatically adjusts the examination to individual variations in heart rate and allows arrhythmia control. The number of beats (2 in the example in **Panel C**) depends on the heart rate recorded during breath-hold training (70–75), and the exact position of the triggered phase (70–80%) is determined online on the basis of the last five heartbeats (real time beat control). Cardiac function analysis (CFA) modulates radiation exposure during different phases of the RR interval (**Panel D**). For the phase of the RR interval deemed favorable for CT angiography, a higher mA is used to ensure good image quality, while mA is reduced to 25% for the remainder of the RR interval. This mode allows evaluation of the coronary arteries with simultaneous functional analysis at a reduced radiation exposure. The number of beats for CFA also depends on the patient's heart rate

Siemens Somatom Sensation and Definition

C. Klessen and K. Anders

Abstract

This chapter describes the acquisition and reconstruction of cardiac CT data sets on Siemens scanners.

10b.1   Preparing the Examination

The vendor recommends performing coronary angiography with the patient in a supine head-first position. Nevertheless, scanning the patient in feet-first position has some advantages: The patient is easier to monitor and can be accessed more quickly in case of an emergency (e.g., contrast medium intolerance or extravasation). Moreover, it is easier to administer intravenous beta blockers or nitroglycerin spray and other medications. Note, however, that the speakers for giving instructions are at the back of the gantry. Thus, the volume must be turned up when examining patients in the feet-first position, especially if they are hard of hearing.

It is important to place the ECG electrodes outside the scan area to reduce image artifacts. Correct electrode placement is illustrated in **Fig. 10b.1**. Moreover, with the Somatom Sensation 64, which uses a unique z-flying focal spot technology with 32 simultaneous detector rows, the ECG electrodes must be in place before the scan protocol is called up in order for the software to recognize the ECG signal. Details of patient preparation for coronary CT angiography on all scanner types are presented in Chaps. 7 and 9.

10b.2   Image Acquisition

Acquisition of a conventional chest topogram (**Fig. 10b.2**) is followed by planning and acquiring two axial control scans (**Fig. 10b.3**). The first control scan is acquired in the plane with the largest transverse extension of the heart and serves to optimize the field of view for the subsequent CT angiogram (**Fig. 10b.3**). To further reduce radiation exposure, this scan may be skipped; the field of view for the CT angiography scan can alternatively be planned on the real-time images acquired during the scan. Optimal spatial resolution is achieved by selecting a small field of view for image reconstruction. The second control scan is obtained to select the scan position for test bolus acquisition (**Fig. 10b.3**). The subsequent test bolus scan consists of a series of images acquired at rate of one image per second (**Fig. 10b.4**). The test bolus consists of 10–15 ml of iodine-based contrast medium, followed by a 30–50-ml saline flush (injection rate: 5 ml s^{-1}) in normal-weight patients. Radiation exposure is minimized by starting the scan 10–15 s after injection and stopping acquisition once the contrast medium peak has been reached. A dedicated software tool, DynEva, is available for automatic analysis of the test bolus series.

M. Dewey, *Cardiac CT*,
DOI: 10.1007/978-3-642-14022-8_11, © Springer-Verlag Berlin Heidelberg 2011

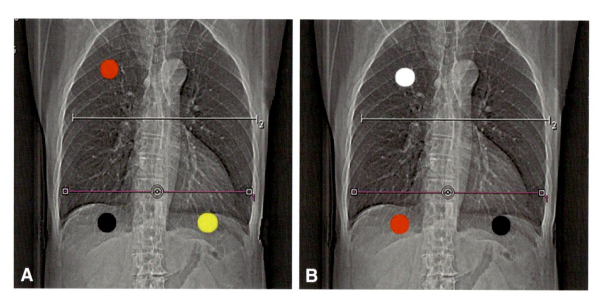

☐ **Fig. 10b.1** Optimal positioning of the ECG electrodes on the chest. **Panel A** shows the IEC standard and **Panel B**: the USA standard

10b

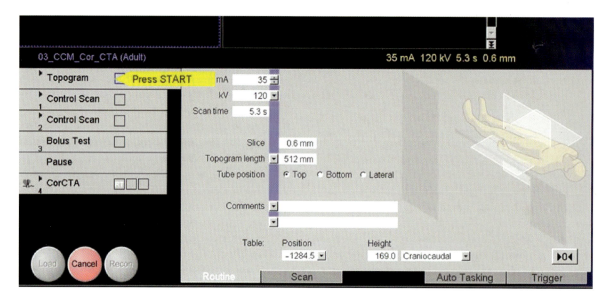

☐ **Fig. 10b.2** The first step is the acquisition of a chest topogram (scanogram), typically acquired from top to bottom. To minimize the scan area, the acquisition can be stopped as soon as the entire heart has been scanned

☐ **Fig. 10b.4** Bolus test scan. The test scan (*red line* in **Panel A**) comprises a maximum of 40 images. It is started 10–15 s after the beginning of the contrast medium injection. The test bolus series can be analyzed visually or with the DynEva software (**Panel B–D**). A region of interest (ROI) is defined in the ascending aorta for analysis (**Panel B**). The time to peak can be read in a table (*arrow* in **Panel C**) after entering the delay used for image acquisition (*arrow* in **Panel D**)

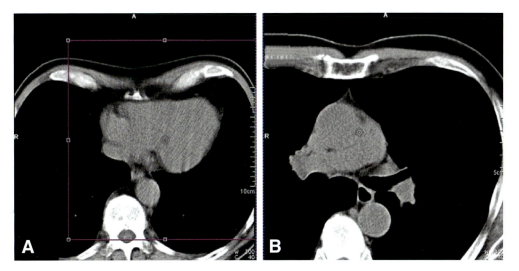

■ **Fig. 10b.3** Acquisition of two control scans. The first control scan (**Panel A**) is positioned at the level of the greatest transverse extension of the cardiac silhouette on the topogram and serves to plan the field of view for the coronary CT angiography scan. The second control scan (**Panel B**) is obtained about 1–2 cm below the tracheal bifurcation to identify the position for test bolus acquisition

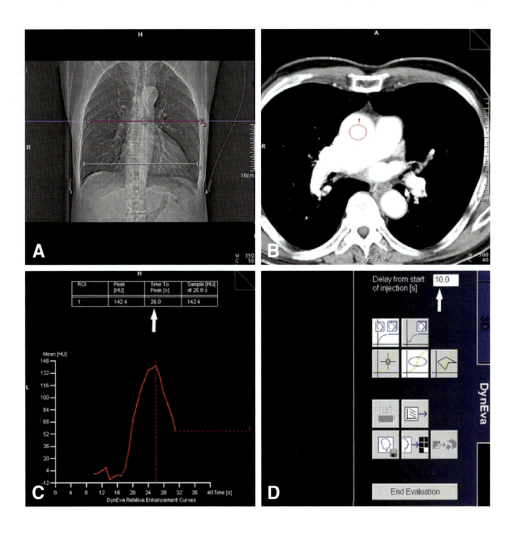

Next, the CT angiography scan, which is acquired from top to bottom, is planned (**Fig. 10b.5**). In patients with a constant low heart rate (≤60 beats per min), prospective ECG dose modulation (ECG pulsing) can be used, thereby reducing the radiation exposure by up to 40–50%. In slender patients, radiation exposure can be considerably reduced by using a 100 kV scan protocol. The scan delay (the time interval between the start of

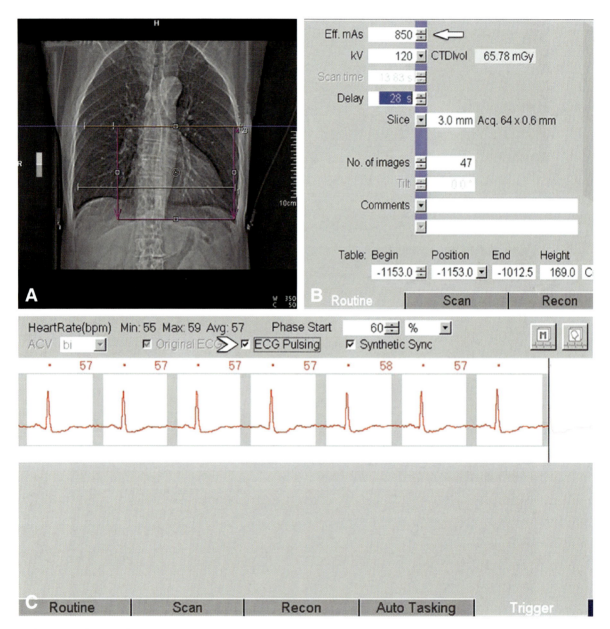

Fig. 10b.5 Planning of the coronary CT angiography scan (**Panel A**). For normal-weight patients, the manufacturer recommends 850 eff. mAs (*arrow* in **Panel B**). In slender patients, radiation exposure can be considerably reduced by using a 100 kV protocol. The highest possible eff. mAs value may be required in obese patients. Finally, prospective ECG dose modulation (ECG pulsing) can be activated from the trigger card of the Syngo menu (*arrowhead* in **Panel C**)

the test bolus injection and image acquisition) is the individual test bolus time plus an additional 3 s. The additional 3 s delay time is needed to obtain optimal arterial contrast in the ascending aorta and the coronary arteries on the one hand and low contrast in the right ventricle and the right atrium on the other, in order to avoid inflow artifacts that may hamper the evaluation of the right coronary artery. To minimize the inferior extension of the scan field, scanning can be

manually discontinued as soon as the real-time images show the entire heart.

10b.3   Image Reconstruction

The first step in image reconstruction is to check the recorded ECG (**Fig. 10b.6**). If there are isolated extrasystoles, the corresponding reconstruction intervals can be

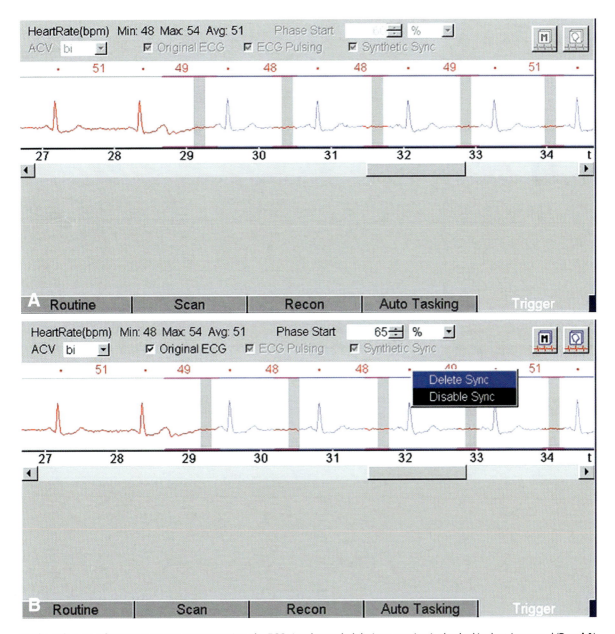

■ **Fig. 10b.6** As a first step in image reconstruction, the ECG signal recorded during scanning is checked in the trigger card (**Panel A**). The minimum, maximum, and average heart rate during the acquisition are displayed on the top of the trigger card. If isolated extrasystoles are present, the corresponding reconstruction intervals can be deactivated or deleted (**Panel B**)

deactivated or deleted for image reconstruction. It is recommended that a preview series be generated at this point on the basis of a reference image at the level of the mid-RCA (segment 2) to identify the most suitable phase for image reconstruction (**Fig. 10b.7**). Next, thick slices and thin slices are reconstructed at the optimal phase of the RR interval determined in this way (**Fig. 10b.8**). Reconstruction is usually done using a soft-tissue reconstruction algorithm (B25f smooth), while a sharper kernel (B 46f) may be used to improve the evaluation of calcified plaques and stents. Alternatively, multiphasic reconstructions (i.e., automatic

reconstruction of multiple phases of the RR interval) can be performed. Multiphasic reconstructions (e.g., 0–90% in 10% intervals) are especially useful if the diagnostic question includes the assessment of ventricular and/or valvular function. In contrast to the situation for the scanners from the other three vendors, the percentage that determines the position of the phase within the RR interval indicates the start, and not the center, of the image reconstruction window (phase). Finally, reconstruction series with a large field of view are computed for assessment of the soft tissue and lungs (**Fig. 10b.9**).

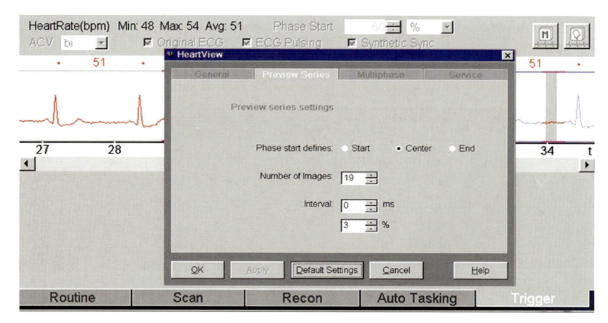

Fig. 10b.7 The user can identify the best time point in the RR interval for image reconstruction by clicking on the "Preview Series" button to generate a series of preliminary images. Such a series may consist for example of 19 images reconstructed at 3% intervals around the start phase. The image selected for generation of the preview series should contain the middle portion of the RCA (segment 2), which is highly susceptible to degradation by motion artifacts

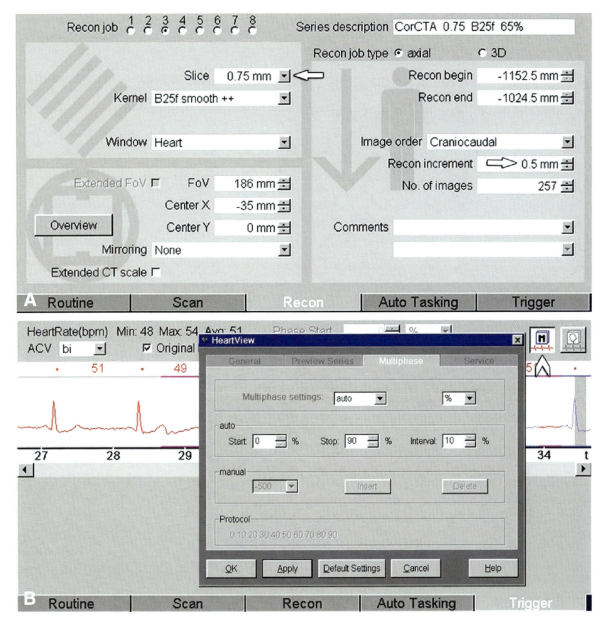

■ **Fig. 10b.8** Next, image series are reconstructed at specific times in the RR interval (**Panels A** and **B**). The time is preselected in the trigger card. As a rule, 0.75 mm images are reconstructed at overlapping intervals (*arrows* in **Panel A**). Alternatively, multiple phases can be automatically reconstructed (in the example shown, from 0–90% of the RR interval at 10% increments). The automatic reconstruction mode is activated by clicking on the multiphase button (*arrowhead* in **Panel B**) and selecting the desired start and stop points as well as the reconstruction interval. Note, however, that the automatic mode generates a large number of images, especially when small intervals are preselected

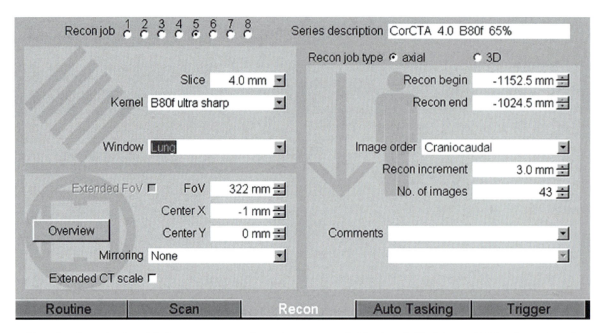

☐ **Fig. 10b.9** For evaluation of the lungs, a reconstruction series is generated with a large field of view and thicker slices, using a lung kernel

10b.4 Dual-Source CT ("Somatom Definition")

The technical background of dual-source CT (DSCT) has been described in Chap. 9. The most important practical advantage of DSCT is the improved temporal resolution resulting in better image quality in patients with higher heart rates and arrhythmia (**Fig. 10b.10**). Although beta blockade is recommended to lower heart rates for DSCT as well, the threshold up to which very good image quality can be expected is increased to about 70 beats per min (in contrast to the 60 beats per min threshold with halfscan reconstruction and 64-row CT). The workflow of scanning using DSCT (Somatom Definition) and the scanner's software is not relevantly different from that of the Somatom Sensation 64. It should be noted that the field of view is limited with dual-source CT because the second gantry has a scan field of only 25 cm. Typical image acquisition parameters are listed in **Table 10b.1**.

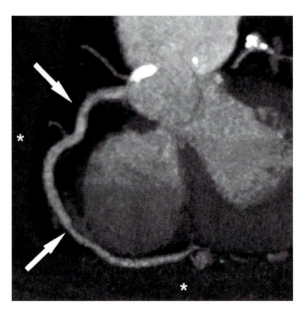

☐ **Fig. 10b.10** Example of an examination with dual-source CT in a patient with a heart rate of 125 beats per min. Maximum-intensity projection of the right coronary artery (*arrows*). Note the surrounding pericardial effusion (*asterisks*) that caused the high heart rate. Used with permission from Achenbach et al., Eur Radiol, 2008

Table 10b.1 Typical data acquisition parameters for first-generation dual-source CT coronary angiography

Parameter	Value
Gantry rotation time	330 ms
Total scan time	7–10 s
Slice width	0.6 mm
Collimation	19.2 mm
Pitch	0.20 for heart rate <50 beats per min 0.22 for heart rate 50–59 beats per min 0.28 for heart rate 60–69 beats per min 0.33 for heart rate 70–79 beats per min 0.39 for heart rate 80–89 beats per min 0.44 for heart rate 90–99 beats per min 0.50 for heart rate ≥100 beats per min
Tube voltage	120 kV 100 kV for patients <85 kg 80 kV for very slim patients
Tube current	e.g., 400 + 400 mA
mAs value per rotation	e.g., 264 mAs (=800 × 0.33); the resulting value is relevant for image quality considerations
Effective mAs value	e.g., 528 mAs (=267 × 0.6/0.3); in this example, a pitch of 0.3 and an ECG pulsing efficiency factor of 0.6 were assumed; the resulting value is relevant for dose considerations
Contrast agent	50–80 ml at 5 ml s⁻¹ (consider 6 ml s⁻¹ in patients >100 kg)
Contrast timing	Test bolus or bolus tracking

Modified and used with permission from Achenbach et al., Eur Radiol 2008

10b.5 Second Generation Dual-Source CT ("Somatom Definition FLASH")

The second generation dual-source CT scanner ("Somatom Definition FLASH") has a wider detector (38.4 mm) and an increased rotational speed of 280 ms. The acquisition window per axial image is thus 75 ms. Furthermore, both X-ray tubes and detectors are arranged at a 95° offset (instead of the previous 90°), which enables the use of a larger detector for the second tube (B-tube) and thus a larger scan field of view (33 cm, Chap. 9). The faster gantry rotation speed, the novel detector arrangement, and finally the use of a larger detector (64 × 0.6 mm, doubled by the use of a dual focal spot) allow cardiac scanning in a nonoverlapping, prospectively triggered spiral mode (FLASH mode) with a pitch of 3.4. Data acquisition can thus be completed within a single heartbeat in patients with heart rates below about 60–65 beats per min. Starting this type of scan at 60% of the RR interval using a craniocaudal scan direction is recommended. This entails visualization of the distal right or left coronary artery branches at a slightly later cardiac phase, e.g., around 80%. Planning of the scan range of coronary CT angiography in the FLASH mode is facilitated by obtaining a noncontrast coronary artery calcium scan (also acquired using a high-pitch spiral). Prior to any FLASH mode scan, a so-called FLASH check has to be performed, which analyzes the patient's ECG recording (obtained during breath-hold) for heart rate stability and RR intervals to determine whether high-pitch scanning is likely to be successful.

Triggered data acquisition without overlap can considerably reduce dose exposure. However, this scan mode so far has been used only in patients with low and stable heart rates. Furthermore, the FLASH mode cannot be used for functional analysis since, as with sequential scan modes, only samples of the cardiac cycle are recorded. Functional imaging requires overlapping spiral acquisition with ECG gating, which of course is also possible – albeit with a higher effective dose. **Fig. 10b.11** shows the scan parameters as displayed by the user interface. **Fig. 10b.12** shows the acquisition window placed according to the patients' recorded ECG with a scan start at 60% of the RR interval. Resulting images of a low-dose examination to rule out relevant coronary artery disease are displayed in **Fig. 10b.13**.

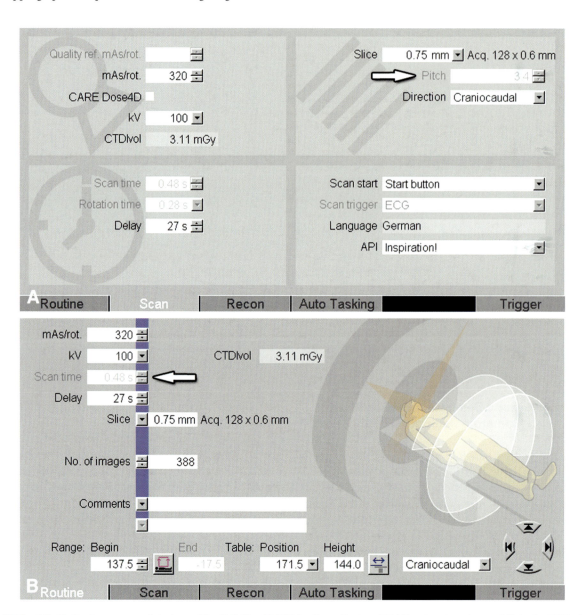

◪ **Fig. 10b.11** Cardiac scan user interface of the Definition FLASH. In slim patients, a 100 kV protocol can be used. Note the CTDI of 3.11 mGy (**Panel A**) and the pitch of 3.4 (*arrow* in **Panel A**). For a scan range of 15.5 cm (Begin: 137.5 mm and End: −17.5 mm), the resulting scan time is 0.48 s (*arrow* in **Panel B**)

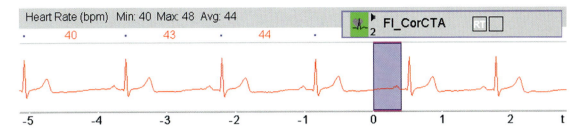

Fig. 10b.12 Cardiac FLASH scan ECG file and data acquisition window. The blue box within the ECG file indicates the tube-on time, during which the entire heart was scanned. Prior to scanning the FLASH check symbol turns green (inset)

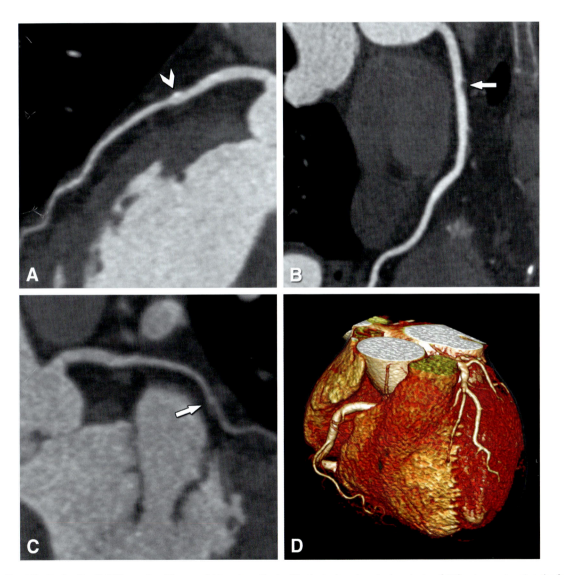

Fig. 10b.13 Cardiac FLASH scan in a 52-year-old female patient with atypical angina at a heart rate of 56 beat per min using the following scanner settings: 100 kV, 320 mAs/rot, CTDIvol 3.10 mGy, resulting DLP 49 mGycm, and scan start at 60% of the RR interval. Small calcified plaque in the left anterior descending artery (**Panel A**, *arrowhead*) and noncalcified, nonstenotic plaque in the right coronary artery (**Panel B**, *arrow*). The small left circumflex artery shows no relevant lesions (**Panel C**); the origin of a side branch (*arrow*) mimics focal wall irregularities on a curved multiplanar reformation. A three-dimensional overview of the case is given in **Panel D**, showing that no relevant motion artifacts are present. No invasive angiography was performed

Philips Brilliance 64 and iCT

O. Klass, M. Jeltsch, and M.H.K. Hoffmann

Abstract

Performing cardiac CT on Philips scanners is described.

10c.1 Preparing and Starting the Examination

After entering the patient's ID, the examiner should select table position, age group, and the desired exam protocol group (**Fig. 10c.1**). The patient is then placed on the CT table in a supine position, and ECG leads are attached. The automatically started ECG viewer enables permanent registration of heart rate and rhythm including calculation of standard deviation and mean heart rate. Details of patient preparation for coronary CT angiography on all scanner types are presented in Chaps. 7 and 9.

Each examination starts with a surview (scanogram) to determine the position of the heart. The localizer scan should be as small as possible while covering the entire heart and is acquired during a single inspiratory breath-

hold. The scan area for a standard coronary CT angiography is often determined using the tracheal bifurcation as the upper reference point. It is also the level of the plane in which the tracker for the bolus timing algorithm is placed. The scan ends about 1–2 cm below the heart (**Fig. 10c.2**). The scanner gantry isocenter line should be properly placed in the center of the heart. Finally, the entire heart is examined with ECG gating during a single inspiratory breath-hold.

The scan is timed to coincide with peak contrast enhancement, derived from the preceding bolus tracking. Bolus tracking is performed by a Locator and a Tracker scan, positioned on the level of the tracheal bifurcation. Pressing "Go" starts the Locator scan, and the system automatically shows the tracker window. A region of interest (ROI) is positioned in the descending aorta (**Fig. 10c.2**). Now bolus tracking and injection of contrast medium must be started at the same time. After a start delay, several transverse sections are successively acquired at the defined level. The scan starts automatically once attenuation enhancement values in Hounsfield units reach a predefined threshold.

10c.2 Prospective Axial Acquisition ("Step & Shoot")

Since the introduction of the new scanner generation (Brilliance iCT) with a rotational speed of 270 ms and a detector width of 8 cm (128 rows), the majority of patients (80%) can be scanned with prospective axial acquisition ("Step & Shoot") with helical retrospective gating being reserved for data acquisition in patients with arrhythmia and high heart rates. As a prospectively gated scan mode, "Step and Shoot" requires a stable heart rate below 65 beats per min. This scan type combines the

M. Dewey, *Cardiac CT*,
DOI: 10.1007/978-3-642-14022-8_12, © Springer-Verlag Berlin Heidelberg 2011

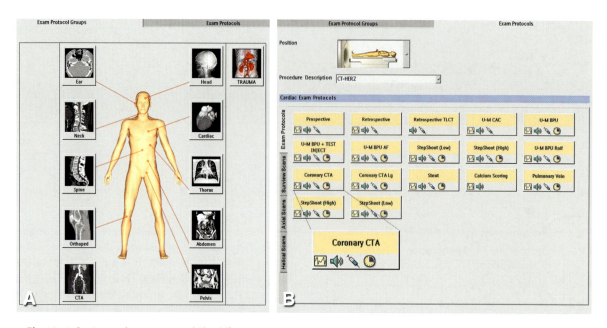

☐ **Fig. 10c.1** Setting up the scan protocol. The different "Exam Protocol Groups" are shown in **Panel A** while **Panel B** details the "Cardiac Exam Protocols" such as "Coronary CTA". Depending on the planned examination, you can select between different protocols (e.g., standard helical "Coronary CTA," "Step & Shoot" mode, or "Calcium Scoring")

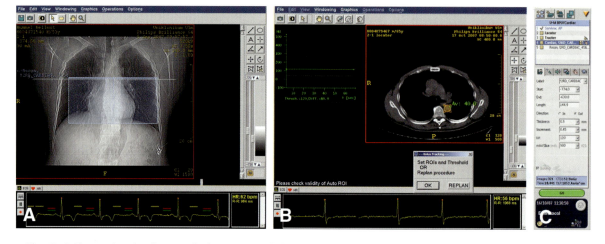

☐ **Fig. 10c.2** The user interface for a standard retrospective helical scan, including the defined field of view and an ECG viewer, is shown in **Panel A**. The *blue box* indicates the preselected scan area and range. For bolus tracking, the ROI is positioned in the descending aorta (**Panel B**). The dose indication box shows the expected dose exposure and scan time (**Panel C**)

advantages of axial and helical scans and relies on sequential axial acquisition. Generally, "Step & Shoot" involves a typical scan sequence that is based on volume acquisition ("Shoot") and table movement ("Step"). Depending on the system used, the heart is covered in four to six (Brilliance 64) or two to three (iCT) axial rotations, combined with prospective triggering (**Fig. 10c.3**). The main advantages of "Step & Shoot" scanning are summarized in **List 10c.1**.

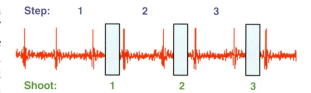

☐ **Fig. 10c.3** The principle of sequential axial acquisition after table movement (Step), combined with prospective ECG gating (triggering)

List 10c.1. Advantages and disadvantages of prospective coronary acquisition

Advantages:

1. Provides a low-dose scan with a dose reduction to one-fourth of that of standard helical scans
2. Image quality is comparable (*or even better with the iCT*) to that of standard helical scans
3. Improved rotational speed of the iCT enables coverage of the whole chest in one breath-hold with "Step & Shoot", e.g., to image coronary artery bypass grafts or to perform a triple rule-out scan
4. Allows each volume to be reconstructed from a single cardiac cycle resulting in a better edge depiction of the coronary arteries
5. Includes an online arrhythmia handling mechanism (**Fig. 10c.4**)

Disadvantages:

1. Limited to patients with stable heart rates below 65 beats per min
2. Lower temporal resolution when compared to helical scans
3. Geometric distortion at the borders of the prospectively acquired slabs (**Fig.10c.5**)

High:

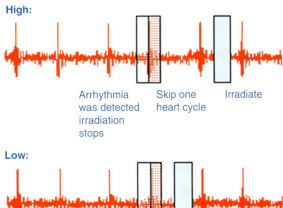

Arrhythmia   Skip one   Irradiate
was detected   heart cycle
irradiation
stops

Low:

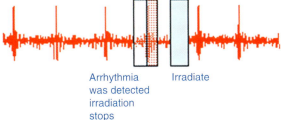

Arrhythmia   Irradiate
was detected
irradiation
stops

◘ **Fig. 10c.4** Two options are available for online arrhythmia handling in the "Step & Shoot" mode. "High" arrhythmia tolerance: When an arrhythmia is detected, irradiation stops immediately; the system waits for one cardiac cycle and then continues exposure in the same table position after the next cycle. "Low" arrhythmia tolerance: When an arrhythmia is detected, irradiation stops immediately; the system continues exposure in the same table position in the cycle immediately following. To prevent excessively long scan times (in the "High" tolerance mode), in a sequence of more than two irregularities, the "High" strategy is automatically changed to "Low"

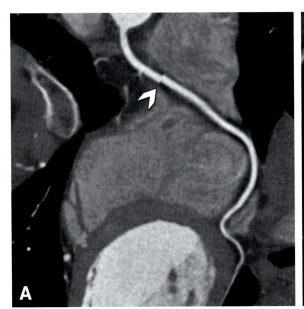

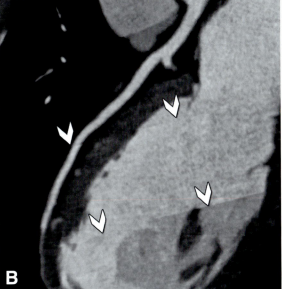

◘ **Fig. 10c.5** Drawbacks of the "Step & Shoot" approach. Curved multiplanar reformations of the right coronary artery with "steps" (*arrowhead* in **Panel A**) and of the left anterior descending coronary artery showing "bands" (*arrowheads* in **Panel B**) as artifacts resulting from geometric distortion at borders of the prospectively acquired slabs

10c.2.1 Scan Protocol

A standardized protocol is used for prospective acquisition (**Table 10c.1**) with 64 × 0.625 mm collimation and a tube rotation time of 400 ms on the Brilliance 64 and 128 × 0.625 mm collimation and a tube rotation time of 270 ms on the iCT. The tube voltage is 120–140 kV, and tube current typically 190–210 mAs. Data are acquired for a full rotation (360°) instead of a half scan plus fan angle, providing greater flexibility in compensating for changes in heart rate.

The planning on the scanogram of the "Step & Shoot" scan is similar to the helical scan with the following differences: the field of view is limited to 250 mm (in both standard and detailed resolutions). This limitation is indicated by a "gray box" that is displayed on the surview image (**Fig. 10c.6**). To make sure that the optimal phase is acquired even under changing conditions, the "Step & Shoot" application has a built-in mechanism that analyzes the patient's heart rate online during the scan, and, if arrhythmia occurs, it responds accordingly. The new reconstruction capabilities of "Step & Shoot" allow the user to select any reconstructed slice thickness and slice increment as in equivalent helical scans. These characteristics are reflected in the values that are defined in the dropdown menus for both "Increment" and "Thickness" fields (**Fig. 10c.6**).

10c.2.2 Dose Indication Box

Since the "Step & Shoot" scan time and irradiation profile are not known in advance (because of potential online arrhythmia handling), the dose indication box is different from that for retrospective image acquisition (**Fig. 10c.2**) to reflect this uncertainty (**Fig. 10c.6**).

10c.2.3 Injection Protocol

The injection protocol for "Step & Shoot" acquisition is identical to that used for current helical acquisition. It is important to emphasize that the minimal post-threshold delay is 7 s, which is the amount of time needed to reach the initial scan position and to build up adequate tube voltage. Another important drawback is that only one cardiac phase can be acquired when using prospective acquisition. The cardiac phase needs to be selected beforehand, and the center of the phase can vary from 40% to 85% of the RR interval. An innovation of the iCT is the option to choose a reconstruction window with a surrounding phase variance of 5% ("padding"), meaning that reconstructions of a preselected phase of 75% can also be done at 70% and 80%.

10c.3 Retrospective Helical Image Acquisition

The retrospectively gated helical acquisition mode, which used to be the standard scan mode for coronary CT angiography, has become the scan mode for "difficult"

□ **Table 10c.1** Typical scan parameters

	Helical scan	Step & Shoot
Total collimation	64×0.625 mm	64×0.625 mm
Rotation time	400 ms	400 ms
Tube voltage	120–140 kV	
Current time product/ tube load	600–900 mAs[a]	150–210 mAs[a]
Pitch	0.2	NA
CTDI$_{vol}$	34–75 mGy[b]	11–22 mGy
Maximum field of view	500 mm	250 mm
Scan duration	Approximately 10 s	Approximately 10 s
ECG synchronization	Retrospective ECG gating	Prospective ECG gating (triggering)
Cycles	NA	4–5
Threshold for bolus tracking	150 HU	150 HU
Postthreshold delay	5–7 s	7 s

NA not applicable

[a]True mA = electrical mA; effective mA = electrical mA divided by pitch

[b] Without temporal dose modulation ("ECG gating")

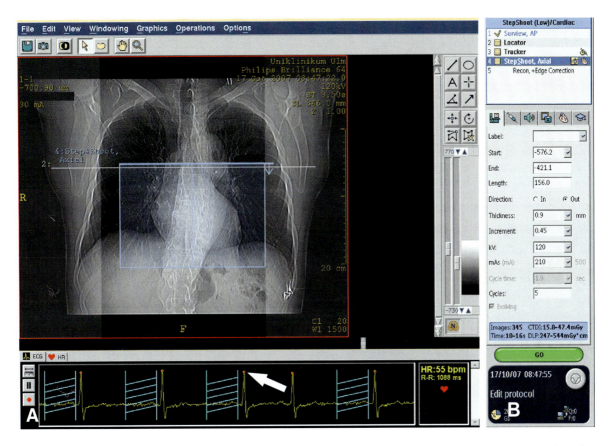

Fig. 10c.6 Limited field of view with "Step & Shoot". The "gray stripes" on both sides of the patient in the scanogram (**Panel A**) reflect the limited field of view (250 mm). To avoid unnecessary radiation exposure an additional lateral scanogram should be obtained only in patients with above-average thoracic diameters. Additionally, prospective ECG triggering with online arrhythmia handling is also shown skipping one RR cycle (*arrow* in **Panel A**). **Panel B** shows the dose indication box, displaying CTDI and DLP values as ranges (e.g., CTDI 15.8–47.4 mGy and DLP 247–544 mGy × cm), where the lowest value represents a case without any arrhythmia, and the highest value a case with severe continuous irregularities. The "Time" field in this box gives the scan time range without irregularities (minimum) and the scan time in the case of continuous irregularities (maximum). The slice increment and thickness are the same as with the helical protocol

patients with high heart rates, a wider range of heart rate variations, and arrhythmias. With the improved temporal resolution of up to 67 ms of the current CT generation, the helical scan mode even allows scanning patients with atrial fibrillation with more or less stable image quality. This is due to the fact that retrospective gating allows multisegment image reconstruction at any arbitrary phase of the cardiac cycle.

10c.3.1 Scan Protocol

A standardized examination protocol (**Table 10c.1**) with 64 × 0.625 mm collimation and a tube rotation time of 420 ms on the Brilliance 64 and 128 × 0.625 mm collimation and a tube rotation time of 270 ms on the iCT is used. The typical tube voltage is 120 kV with a tube current of 600–900 mAs, depending on patient size, body mass index, and thoracic diameters in the scan area. A standard patient with 75 kg body weight is scanned with 120 kV and a tube voltage of 800 mAs. A separate dose indication box gives the expected dose exposure and scan time (**Fig. 10c.2**).

After the scan is completed, preview images are presented and can be centered and zoomed to the optimal size. Philips also offers an option for editing of the ECG wave as well as off-line arrhythmia handling prior to the start of reconstruction (**Fig. 10c.7**).

10c.4   Reconstruction

Image reconstruction is performed using comparable parameters for retrospectively and prospectively acquired data (**Table 10c.2**), with cardiac standard filters XCA-D during mid-diastole and end-systole of the cardiac cycle (**Fig. 10c.8**). Philips uses an adaptive multisegment reconstruction algorithm for retrospectively acquired data integrating 3D voxel-based backward projection of the cone beam. Image reconstruction using the raw data

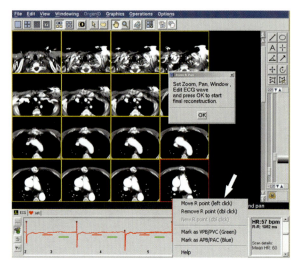

Fig. 10c.7 Preview images shown after completion of scan acquisition. Images can be centered and zoomed to the optimal size. Prior to starting final image reconstruction the ECG of the acquired scan can be manipulated using the off-line arrhythmia handling software as shown in the pop-up window (*arrow*)

□ Table 10c.2 Typical reconstruction parameters

	Prospective helical scan	**Step & Shoot**
Reconstruction filter kernel	Xres Standard (XCA-D)	Xres Standard (XCA-D)
Reconstruction field of view	Approximately 200 mm	Approximately 200 mm
Matrix	512×512	512×512
Slice thickness	0.9 mm	0.9 mm
Reconstruction increment	0.45 mm	0.45 mm
Reconstructed ECG intervals[a]	Normally 40 and 75%, for functional analysis 0–90% equally spaced by 10%	Normally 75% (40–85%)

[a] Percentages indicate the center of the image reconstruction interval

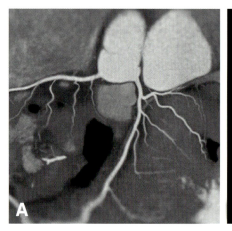
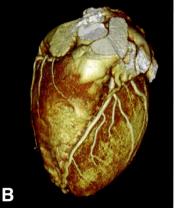
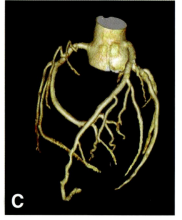

□ Fig. 10c.8 Reconstructions from a "Step & Shoot" examination: two-dimensional map (**Panel A**), volume-rendering of the heart (**Panel B**), and the extracted coronary tree (**Panel C**) reconstructed at 75% of the R-R cycle using an XCA-D filter

from up to five segments from consecutive cardiac cycles improves the theoretical temporal resolution. A coronary artery will be reconstructed from partial raw data from several consecutive RR intervals. This reconstruction principle is applied separately for each voxel.

Left/right ventricular analysis requires ECG intervals equally spaced by a maximum of 10%. It is advisable to perform an additional reconstruction of the raw data in a lung-adapted window setting using maximum fields of view.

General Electric Light Speed VCT and Discovery CT750HD

L. Lehmkuhl and E. Martuscelli

Abstract

This chapter describes how cardiac CT is performed on General Electric scanners.

10d.1 Electrode Placement and ECG

10d.1.1 Electrode Placement

It is recommended that the electrodes not be placed over muscle, scar tissue, or hair; the proper placement is medially over the clavicle to avoid the muscle tissue when the arms are raised over the head. It is very important to ensure good skin contact. Details of patient preparation for cardiac CT and of the examination procedure on all scanner types are presented in Chaps. 7 and 9.

Figure 10d.1 shows proper lead placement using the IVY ECG monitor: First raise the patient's arms above the head, and then position the leads as shown. Place the two upper leads directly on the patient's clavicle. This placement ssssprovides the best signal for the IVY monitor. To avoid incompatibilities, do not use patient monitoring electrodes that may be available from other departments in your facility. The electrodes recommended by General Electric (GE) are Dyna/Trace 1500 by Conmed.

10d.1.2 ECG Monitor

Turn on the ECG machine and make sure that there are good connections to the gantry and leads. A good connection is confirmed if "CONNECTED" appears in the upper right display area of the monitor. Otherwise, check to make sure that the cable connecting the ECG machine to the backside of the gantry is plugged in properly and that the same cable is connected to the ECG machine. In case of low signal, check the electrode placement and choose an alternative position if needed (**Fig. 10d.1**). If there is "noise" within the ECG wave, it is recommended that you do not scan until this condition is corrected.

10d.2 Scan Preparation

10d.2.1 Breathing Instructions

Prior to the scan, have the patient practice the automatic breathing instructions. Scanning is sufficiently rapid that it is not necessary for the patient to hyperventilate. The scanning time should be no longer than 5–8 s on average. Let the patient take one breath in, blow it out, then

M. Dewey, *Cardiac CT*,
DOI: 10.1007/978-3-642-14022-8_13, © Springer-Verlag Berlin Heidelberg 2011

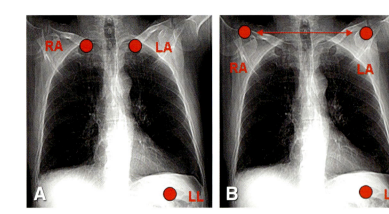
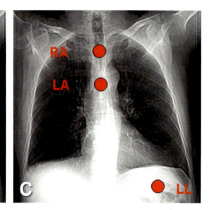

◘ **Fig. 10d.1** ECG electrode placement. **Panel A** shows a scanogram depicting the recommended ECG lead placement for best signal clarity. If the signal is low or the QRS peak is not noticeably stronger than the other ECG wave segments, using one of the two alternate positions (**Panels B** and **C**) may improve the ECG signal and its detection

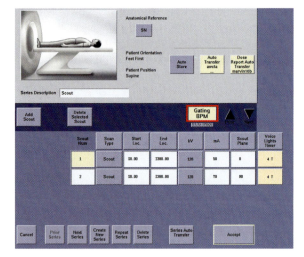

◘ **Fig. 10d.2** Planning the scout (scanogram) acquisition. Make sure that "Active Gating" (see *red frame*) has been selected when taking the two scout views (AP and lateral). The cardiac breathing protocol should be used for the scout scans and all subsequent scans

take a breath in and hold it, while you watch the ECG monitor and take note of the patient's heart rate during breath-holding. A patient who has any difficulty holding his or her breath may be put on 2–4 l min⁻¹ of oxygen via a nasal cannula. Oxygen administration may also help to lower the heart rate.

When recording the breathing instructions for cardiac CT that are programmed in the scanner, make sure to give the breathing instructions slowly. The breathing instructions should be no shorter than 10 s. When recording the instructions, and after you say, "take a breath in and hold it," be sure to wait for 3–5 s (of silence) prior to clicking on the "stop recording" button. This delay will give the patient enough time to hold his or her

breath before the actual start of the scan and for the heart rate to stabilize; otherwise the patient may still be breathing in during the first several slices, which could lead to motion artifacts on the images.

10d.2.2 Scout Scans

The following steps, summarized in **List 10d.1**, should be performed to choose the correct scan protocol and to acquire the scout scans.

List 10d.1. Choice of protocol and scout acquisition

1. Landmark the patient at the sternal notch
2. Select "new patient" and enter patient data
3. Select the anatomical area (chest)
4. Select the snapshot (cardiac) protocol from the main menu
5. On the scout screen, check to make sure you are in "Active Gating" mode and that the gating is fine, then take the scout views
6. Use the cardiac breathing protocol for the scout scans and all subsequent scans (**Fig. 10d.2**)
7. Monitor the patient's heart rate during the breath-hold[a]
8. When the two scout scans are completed, select "next series" to display the next step of the protocol

---

[a] The body's natural physiologic response during breath-hold is to reduce the heart rate by approximately 5 beats per min. Knowing what the patient's heart rate does during the breath-hold will help you determine what scanning mode to use during the cardiac scan (**Fig. 10d.3**).

If the heart rate is not displayed on the screen and you have a "red" gating box, the scanner is not reading the patient's waveform. To correct this problem, try the following: (1) click on the red "Gating" box and turn off the gating, then turn it back on; (2) check all connections between the gantry and the ECG machine; and (3) check once again for proper placement of the leads on the patient.

10d.3 Scan Modes, Bolus Timing, and Image Acquisition

10d.3.1 CT Coronary Angiography Scan Modes

There are three different modes for retrospectively gated reconstruction that can be used for image acquisition, depending on the patient's heart rate. These modes are described in **Fig. 10d.3**. Alternatively, in patients with

low and stable heart rates, prospectively ECG-gated (i.e., triggered) axial acquisitions (nonhelical) can also be performed; this approach has the advantage of reducing the radiation exposure.

10d.3.2 Bolus Timing

To calculate the exact arrival time of the contrast medium in the coronary arteries, the test bolus protocol described in **Table 10d.1** is recommended. View the scout and place an axial monitoring scan 1 cm below the carina. If a noncontrast localizer series was previously done (e.g., for calcium scoring), you may also scroll through these images and determine the location for the axial monitoring scan by manually typing the location into the View/Edit screen.

If you have a dual-head injector, it is recommended that you follow the contrast test bolus with a 20-ml saline chaser. Scan the patient with the cardiac breathing protocol and note the heart rate during the scan.

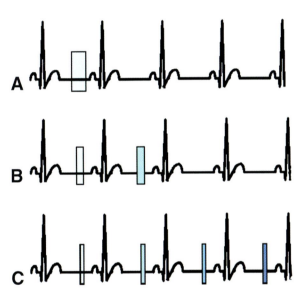

□ **Fig. 10d.3** Alternative retrospective cardiac reconstruction methods. **Panel A** shows the "SnapShot Segment Mode" (half-scan): heart rate, 30–74 beats per min; one sector; reconstruction window, 175 ms; a retrospectively gated reconstruction using data from 2/3 of a gantry rotation to create an image from one cardiac cycle. **Panel B** shows the "SnapShot Burst Mode" (multisegment): heart rate, 75–113 beats per min; two sectors; reconstruction window, ~87 ms; a retrospectively gated reconstruction using data from up to two cardiac cycles within the same cardiac phase to create an image at a given table/anatomic location. **Panel C** shows the "SnapShot Burst Plus Mode" (multisegment): heart rate, >113 beats per min; two, three, or four sectors; reconstruction window, 44 ms; stable heart rates; a retrospectively gated reconstruction using data from up to four cardiac cycles within the same cardiac phase to create an image at a given table/anatomic location

□ **Table 10d.1** Parameters of the test bolus scan

Parameter	Value
Rotation time	0.5 s
Interval	0
Thickness	5 mm
Prep delay	5 s
Interscan delay	1.5 s
SFOV	Large
DFOV	25 cm
kV	120
mA	40
No. of scans	14
Contrast agent amount	15 ml
Injection rate	5 ml s⁻¹, or the same injection rate as for the cardiac angiogram

DFOV display field of view. This term describes the central part of the scan field of view, which is chosen for image reconstruction. *SFOV* scan field of view. This term describes the maximum diameter of the acquired scan area that can be used for image reconstruction

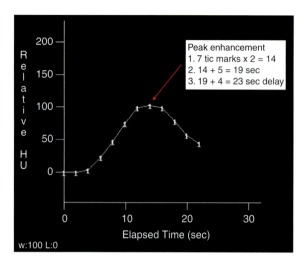

Fig. 10d.4 Time-to-peak curve derived from the test bolus acquisition. On the graph image, count each tic mark on the line graph to the peak of the curve, multiply the number of tic marks by 2, and then add 5 s. Remember that image no. 1 is at 5 s and the tic marks are 2 s apart. This time represents the time it takes for the contrast agent once injected to reach the root of the aorta, where the coronary arteries arise (time-to-peak enhancement). Once you have the time-to-peak enhancement, add an additional 4 s (to allow for filling of the distal coronary vessels); this number is now the pre-scan delay or prep group delay for the cardiac CT exam. In brief, prep delay is calculated as follows: (number of tic marks × 2) + 5 s + 4 s; alternatively, it can be expressed as: peak + 9 s. This bolus time is a key parameter to use for the gated cardiac acquisition.

Once all of the test bolus images are reconstructed, highlight the view port in which they are loaded, select the measurement icon on the "Exam Rx Desktop," then select "MIROI" (Multi-Image Region of Interest). Select the elliptic ROI from the pop-up box on the screen, and place the ROI in the ascending aorta and size it to fit completely within the aorta. Then click OK on the pop-up box and calculate the bolus arrival time as described in **Fig. 10d.4**. Click on "Next series" to display the gated cardiac helical acquisition protocol. Enter in the prep delay, based on the test bolus. Alternatively, a bolus tracking technique can be selected by clicking on "Smart Prep." For bolus tracking, a threshold of 120–150 HU is recommended for initiation of the subsequent helical scan (**Fig. 10d.5**).

10d.3.3 Image Acquisition

Prescribe the location of the scan on the scout using graphic Rx, or type in the start and end locations using explicit Rx, on the basis of the noncontrast localizer images. Use the scan parameters described in **Table 10d.2**. Choose detector coverage, helical thickness, and rotation time as shown in **Fig. 10d.6**.

Just prior to scanning the patient, it is very important to check the ECG trace on the scanner console to make sure that you are properly gating and that the scanner is triggering on the appropriate segment of the

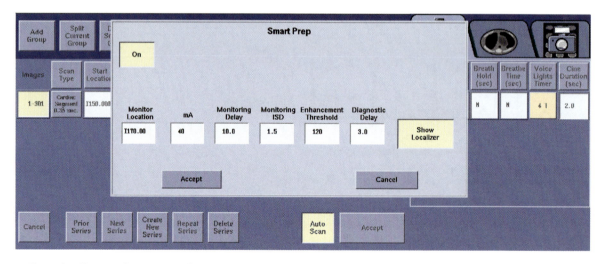

Fig. 10d.5 Choosing the parameters for bolus tracking ("Smart Prep"). An enhancement threshold of 120–150 HU is recommended

▣ Table 10d.2 Image acquisition parameters

Scan parameter	Value	Comment
Scan type	Cardiac helical	
Rotation time	0.35 s	
Start location	–	Based on the scout scans
End location	–	Based on the scout scans
Coverage	Entire heart	
Slice thickness	0.625 mm	See **Fig. 10d.6**
Slice interval	0.625 mm	No overlap (overlap results in more artifacts)
SFOV	Cardiac large	See **Table 10d.3**
DFOV	25 cm	Adjustable as desired to contain coronaries
mA	See **Table 10d.4** and **Fig. 10d.7** for recommended values (adjust these as appropriate for your clinical needs)	ECG modulation can lead to a dose decrease of up to 50% in low stable heart rates; see **Fig. 10d.8** for further instructions
kVp	120	
Pitch	–	The pitch is automatically set by the software, based on the patient's heart rate
Reconstruction type	Standard	
Cardiac noise reduction filters	C1, C2, or C3	These filters allow dose reductions of up to 30% on topof the ECG modulation dose reduction while preservingimage quality

DFOV display field of view; *SFOV* scan field of view

ECG wave. You should see a "RED" line on the R peak of the QRS complex on the patient's ECG wave. If you do not see the "RED" line on the R peak but rather somewhere else, make the appropriate adjustments to the electrode placement or monitor settings to ensure proper gating on the R peak. The "white" area represents the reconstruction window of 75% in the RR interval used for the reconstruction of the first set of images. The ECG trace on the console refreshes every 2 s.

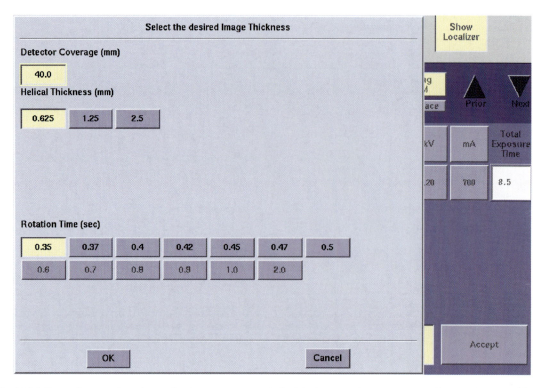

Fig. 10d.6 For cardiac scanning, choose the detector coverage, helical thickness, and rotation time as shown in this screenshot

10d

Table 10d.3 Different cardiac scan fields of view

SFOV	Bowtie filter	DFOV (cm)[a]
Cardiac small	Small	9.6–32
Cardiac medium	Medium	9.6–36
Cardiac large	Large	9.6–50

DFOV display field of view; *SFOV* scan field of view
[a] The standard DFOV for cardiac CT using GE scanners is 25 cm

Table 10d.4 Recommended mA values for ECG modulation

Body weight	Minimum mA value	Maximum mA value
<60 kg (<132 lb)	100	450
60–80 kg (132–176 lb)	250	550
>80 kg (>176 lb)	400	750

If no modulation is desired, the scan should be acquired with the maximum mA value

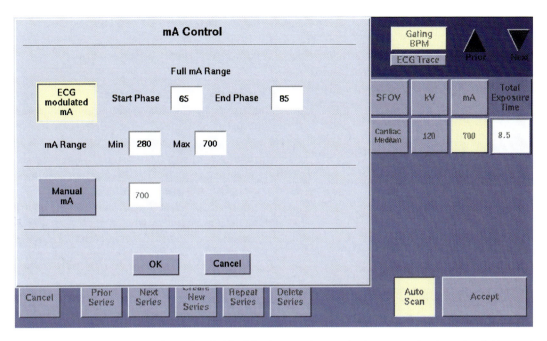

Fig. 10d.7 Adjusting the mA setting for cardiac CT. The full mA range phase and mA range can be chosen by clicking on the "mA" button. ECG modulation can be switched off by clicking on the "Manual mA" button. "Min" and "Max" define the mA range of the modulation, whereas "Start phase" and "End phase" describe the part of the RR interval to which the maximum mA is applied. Recommended mA values are listed in **Table 10d.4**

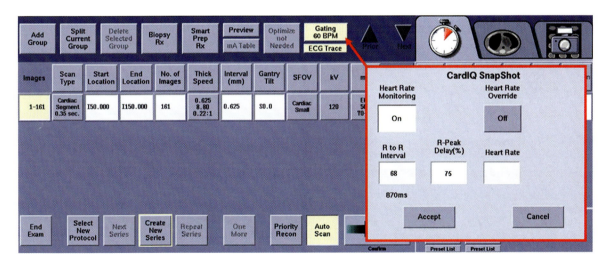

Fig. 10d.8 Before starting the scan, make sure that the reconstruction phase is centered at 75%. The "Heart Rate Override" button allows you to use a lower pitch than suggested by the software

10d.4   Image Reconstruction

Once the scan is completed, select "retro recon." Select the phase button and process the images from 70% to 80% of the RR interval with an incremental step of 10% in the mode in which the images were acquired. These images (displayed as complete series) will be used if the heart is not frozen at 75% of the RR interval from the initial scan. The images can also be processed from any other point within the RR interval (**Fig. 10d.9**) to make it possible to see images from systole to diastole. If the RCA is not frozen in the 70–80% phase range, it is best to reconstruct the phases centered at 40–55% (end-systole)

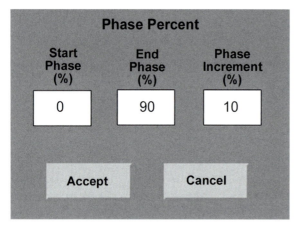

■ **Fig. 10d.9** Reconstruction at different phases

10d.5   Discovery CT750 HD

10d.5.1 Technical Characteristics

The last-generation GE scanner is characterized by a better in-plane spatial resolution (0.23 mm). This improvement is due to (1) new detector material (gemstone) able to provide a primary speed of 0.03 μsec and an afterglow of only 0.001% and (2) a new data acquisition system, which allows acquiring 2.5 times more views. Also, this scanner features a new generator tube supporting ultrafast kV switching for dual-energy imaging and can reconstruct images using adaptive statistical iterative reconstruction (ASIR), reducing noise by 50–70%.

10d.5.2 Image Acquisition and Specific Reconstruction Kernels

Coronary CT should be done in the high-resolution mode (**Fig. 10d.10**). Prospective (axial) acquisition can be selected using the snapshot segment cine mode. Retrospective helical acquisitions with the HD 750 can also be done using (a) single segment (SnapShot), (b) dual-segment (SnapShot Burst), or (c) three to four segments (SnapShot Burst Plus, **Fig. 10d.3** and **10d.10**). The recommended scanning parameters and tube settings for the prospective and retrospective modes are summarized in **Table 10d.5** and **10d.6**. To take advantage of the high-definition mode the use of specific kernels (HD standard

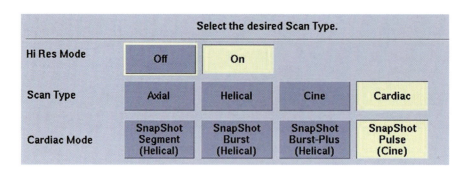

■ **Fig. 10d.10** Choosing the high-definition option: the high definition is indicated as Hi Res Mod (high resolution modality) option. The label of the HD modality is right above the Scan Type. After choosing cardiac scanning, the axial reconstruction algorithm (step and shoot) can be selected with SnapShot Pulse (Cine). The helical reconstruction algorithm can be planned selecting "SnapShot Segment" (Helical), "SnapShot Plus" (Helical), or "SnapShot Burst-Plus" (Helical)

and HD details) is mandatory (**Fig. 10d.11**). Cardiac CT reconstruction should be done using the adaptive statistical iterative reconstruction (ASIR) algorithm although this takes slightly longer than standard filtered backprojections (35 s vs. 16 s for 10 images). The ASIR level should only be 40% since a combination of filtered backprojection and a certain level of ASIR provides a compromise between adequate noise reduction and retaining the more typical appearance of CT images.

▪ Table 10d.5 Image acquisition parameters with the 750HD CT scanner

Scan type	Helical	Axial
Rotation time (s)	0.350	0.350
Slice thickness (mm)	0.625	0.625
Slice interval (mm)	0.4	0.625
SFOV	Cardiac small	Cardiac small
DFOV	Adjust as small as possible	Adjust as small as possible
Pitch	0.16–0.24 (automatically selected by the scanner)	
Reconstruction type	HD standard	HD standard
ASIR	40%	40%
Padding		Automatic: based on heart rate Manual: 0–200 ms

DFOV display field of view; *SFOV* scan field of view

▪ Table 10d.6 Recommended kV and mA values with the 750HD CT scanner

Acquisition mode	Helical[a]		Axial	
	Tube current	Tube voltage	Tube current	Tube voltage
BMI <20	150–400 mA	80–100 kV	400 mA	80–100 Kv
BMI 20–≤25	150–500 mA	100 Kv	500 mA	100 Kv
BMI 25–29	150–750	100 Kv	750 mA	100 Kv
BMI >29	150–625 mA	120–140 Kv	625 mA	120–140 Kv

[a] Using tube current modulation

▪ Fig. 10d.11 Choosing the cardiac scan type and the high-resolution option, the user can select the "HD Std" kernel or the "HD Detail" kernel. HD Detail allows having higher spatial resolution but is also noisier than HD Std and may thus be best suited for stent analysis and heavily calcified vessels

10d.5.3 Adaptive Gating and ECG Editor

One of the most important features of HD CT is the adaptive gating system in the SnapShot Pulse mode. When this prospectively gated acquisition mode is used, the scanner is able to stop and skip a premature heartbeat and wait for the next normal cardiac cycle to acquire data. Before scanning in the SnapShot Pulse mode, the operator can choose the maximum number of extrasystoles to be skipped during acquisition. In the cardiac retro recon, the HD scanner provides an ECG editor (**Fig. 10d.12**), which allows manipulating the position of the reconstruction window within the cardiac cycle in case of premature contractions. Typical images obtained using this scanner and reconstruction are shown in **Fig. 10d.13**.

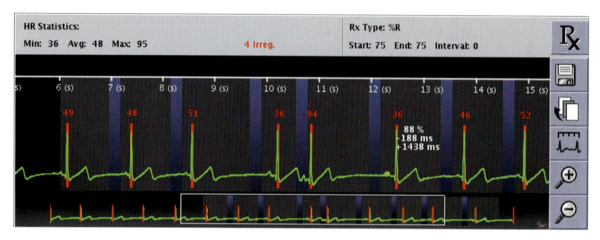

Fig. 10d.12 The ECG editor allows one to move the reconstruction window along the cardiac cycle to reduce artifacts and is available in both retrospective helical and prospective (pulse) acquisitions. In the pulse mode, the width of padding somewhat limits the range through which the reconstruction window can be moved. The position of the recon window can be adjusted by dragging the corresponding R peak (*red line*)

10d

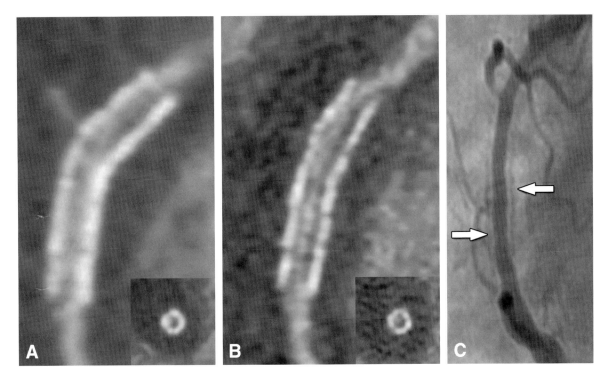

■ **Fig. 10d.13** Typical images obtained with the *Discovery CT750 HD in a* 50-year-old male patient for stent patency evaluation. **Panel A** shows a curved multiplanar reformation of the inital examination with the Lightspeed VCT XT (cross-section, *inset*); after 7 months the study was repeated on the Discovery CT 750 HD (**Panel B**). With depiction of intimal hyperplasia without significant stenosis. Conventional coronary angiography confirmed the presence of intimal hyperplasia (*arrows* in **Panel C**). Image courtesy of J.-L. Sablayrolles, Paris

Reading and Reporting

L.J.M. Kroft and M. Dewey

Abstract

In this chapter, we describe how to read and report cardiac CT angiography studies.

11.1 Reading

11.1.1 Selecting Cardiac Phases

With current prospective electrocardiogram (ECG) gating techniques ("step-and-shoot") that substantially reduce patient dose, image acquisition is performed during a limited portion of the RR interval. Depending on the acquisition interval width (e.g., 70–80%, or 30–80%), "padding" for image reconstruction can be performed within the acquired range. It is important to select the phase(s) with the sharpest coronary artery depiction to maximize the number of coronary segments rendered without motion artifacts. If acquisition is restricted to the smallest acquisition interval possible for image reconstruction (e.g., center of the phase predefined at diastole at 75% of the RR interval for slow heart rates below 60 beats per minute), padding is not possible and image reconstruction can be performed at the predefined 75% phase only. With acquisition at a wider interval during the cardiac cycle, the best phase can be manually selected by visual inspection of different reconstructions from the acquired interval. Another approach that has recently become available is motion mapping, which automatically identifies the phases with the least overall motion (**Fig. 11.1**). Various automatic phase selection software tools are now available for use in clinical practice. If the phases reconstructed using any of these methods are not sufficient for making a reliable diagnosis, further reconstructions (e.g., from the 10 reconstructions rendered at 10% intervals throughout the RR interval) may be reviewed, although this requires acquisition of the full cardiac cycle (**Fig. 11.2**).

However, even after all the desired phases are reviewed, a coronary artery segment may occasionally still prove to be of nondiagnostic quality, e.g., because of artifacts resulting from very high or irregular heart rates or patient movement.

If a stenosis is seen in any phase, this finding should be confirmed by excluding motion artifacts. This confirmation can be accomplished in two ways: (1) by correlating the results with those for the same coronary segment in another phase, and/or (2) by reviewing the axial images in lung window settings in order to detect potential motion in the image (e.g., at the heart–lung border).

M. Dewey, *Cardiac CT*,
DOI: 10.1007/978-3-642-14022-8_14, © Springer-Verlag Berlin Heidelberg 2011

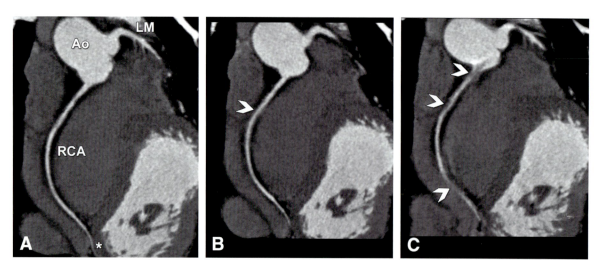

Fig. 11.1 Improved depiction of the right coronary artery (RCA) on curved multiplanar reformations using motion mapping with automatic identification of the phase with least motion during mid-diastole (**Panel A**), when compared with standard reconstructions centered at 70% (**Panel B**) and 80% (**Panel C**) of the cardiac cycle, which show minimal (**Panel B**) and more severe (**Panel C**) motion artifacts (*arrowheads*). Note the excellent visualization of the distal vessel segment with automatic phase selection (*asterisk* in **Panel A**). *Ao* aorta; *LM* left main coronary artery

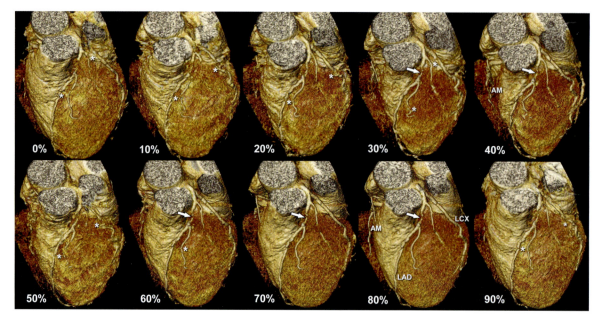

Fig. 11.2 Three-dimensional volume-rendered reconstructions of the coronary arteries (left anterosuperior views) shown for 10 image reconstruction intervals throughout the entire cardiac cycle (centered at 0–90%). There is a significant stenosis (*arrow*) of the proximal left anterior descending coronary artery (LAD), which is best seen at 70% and 80% but also at 40%. In comparison, however, the left circumflex coronary artery (LCX) is best seen at 70% and 80%. There are multiple motion artifacts in the other reconstruction intervals (marked with *asterisks*), rendering these phases nondiagnostic (artifacts were identified using the axial source images). Interestingly, the right coronary artery with its acute marginal (AM) branch is well depicted during mid-diastole (80%) as well as end-systole (40%). In many cases, the right coronary artery is best seen at end-systole (especially at higher heart rates)

If no stenoses are seen and image quality is good, it is not necessary to go through all the reconstructed coronary artery phases. The comprehensive assessment of a cardiac CT study on a workstation takes time and concentration.

11.1.2   Systematic Approach

The review of a cardiac CT data set focuses on the coronary arteries but should also comprise assessment for other cardiac findings and extracardiac findings. As in all radiological examinations, a systematic approach is pivotal to a comprehensive evaluation of all anatomical regions (**List 11.1**). Easy evaluation of the coronary arteries is now possible by reading (semi)automatic curved multiplanar reformations, which are crucial for

---

List 11.1. Systematic approach to reading cardiac CT studies[a]

1. Obtain a quick overview of the gross anatomy, e.g., by looking at three-dimensional renderings
2. Assess the individual coronary arteries and major side-branches by using reconstruction tools and viewing original slices, preferably simultaneously[b]
3. Evaluate the cardiac extracoronary structures[c]
4. Evaluate extracardiac organs[d]

---

[a] The approach may vary with the workstation used.

[b] Double-oblique orthogonal reconstructions, thin-slab maximum-intensity projections, and curved multiplanar reformation are very helpful displays for evaluating the major coronary arteries and their large side-branches. Any pathology detected on such advanced reconstructions should be confirmed on original axial, coronal, or sagittal slices.

[c] This includes the cardiac valves, the myocardium, the atrial, and ventricular cavities (e.g., for presence of intracavitary thrombus), evaluation of (left) ventricular function, the pericardium, and the aortic root.

[d] This includes assessment of all organs other than the heart and has to be performed on large fields of view. Evaluate the large vessels (e.g., the aorta for dissection or aneurysm and the pulmonary arteries for presence of emboli), mediastinum, hila, lungs, chest wall and breasts, abdominal organs, and bones.

---

detecting pathology. However, the findings should always be confirmed on the original slices in axial and/or orthogonal orientations. Reading is improved when curved multiplanar reconstructions, double-oblique reconstructions, and source images can be evaluated simultaneously. Thin-slab (3–5 mm) maximum-intensity projections are usually very helpful in evaluating the continuity of the coronary arteries.

Among patients with suspected coronary artery disease, only 5% have obstructive ($\geq$50% diameter reduction) stenoses in distal segments or minor side branches without a more proximal stenosis (**Fig. 11.3**). Thus, major branches and side branches as well as bifurcations are first places to look when searching for significant stenoses. Prestenotic dilatation of the vessel lumen is an interesting indirect indicator of a significant stenosis located distally, and its recognition is critical. Furthermore, aneurysms of the coronary arteries are present in 5% of patients with atherosclerotic coronary artery disease but can also be present in patients without significant stenoses (**Fig. 11.4**).

If images look very poor on every reconstruction despite adequate contrast and compliance of the patient during the examination, one should inspect the recorded ECG tracing for irregularities, such as premature ventricular contraction, extrasystoles, or atrial fibrillation, or search for postprocessing errors by looking at the phases selected for image reconstruction. Using ECG editing, image degradation due to ECG irregularities can often be overcome by deleting or adding R waves for triggering and rereconstructing image data without scanning the patient again (**Fig. 11.5**).

11.1.3   Source Images

Reading cardiac CT datasets requires knowledge of coronary and cardiac anatomy (Chap. 3). The axial source images represent the basic reconstructions that contain all information available in the three-dimensional dataset. Conclusions and final diagnoses should always be based on standard slices in the axial and orthogonal planes (which is possible because of isotropic voxel size in CT). Scrolling through the slices back and forth on a workstation is the best way to look at the source images. Additional information can be obtained from thin-slab maximum-intensity projections (see below) and double-oblique positioning of slices along or orthogonal to lesions.

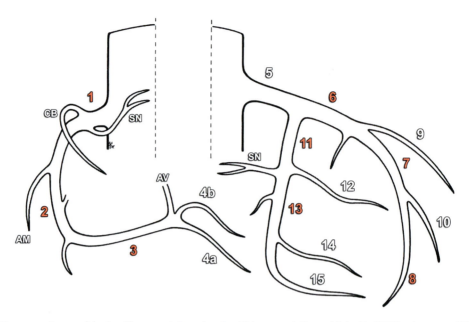

Fig. 11.3 Coronary artery model using 17 segments based on the AHA segmentation published in 1975 by Austen et al. The segments which account for more than 5% of percutaneous coronary interventions each and are thus of major relevance in reading cardiac CT have pink numbers (1–3, 6–8, 11, and 13). The left main coronary artery (segment 5) is also of great relevance and in about 3% of cases obstructive stenoses are found here; they are mainly treated with bypass grafting (about two thirds of cases) and less commonly with percutaneous coronary intervention. It is important to note that it is very rare to detect an isolated distal obstructive (≥50%) stenosis without a significant proximal lesion in a patient. Nevertheless, also side branches and distal segments (as small as 2 mm in diameter) need to be searched for significant stenoses that might be amenable to treatment. Bifurcations are other important sites to look for stenoses when ruling out coronary artery disease. The right coronary artery consists of 5 segments (1–4a/b), with the distal segment (4) being further subdivided into 4a (posterior descending artery, PDA) and 4b (right posterolateral branch) in right-dominant circulation. The left anterior descending coronary artery consists of segments 6–10, with the two diagonal branches being segments 9 and 10. The left circumflex coronary artery consists of segments 11–15, with the two (obtuse) marginal branches being segments 12 and 14. In case of right-coronary dominance, at least one right posterolateral branch (segment 4b) is present and supplies the inferolateral myocardial segments. If the left coronary artery is dominant, the distal left circumflex ends as the posterior descending coronary artery (segment 4a). In case of codominance, segment 4a is part of the right coronary, and the distal left circumflex ends as a posterolateral branch (4b) after giving off two marginal branches. *AM* acute marginal branch; *AV* atrioventricular node branch; *CB* conus branch; *SN* sinus node artery. Modified from Austen et al. Circulation 1975

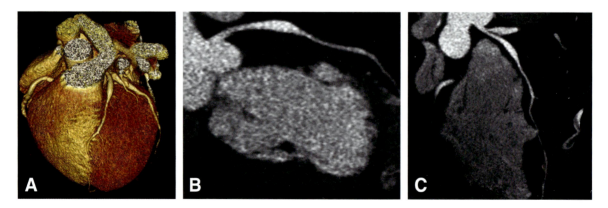

Fig. 11.4 Dilation without significant coronary stenosis. Volume-rendered image (**Panel A**) and multiplanar reconstructions (**Panels B** and **C**) of the left anterior descending coronary artery in a 47-year-old male with atypical chest pain. The patient had no coronary artery stenoses but did have dilating coronary artery disease. Note the dilation in the proximal left descending coronary artery. There is some focal myocardial bridging, and the right and left circumflex coronary arteries were also dilated (not shown)

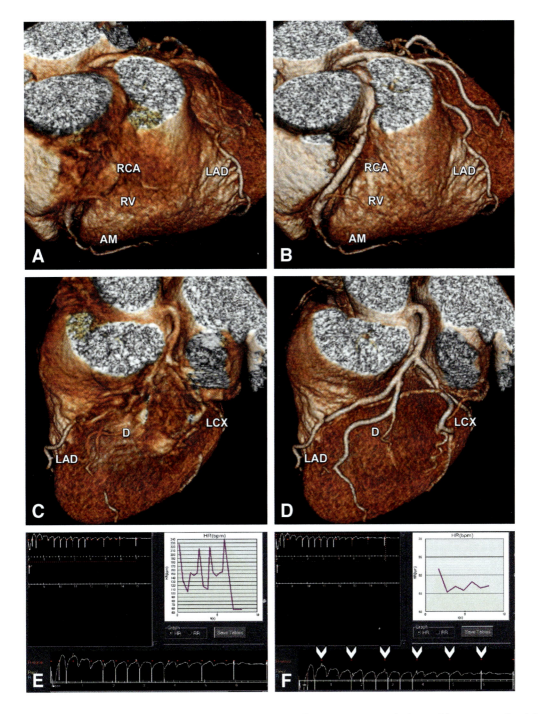

◻ Fig. 11.5 Use of ECG editing significantly improves the image quality of reconstructions on the basis of the same raw data (without rescanning the patient). The left side (**Panels A**, **C**, and **E**) shows the results before editing, and the right side (**Panels B** and **D**) the three-dimensional reconstructions obtained after ECG editing. The entire course of the coronary arteries is blurred before ECG editing because of extrasystoles during scanning (**Panel E**, differentiating supraventricular and ventricular extrasystoles was not possible using this data and Holter ECG was recommended). Excluding the arrhythmic peaks and using only the typical R-wave peaks for editing (*arrowheads* in **Panel F**) greatly improves the images of both the right (**Panel B**) and the left (**Panel D**) coronary artery system. The right-hand corner *insets* in **Panels E** and **F** show the unedited and edited heart rate courses over time that were used for image reconstruction. *AM* acute marginal artery; *D* diagonal branch; *LAD* left anterior descending coronary artery; *LCX* left circumflex coronary artery; *RCA* right coronary artery; *RV* right ventricular branch

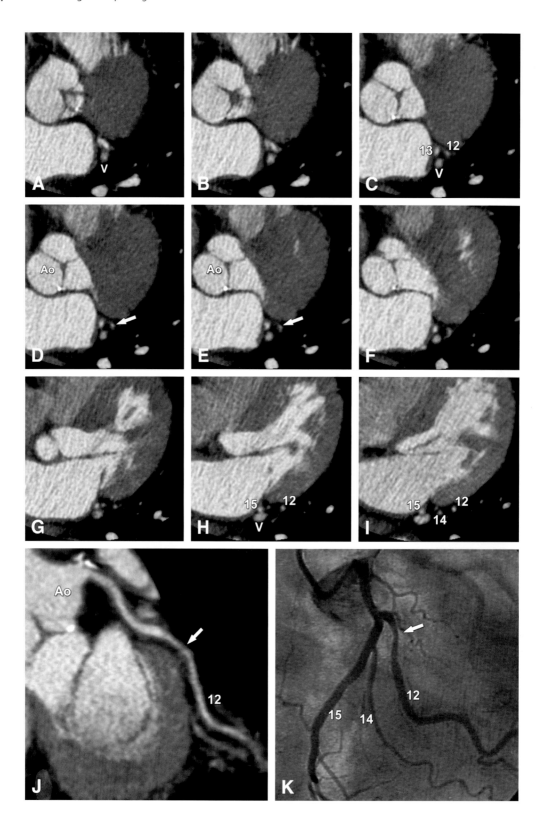

Compared with the source images, all other reconstructions such as curved reformations, maximum-intensity projections, angiographic emulations, and volume rendering (**List 11.2**) tend to reduce the information content and may even obscure relevant information. The main advantage of these reconstructions, which can be prepared by the technician, is that they make evaluation of the coronary arteries much easier because large vessel segments are displayed in a single image. This wide view can be beneficial in detecting abnormalities such as short coronary stenoses or wall irregularities (**Fig. 11.6**). Also, reconstructed images can be useful for demonstrating results during multidisciplinary team meetings. Printouts showing the reconstructed coronary arteries can be sent to the referring physicians as summaries of image findings and images stored in the picture archiving and communication system can be used for demonstration in interdisciplinary conferences.

11.1.4 Curved Multiplanar Reformations

Curved multiplanar reformations are generated using a centerline along the coronary vessel path and show large parts of the coronary vessel lumen in a single image (**Figs. 11.6** and **11.7**). Depending on the workstation used, the curved multiplanar reformations may be rotated around their centerlines, thereby rotating the

coronary artery lumen around its longitudinal axis and greatly improving the visual estimation of the severity of the stenosis. The curved multiplanar reformations also allow rendering cross-sectional images orthogonal to the vessel course, which further facilitates the quantification of the percent diameter stenosis (based on reference and stenosis diameters, **Fig. 11.8**).

Continuously improving automatic vessel detection and segmentation tools are available for the creation of curved multiplanar reformations. These automatic software tools are currently available on all competitive workstations and allow diagnostic accuracy to be maintained while relevantly reducing analysis time. When using one of the currently available reconstruction tools, however, the user must be aware of two limitations of automatic segmentation that can lead to false-positive or false-negative lesions: First, the automatic vessel probing tools do not always entirely follow the course of the coronary vessels (especially if these are very tortuous). The resulting images may suggest stenoses on the curved multiplanar reformations that are, however, usually readily identified as artifacts (**Fig. 11.9**). The centerline should be checked (e.g., on three-dimensional renderings) when stenoses are suggested (**Fig. 11.9**), and the findings should be confirmed on the original images. The second common limitation of automatic vessel detection is that the most proximal segment of the coronary artery may not be completely probed. Significant proximal stenosis can thus be missed if one looks only at the automatically probed vessel segments. However, this limitation is also easily overcome by manually or automatically adding the vessel portions that have been missed by the automatic tool (**Fig. 11.10**). Fully automated computer-aided diagnosis systems for coronary CT angiography have become available recently (**Fig. 11.11**). These are currently being validated for clinical use and may have the potential to be used as a second reader to increase sensitivity, especially when a less experienced reader is interpreting the scan.

In addition to motion artifacts resulting from a rapid or irregular heartbeat, heavily calcified coronary segments pose the greatest challenge because they obscure the coronary artery lumen (**Fig. 11.12**). Heavily calcified segments may not be evaluable, although severe calcifications do not per se exclude evaluation. In this situation,

◘ Fig. 11.6 Short coronary artery stenosis of the first obtuse marginal artery (segment 12) that might be missed on axial images (**Panels A–I**), which show the stenosis on only two consecutive slices (*arrow* in **Panels D** and **E**). In contrast, this 75% diameter stenosis (as measured on quantitative coronary angiography) is easily detected on a curved multiplanar reformation (*arrow* on **Panel J**), demonstrating the advantage of such reconstructions along the vessel course. There is good agreement of the CT finding with conventional coronary angiography (**Panel K**). *V* cardiac vein

11

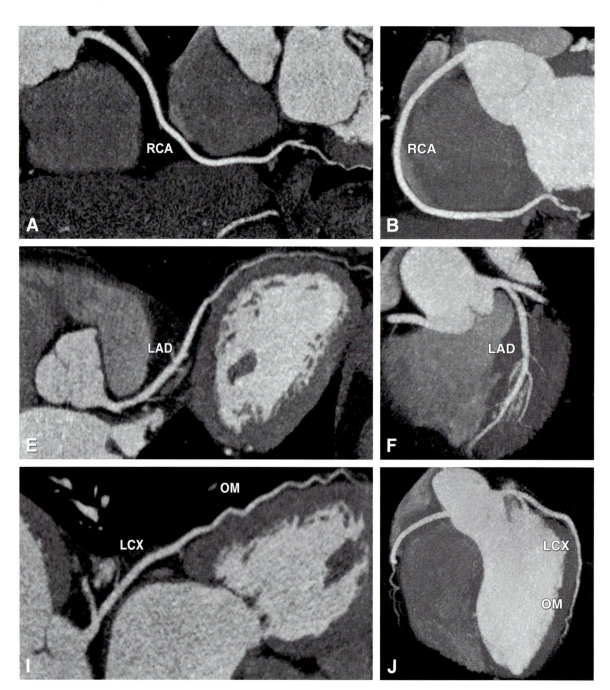

□ **Fig. 11.7** Normal coronary arteries as seen on curved multiplanar reformations (*first column*), maximum-intensity projections(*second column*), and three-dimensional volume-rendered reconstructions (*third column*) of multislice CT using 64 simultaneous detector rows. There is good correlation with conventional coronary angiography (*last column*). The results are shown separately for the right coronary artery (RCA, **Panels A–D**), left anterior descending coronary artery (LAD, **Panels E–H**), and left circumflex coronary artery (LCX, **Panels I–L**). Curved multiplanar reformations allow estimation of the percent diameter stenosis from two perpendicular directions along the long axis or from orthogonal cross-sections and also the detection of coronary artery plaques, with evaluation of their composition. Maximum-intensity projections give a nice overview of the entire vessel but may obscure stenoses because of their projectional nature. Three-dimensional reconstructions provide an overview of long segments of the coronary arteries but should not be used for reading cases. Please note that there is right coronary artery dominance in this patient, with the right coronary giving off the posterior descending artery (PDA), as well as a large right posterolateral artery (RPL, inferior view of the heart in the *inset* in **Panel C**). *OM* obtuse marginal artery

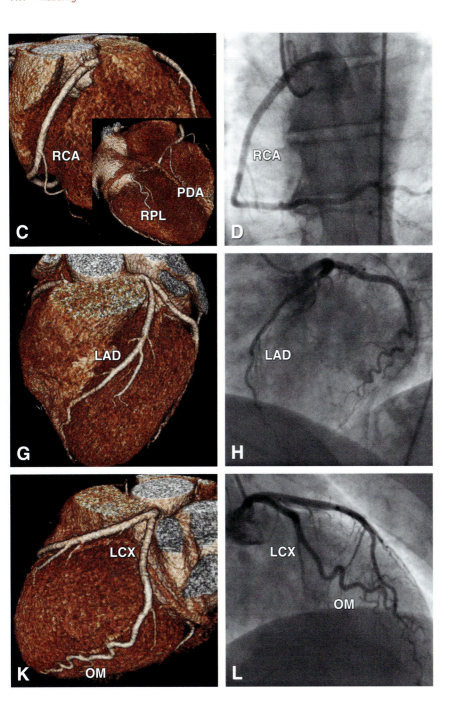

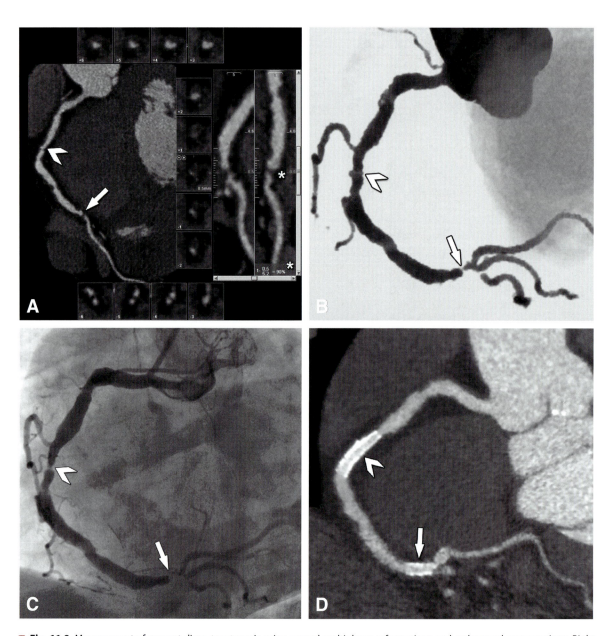

Fig. 11.8 Measurement of percent diameter stenosis using curved multiplanar reformations and orthogonal cross-sections. Right coronary artery with a high-grade stenosis at the crux cordis (*arrow* and *asterisk* in the perpendicular longitudinal views in **Panel A**). The reference vessel diameter is measured proximal and distal to the lesion, and the stenosis diameter is measured within the lesion on orthogonal cross-sections (*squared insets* in **Panel A**). From these measurements (automatic or by caliper) the percent diameter stenosis (in this case 90%) is calculated (*asterisk* in **Panel A**). There is good correlation with angiographic emulation of CT (**Panel B**) and conventional coronary angiography (**Panel C**) regarding this high-grade coronary artery stenosis. A second stenosis is present in segment 2 of the right coronary artery, which was calculated to be a 75% diameter stenosis on quantitative analysis (*arrowhead* in **Panels A–C**). Both stenoses were treated with stent placement and there was no significant in-stent restenosis on a cath view reconstruction of the follow-up CT (**Panel D**)

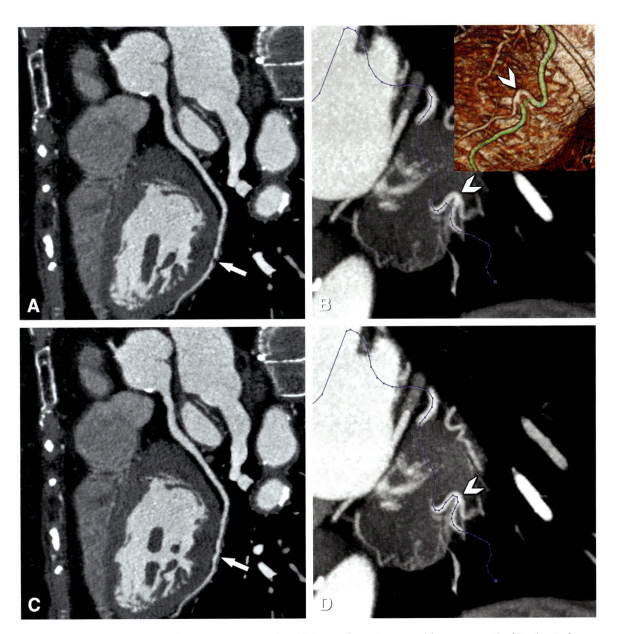

◘ Fig. 11.9 Coronary artery pseudostenosis on a curved multiplanar reformation, caused by an automatic detection tool error. Pseudostenosis on the curved multiplanar reformation along the left circumflex coronary artery (*arrow* in **Panel A**) is caused by a short-track route of the automatic probing tool. This error in vessel tracking (*arrowhead*) is easily recognized on a maximum-intensity projection (*blue centerline* in **Panel B**) and in the *green centerline* on a three-dimensional reconstruction (*inset* in **Panel B**). After manual correction of the centerline (*arrowhead* in **Panel D**) the curved multiplanar reformation shows the actual course of the left circumflex coronary artery, which is unremarkable and continuous (**Panel C**)

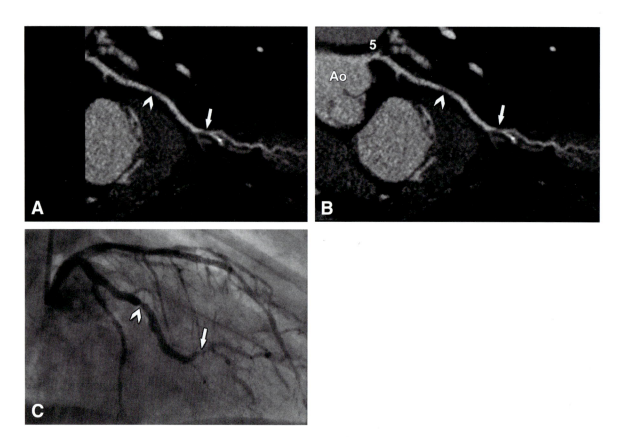

▪ **Fig. 11.10** The proximal vessel segment is sometimes missed by the automatic probing tool. Using such a curved reformation (**Panel A**), proximal stenoses cannot be excluded and, as illustrated here, manual extension of the *centerline* to the aorta (Ao) is necessary to visualize the entire vessel (**Panel B**) including segment 5 (left main coronary artery). There is a nonsignificant (*arrowhead*, 40%) and a significant stenosis in the first obtuse marginal branch (*arrow*, 70%), with good correlation with conventional coronary angiography (**Panel C**)

▪ **Fig. 11.12** Severe coronary calcifications can hamper the interpretation of CT coronary angiography. In this 82-year-old male patient, there are severely calcified plaques (*asterisks*) along the major course of the right coronary artery (**Panel A**) and left anterior descending coronary artery (**Panel B**). The resulting blooming artifacts obscure the coronary artery lumen, rendering the affected coronary artery segments nondiagnostic. These calcifications were found to cause only short significant stenoses (*asterisk*) in conventional coronary angiography (**Panel D–E**). There are additional less-pronounced calcifications in the left circumflex coronary artery (*arrow* in **Panel C**), but these likewise preclude a definitive diagnosis regarding the presence of significant coronary artery stenosis. Conventional coronary angiography shows moderate stenosis of the left circumflex coronary artery (**Panel F**). Using stent kernels for severely calcified lesions might help to reduce the artifacts, although this approach results in higher noise levels that may also hamper evaluation. Specific window-level settings might be an option for analysis of both calcified and noncalcified plaques (**Fig. 11.13**). Note that there is also a short ostial stenosis of the right coronary artery (*arrow* in **Panels A** and **D**). *Ao* aorta

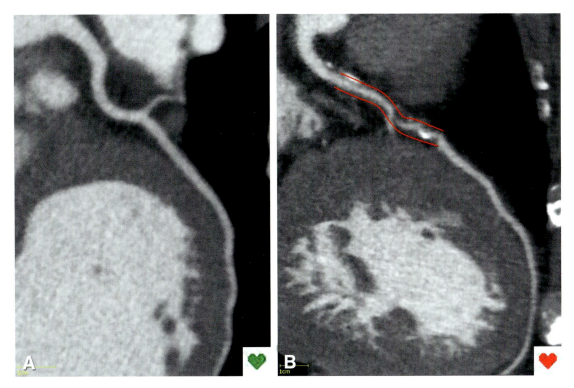

Fig. 11.11 Fully automated computed-aided diagnosis system for coronary CT angiography. This software (RCADIA, Cor Analyzer) allows automatic identification of patients without stenosis (**Panel A**) and with coronary stenosis (**Panel B**), who are indicated by green and red heart icons (*inset*), respectively

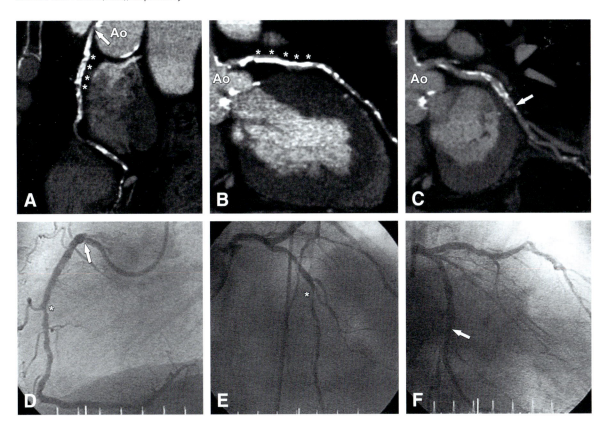

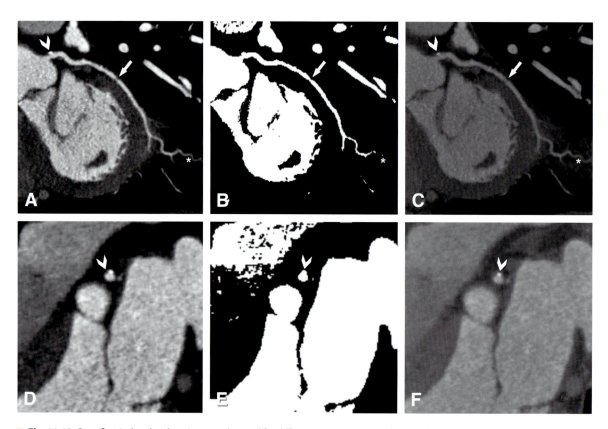

▫ **Fig. 11.13** Specific window-level settings may be used for different coronary artery plaques. The *upper row* presents curved multiplanar reformations along the left circumflex coronary artery, and the *lower row* presents cross-sections orthogonal to the left main coronary artery (as indicated by the direction of the *arrowhead* in **Panel A**). Noncalcified coronary plaques and outer vessel boundaries are best visualized using a window representing 155% of the mean density within the coronary lumen and a level representing 65% of the mean density within the lumen as described by Leber et al. (Chap. 14). (**Panels A** and **D**; this is very commonly equal to 600–700/250–300 HU settings). The noncalcified plaque in the left main coronary artery is nicely seen on the cross-section in **Panel D** (*arrowhead*), and distal vessel segments are depicted on the curved multiplanar reformation using these settings (*asterisk* in **Panel A**). Optimal measurement of the coronary lumen, however, is obtained by keeping the level constant at 65% of the mean lumen density while reducing the window width to 1 (**Panels B** and **E**). Using these settings yields the most accurate measurement of the diameter stenosis in comparison to intravascular ultrasound (in this case 55% diameter reduction) as recently shown by Leber et al. The drawbacks of these settings include the fact that distal vessel segments are not seen as well (*asterisk* in **Panel B**), and calcified plaques are no longer discernible from the lumen (*arrowhead* in **Panel E**). Using more bone-window-like settings (e.g., 1,300/300 HU here), as shown in the last column, reduces the artifacts caused by calcifications and results in less overestimation of calcified coronary plaques than when standard settings are used (*arrowhead* in **Panels C** and **F**)

visualization of coronary stenoses can be improved by using specific window-level settings (**Fig. 11.13**).

11.1.5 Maximum-Intensity Projections

Maximum-intensity projections can be varied in projection thickness and give a nice overview of vessel continuity and course in a single image (**Fig. 11.7**). In particular, thin-slab maximum-intensity projections (3–5 mm) are very useful for quickly depicting coronary artery disease. By scrolling through a dataset of thin-slab maximum-intensity projections (e.g., of axial source images), side branches are easily visualized and more side-branches can be recognized than on three-dimensional reconstructions. However, low-grade stenoses

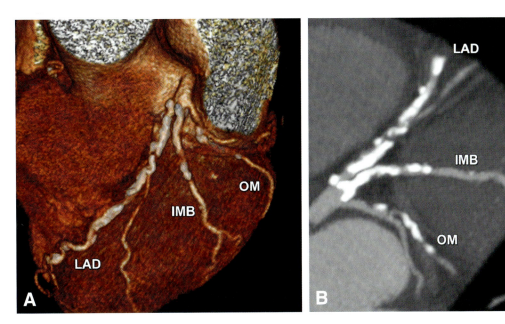

Fig. 11.14 Three-dimensional reconstructions (**Panel A**) and maximum-intensity projections (**Panel B**) do not allow the assessment of severely calcified coronary artery plaques, as shown here in the left anterior descending (LAD), intermediate branch (IMB), and obtuse marginal branch (OM). Because of the projectional nature of maximum-intensity projections, calcified plaques can even be overemphasized (i.e., blooming; **Panel B**). Such blooming artifacts are less pronounced on curved multiplanar reformations and standard two-dimensional images with bone-window-type settings (**Fig. 11.13**). In this patient, conventional coronary angiography revealed significant stenoses in all three vessels

may be overlooked. The main drawback of reading maximum-intensity projections is that heavily calcified stenoses present with exaggerated blooming artifacts (**Fig. 11.14**).

11.1.6 Volume Rendering and Angiographic Emulation

Volume-rendered and angiographic three-dimensional reconstructions are elegant methods for the display and presentation of findings (**Figs. 11.2, 11.5, 11.7, 11.8,** and **11.15**) to referring physicians, patients, and colleagues during interdisciplinary meetings (Chap. 19). Interestingly enough, referring physicians have been reported to prefer angiographic emulations to standard curved multiplanar reformations, while simultaneously identifying the limited visibility and assessability of coronary plaques on these images as a main drawback. Coronary interventionalists may also prefer angiographic emulations of CT data, since they are used to viewing coronary arteries in predefined angiographic projections. Angiographic emulations look much like the interventional

angiographic images, and if the desired angled projections are generated, these images may serve as improved anatomic roadmaps for guiding interventions. Making a diagnosis using only three-dimensional reconstructions is not recommended because of the abovementioned limitations.

11.1.7 Typical Artifacts

It is necessary to understand the technical limitations of CT that affect image quality in coronary angiography. The recognition of artifacts that can simulate coronary artery stenoses is particularly critical. The most important artifacts encountered in cardiac CT are summarized in **List 11.3**.

List 11.3. The most important artifacts in cardiac CT

1. Blooming artifacts caused by calcifications
2. Motion artifacts causing blurring
3. Low-contrast artifacts

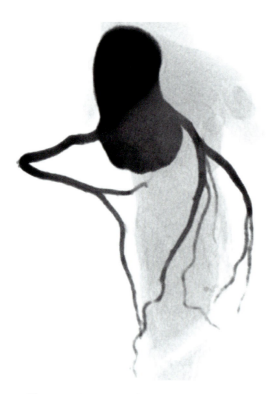

◘ Fig. 11.15 An angiographic emulation of the entire coronary artery tree shows no significant stenoses. The advantage of this type of reconstruction is the striking similarity to conventional angiography, which helps interventionalists rapidly grasp the type and location of coronary lesions before performing invasive procedures. The drawback is that only the lumen and not the underlying plaque is seen on these images (**Fig. 11.8**)

Artifacts have major implications for cardiac CT. Although spatial and temporal resolution has been greatly improved with 64-row CT scanners when compared with earlier scanners, artifacts are still a major problem. Such artifacts, which generally result from inappropriate motion, can preclude the evaluation of parts of the coronary arteries, as is still the case in 3–12% of coronary artery segments imaged by 64-row CT scanners. Moreover, artifacts are the main cause of false-positive and false-negative diagnoses regarding the presence of coronary artery stenosis, with misinterpretation being generally attributable to the presence of coronary artery calcifications (**Figs. 11.12** and **11.14**). Other important causes of misinterpretation are motion artifacts and poor contrast-to-noise ratio in obese patients.

Nearly all artifacts in CT are caused by limitations related to spatial resolution, temporal resolution, noise, and the reconstruction algorithms used. Artifacts cause blurring, blooming, streaks, missing data, discontinuities, and poor contrast enhancement.

Spatial resolution is the ability to visualize small structures in the scanned volume and is considered in three dimensions. Important parameters of spatial resolution are voxel size and geometric unsharpness. In the *x-y* plane, a pixel size of 0.35×0.35 mm^2 can be obtained with a reconstructed field of view of 180 mm and a 512^2 pixel matrix. The greatest improvement introduced by the current generation scanners is that volumes with smaller section thickness in the *Z*-axis can be obtained. With 64-row CT, 64×0.6 mm or 64×0.5 mm collimations are achieved. Geometric unsharpness depends on factors such as focal spot size, detector size, and scanner geometry. Limitations in spatial resolution cause partial volume artifacts as a result of the attenuation coefficient in voxels that are heterogeneous in composition. Resulting artifacts include blooming and blurring, especially in the presence of calcifications (**Figs. 11.12** and **11.14**).

Temporal resolution is the ability to resolve rapidly moving objects and is strongly related to coronary artery size and motion. With the ECG-synchronized scanning techniques and rapid rotation times available today, it is possible to obtain "frozen" images by using half-scan or adaptive multisegment reconstruction at the cardiac phase with the least motion. If the cardiac rest phase is shorter than the scanner's image reconstruction window, motion artifacts occur, but images usually still have adequate diagnostic quality if the artifacts are slight (**Fig. 11.1**). Depending on the heart rate, image quality is generally best in diastole or at late systole (**Fig. 11.2**). Overall, image quality is better in patients with low and stable heart rates. For this reason, beta blocker administration is recommended to lower and stabilize the heart rate. For heart rates <65 beats per min, image quality is usually best at mid-diastole, whereas for heart rates >75 beats per min, the best image quality shifts to systole. At low heart rate, a single time-phase reconstruction is usually enough to visualize all the coronary artery segments with diagnostic quality. At high heart rates, additional reconstructions may be necessary. In conclusion, limitations in temporal resolution cause blurring that may hamper the coronary artery evaluation. The smaller the coronary artery size the greater the effect of motion on the diagnostic image quality.

Respiratory motion can seriously degrade the image quality (**Fig. 11.16**). With scan times of 8–12 s on current 64-row CT scanners, patients are usually able to hold their breath during scanning.

Image noise is mainly dependent on the number of photons used to make the image. Large chest sizes result in higher image noise, which can be reduced by adjusting the dose settings (kV, mA) to account for the patient's size (Chaps. 9 and 10). Contrast is improved by using iodinated contrast agents. Other influencing factors are the kV setting used and whether patients are adequately instructed on how to hold their breath. (The Valsalva maneuver should be avoided because it impairs contrast agent flow to the heart.) At the workstation, window-level settings can optimize image contrast. Artifacts caused by noise and contrast-to-noise limitations result in poor overall image quality (high noise-level images) and images with low contrast (**Fig. 11.17**).

Reconstruction algorithms also cause artifacts. Spiral acquisition may cause geometric distortion, resulting in dark shadows near the coronary arteries that should not be confused with noncalcified plaques (**Fig. 11.18**).

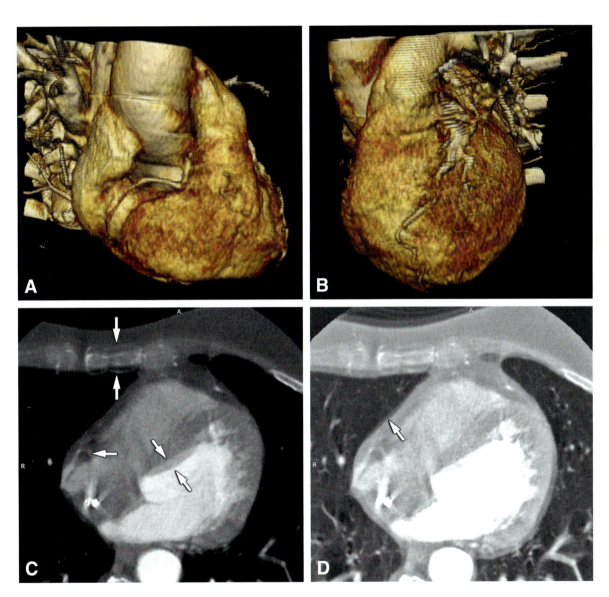

◻ **Fig. 11.16** Severe respiratory motion artifacts. Volume-rendered images (**Panels A** and **B**) and axial source images using soft tissue setting (**Panel C**) and lung window-level setting (**Panel D**) in a 46-year-old female patient who panicked during contrast agent injection and was then unable to hold her breath during scanning. The right coronary artery (**Panel A**) and left coronary artery (**Panel B**) were not evaluable. Note the motion visible in the area of the sternum, right coronary artery, and interventricular septum (*arrows* in **Panel C**). Breathing is also clearly indicated by blurring of the vascular structures and cardiac double contour in the lung setting (*arrow* in **Panel D**). Note that the coronary arteries are not well visualized (**Panels A–C**). The movement of body structures due to breathing resulted in a nondiagnostic scan

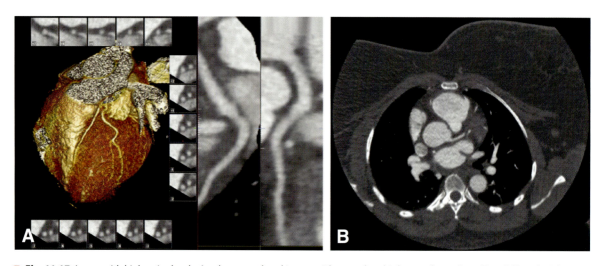

Fig. 11.17 Issues with high noise levels. A volume-rendered image with curved multiplanar reformations (**Panel A**) and axial source images using soft tissue setting (**Panel B**) in a 65-year-old very obese female patient. The image is noisy and of moderate quality despite the use of higher kV and mA settings (135 kV and 350 mA) to increase the radiation dose. Only the proximal parts of the coronary arteries can be evaluated well. Compare the image quality in **Panel A** with that of other figures (e.g., **Fig. 11.7**). Small side-branches are not visible in this overweight patient

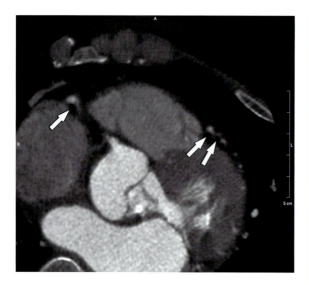

Fig. 11.18 Artifacts resulting from coronary artery motion and geometric distortion appear as *dark spots* adjacent to the right coronary artery and the left anterior descending coronary artery, including its diagonal branches (*arrows*). These artifacts should not be confused with noncalcified coronary artery plaques

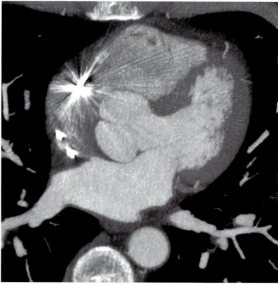

Fig. 11.19 Beam-hardening artifacts in a patient with a pacemaker lead (metal artifact) obscuring the right coronary artery. The patient had no coronary artery stenosis. Note the dilated aortic root with a maximum size of 4.7 cm

Other artifacts related to limitations in reconstruction algorithms are beam-hardening artifacts (e.g., resulting from high-density contrast agent injection) causing dark bands, as well as metal objects causing complex artifacts, including beam-hardening and partial-volume artifacts (**Fig. 11.19**). Fully automated reconstruction tools used during postprocessing can also result in image artifacts (**Figs. 11.9** and **11.10**). An irregular heart rate during scanning, such as that resulting from premature atrial contraction, can lead to erroneous phase selection during that abnormal heartbeat, which may cause blurring or even pseudostenosis (**Fig. 11.20**). We recommend

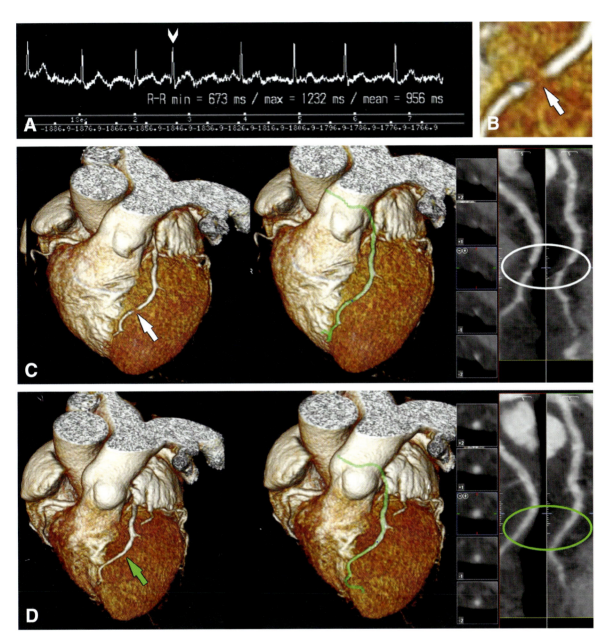

Fig. 11.20 Artifacts caused by irregular heart rate during scanning. CT coronary angiography in a 73-year-old female patient with suspected acute coronary artery syndrome. Premature atrial contraction after the third R-peak (*arrowhead*), followed by a compensatory long pause before the next R-peak (**Panel A**). Automatic reconstruction centered at 75% of the RR interval was performed with subopti-mal time points relative to the R-peaks at the location of the short RR interval, giving rise to a coronary artery pseudostenosis (*arrow* in **Panels B** and **C**). Reconstruction at an optimal time point (ECG editing) resulted in normal image quality and elimination of the pseudo-stenosis (*green arrow* and *circle* in **Panel D**)

checking the ECG during image interpretation to recognize heart rate irregularities that may cause these types of artifacts, which can be eliminated by manual ECG editing (**Figs. 11.5** and **11.20**). If pathology such as coronary artery stenosis is identified on postprocessed images, the findings should always be confirmed by reviewing the original data set (axial and/or orthogonal source images).

11.1.8   Cardiac Function

In addition to the location and severity of coronary artery stenoses and the presence of diabetes mellitus, left ventricular ejection fraction (above vs. below 50%) is of pivotal importance in determining the most suitable therapy for patients (percutaneous coronary intervention vs. coronary artery bypass grafting, **Fig. 11.21**).

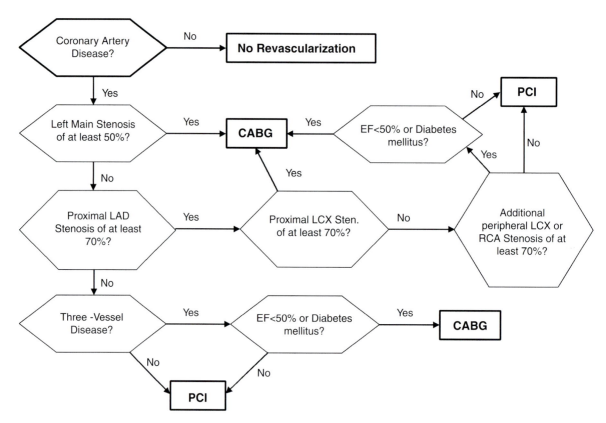

◘ **Fig. 11.21** Flowchart for the management of patients with suspected coronary artery disease, according to current guidelines. Interventional treatment is indicated when the percent diameter stenosis is at least 70%, or 50% for the left main coronary artery. Whether coronary artery bypass grafting (CABG) or percutaneous coronary intervention (PCI) should be performed is influenced by the presence of left main disease or left main equivalents as well as global left ventricular cardiac function (ejection fraction, EF) and the presence or absence of diabetes mellitus. This situation highlights the importance of locating coronary stenoses and assessing left ventricular global cardiac function by CT. The guidelines on which this flowchart is based were established by the American College of Cardiology/American Heart Association for conventional coronary angiography: (1) "For the Management of Patients With Chronic Stable Angina" (Gibbons et al. Circulation 2003), (2) "Update for Coronary Artery Bypass Graft Surgery" (Eagle et al. Circulation 2004), and (3) "For Percutaneous Coronary Intervention" (Smith et al. JACC 2001). Recommendations I and Level of Evidence A and B were included in creating the flowchart. *LAD* left anterior descending coronary artery; *LCX* left circumflex coronary artery; *RCA* right coronary artery. With permission from H. Hoffmann et al. Acad Radiol 2007

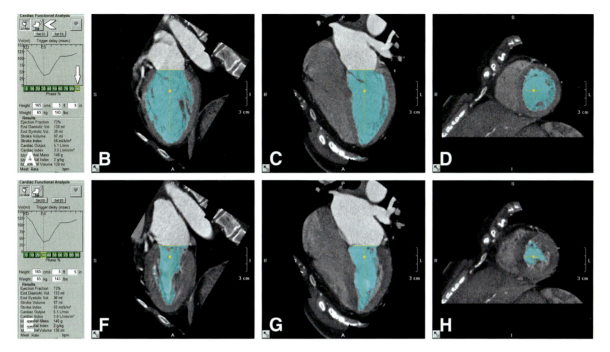

□ **Fig. 11.22** Fully automated cardiac function analysis software (Vitrea, Vital Images). Diastolic frames are shown in the *upper row* (**Panels A–D**) and systolic frames in the *lower row* (**Panels E–H**). This software tool automatically identifies the cardiac axes with the two-chamber (**Panels B and F**) and four-chamber view (**Panels C and G**) as well as the cardiac short axis (**Panels D and H**). The orientation of the left ventricular cardiac axis (marked in *yellow*) and the level at the border of the left atrium and left ventricle can be manually changed. The left ventricular blood pool (excluding the papillary muscles) is also automatically identified and marked in **light blue**. Using the edit function (*arrowhead* in **Panel A**) makes it possible to manually change the automatically defined endo- and epicardial contours in the short-axis views. The end-diastolic time frame is mostly centered around 90% or 0% of the cardiac cycle (**Panel A**, *arrow* at 90%), whereas the end-systolic time frame is mostly at 30% or 40% (**Panel E**). Analysis of 10 image reconstruction intervals serves to calculate a left ventricular volume curve over time (**Panels A and E**). Ejection fraction, end-diastolic and end-systolic volumes, stroke volume, and myocardial mass are calculated automatically (**Panels A and E**). If the patient's weight and height and the heart rate are given, the software will also calculate stroke index, cardiac index, cardiac output, and myocardial index (**Panels A and E**)

Also, left ventricular ejection fraction has been shown to be the most important prognostic factor for cardiac events and death that can be derived from diagnostic testing. Cardiac function analysis may be performed as part of cardiac CT, and preferably with using ECG-triggered dose modulation techniques to limit patient dose (Chap. 15). Automatic or semiautomatic software tools can be used to derive left ventricular volumes and ejection fraction (**Figs. 11.22 and 11.23**). Software tools allow manually changing the contours if the automatically detected contours are not sufficiently accurate. Quantitative analysis of regional cardiac function is facilitated by using bull's eye plots, which are available on many workstations (**Fig. 11.24**). Another convenient approach is to evaluate regional cardiac function by looking at cardiac short-axis and long-axis views in cine mode (using 10 reconstructions throughout the cardiac cycle). The cine mode is sssalso useful for the assessment of cardiac valves (Chap. 16) in different orthogonal or long-axis views (**Figs. 11.25 and 11.26**).

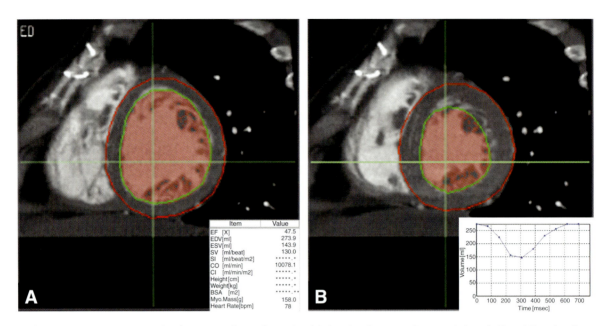

Fig. 11.23 Semiautomatic cardiac function analysis software (Toshiba) with a short-axis slice at end-diastole (**Panel A**) and end-systole (**Panel B**). The *green* and *red contours* in these images represent the automatically generated endo- and epicardial contours, respectively. Note that not all of the area surrounded by the *green line* is assigned to the left ventricular volume, as only pixels with a certain manually adjustable minimum Hounsfield unit density are recognized as part of the blood pool (colored *pink* in the images). In this way, the papillary muscles are excluded from the blood pool. In the *inset* in **Panel A**, the results of global left ventricular function analysis are displayed; the *inset* in **Panel B** shows a volume curve, with end-diastole and end-systole represented by the largest and smallest left ventricular volumes, respectively. This semiautomatic analysis tool, although not optimized for this purpose, is also easier to use for right ventricular function assessment than the current fully automated approaches

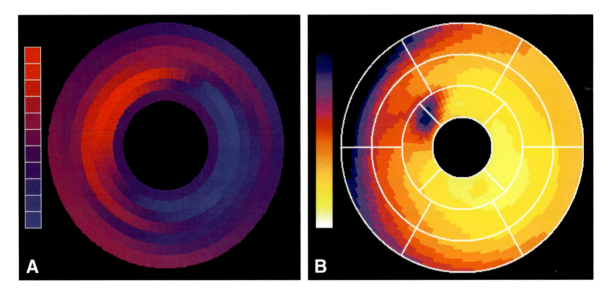

Fig. 11.24 Regional quantitative cardiac function analysis using bull's eye plots of cine magnetic resonance imaging (**Panel A**) and multislice CT (**Panel B**) in a patient with regional hypokinesia in the apical anteroseptal segments (segments 13 and 14, see Chap. 3). This regional wall motion deficit is identified by an analysis of relative wall thickening during systole, and is easily identified by the coloring (*red* in **Panel A** and *dark blue* in **Panel B**), which is different from that of normal segments. In CT (**Panel B**), the borders of the myocardial segments are used as an overlay to facilitate the assignment of findings

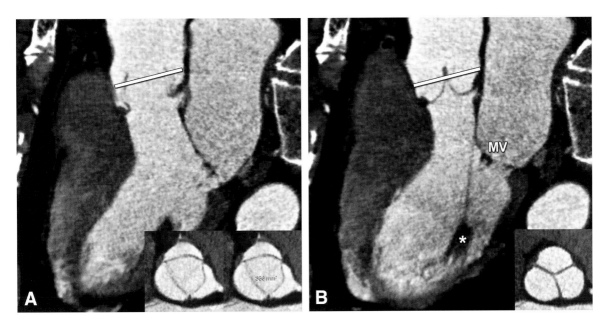

◘ **Fig. 11.25** Assessment of the aortic valve using CT in a long-axis three-chamber view during systole (**Panel A**) and diastole (**Panel B**). In this patient, the aortic leaflets are unremarkable; in particular there are no calcifications. During systole, the aortic valve area measures over 3.5 cm² (see *insets* in **Panel A**, which are oriented along the *white line* in **Panel A**). During diastole there is complete closure of the aortic valve leaflets (**Panel B**), and there is no aortic regurgitation area visible (*inset* in **Panel B**). Note the closed aortic leaflets showing the Mercedes-Benz sign in this *inset*. *Asterisk* papillary muscles; *MV* mitral valve

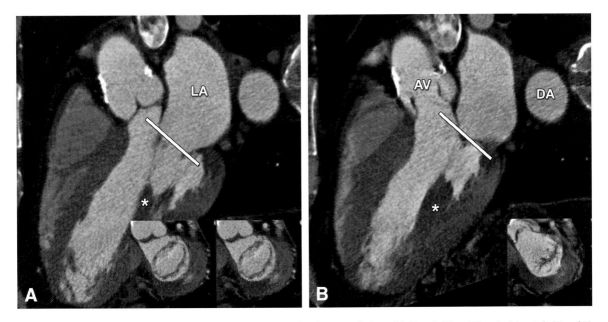

◘ **Fig. 11.26** Assessment of the mitral valve in a long-axis three-chamber view during mid-diastole (**Panel A**) and mid-systole (**Panel B**). In this patient, the mitral valve leaflets are unremarkable; in particular there are no calcifications. During mid-diastole, the mitral valve area measures over 6 cm² (see *insets* in **Panel A**, which are oriented along the *white line* in **Panel A**). During systole there is complete closure of the mitral valve (**Panel B**), and there is no mitral regurgitation area visible (*inset* in **Panel B**). Please note the calcifications of the ascending aorta. *Asterisk* papillary muscles; *AV* aortic valve; *DA* descending aorta; *LA* left atrium

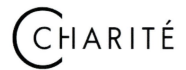 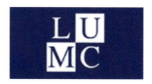

Coronary CT Angiography

History:

- Suspected coronary disease, atypical angina pectoris, equivocal stress ECG

Technique:

Multislice computed tomography with ECG-gated acquisitions through the heart after IV bolus injection of 80 ml of Xenetix 350 in multislice technique (64*0.5 mm slices). Premedication with 1.2 mg sublingual nitroglycerin and an intravenous beta blocker (10 mg Beloc Zok). Retrospective reconstruction using adaptive multisegment reconstruction at 10 time points (0-90%) at 10% intervals throughout the cardiac cycle. 3D and MPR postprocessing at 80% of the cardiac cycle.

Findings:

Very good image quality. Right coronary artery dominance.

LMA: No significant stenoses or plaques.

LAD: No significant stenoses or plaques.

LCX: No significant stenoses or plaques.

RCA: No significant stenoses or plaques.

Left ventricular EF 62.9; EDV, 113.2; ESV, 42.0; SV, 71.2; MM, 131.4 g. No regional akinesia.

Unremarkable appearance of the regions of the lungs visualized.

Overall impression:

Based on this CT of the heart, significant coronary stenosis can be excluded (images and CD attached). Normal left ventricular function.

◘ **Fig. 11.27** Example of a report of a cardiac CT study in a patient in whom no significant stenoses were found and cardiac function was normal

◘ **Fig. 11.28** Example of a report of a cardiac CT study in a patient in whom significant coronary stenoses were found. Global and regional left ventricular function were also markedly reduced. Plaque volume and density measurement results are given here as an example to illustrate how they can be reported. Note that it is not generally necessary to report coronary plaque findings in such detail (Chap. 14)

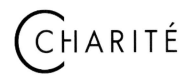 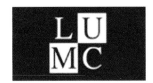

Coronary CT Angiography

History:

- Status post MI 20 years earlier, no angina pectoris, hypertension; obesity; nuclear stress test: anterior ischemia and posterior infarction; exercise ECG: normal; no invasive tests; coronary artery stenosis?

Technique:

Multislice computed tomography with ECG-gated acquisitions through the heart after IV bolus injection of 80 ml of Xenetix 350 in multislice technique (64*0.5 mm slices). Premedication with 1.2 mg sublingual nitroglycerin and an intravenous and oral beta blocker (100 mg Esmolol and 50 mg Atenolol). Retrospective reconstruction using adaptive multisegment reconstruction at 10 time points (0-90%) at 10% intervals throughout the cardiac cycle. 3D and MPR postprocessing at 40 and 70% of the cardiac cycle.

Findings:

Good image quality. Balanced coronary distribution.

LMA: Noncalcified plaque (HU: 15; vol : 32 mm^3). Extends to proximal LAD (segment 6), where it causes significant stenosis.

LAD: Significant stenosis 12 mm in length in segment 6 (60% diameter reduction) due to a noncalcified plaque (HU: 38; vol.: 42 mm^3). Additional noncalcified and nonsignificant (30%) stenosing plaque (HU: 38; vol.: 7 mm^3) in segment 7.

LCX: Noncalcified plaque (HU: 33; vol.: 48 mm^3) in segment 11 without significant stenosis. Segment 13 shows subtotal occlusion (about 95% proximally) due to a noncalcified plaque (HU: 35; vol.: 16 mm^3).

RCA: Reliable evaluation down to the distal portion of segment 2: no significant stenosis. There are two motion artifacts affecting the proximal portion of segment 3, which degrade evaluation of a segment of about 10 mm. No stenoses and plaques further downstream.

Unremarkable appearance of the regions of the lungs visualized.

Left ventricular myocardial function: EF, 35; EDV, 113; ESV, 73; SV, 40; MM, 118 g. Global hypokinesia, posteromedial akinetic areas (segment 10) after history of posterior MI.

Overall impression:

2-vessel coronary artery disease with significant stenoses in segments 6 (LAD) and 13 (LCX) (see attached images). The stenosis in the proximal LAD is very likely responsible for the anterior ischemia found on nuclear imaging. 10 mm long nondiagnostic (unevaluable) portion of segment 3 of the right coronary artery. Reduced left ventricular EF in the presence of marked global hypokinesia and posterior akinesia. Invasive coronary angiography recommended.

List 11.4. Pivotal elements of a cardiac CT report[a]

1. Clinical history, symptoms, and question to be answered[b]
2. Technical details of the CT protocol used and image quality
3. Description of findings
4. Overall impression and recommendations for further testing if necessary

---

[a] The elements are basically the same as for general radiological (CT) reports.

[b] To explain why an examination with radiation exposure was necessary.

Examples of reports of cardiac CT studies are shown in **Figs. 11.27** and **11.28**.

11.2   Reporting

11.2.1   Structured Reporting

Reports of cardiac CT studies should be precise and concise. Using a structured reporting technique ensures that no important aspects are overlooked and also improves consistency (Stillman et al. J Am Coll Radiol 2008). The important elements of a cardiac CT report are summarized in **List 11.4**.

In 2006, the American College of Radiology (ACR) published a practice guideline (Jacobs et al. J Am Coll Radiol 2006) on the conduct and interpretation of cardiac CT studies. This guideline describes how cardiac CT studies should be interpreted and the findings documented. Another, more general ACR practice guideline (Kushner et al. J Am Coll Radiol 2005) describes the steps involved in reporting and communicating diagnostic imaging findings. In 2009, the SCCT published its guidelines for the interpretation and reporting of coronary CT angiography (Raff et al. JCCT 2009).

11.2.2   Medical History, Symptoms, and Questions to be Answered

Only the pertinent facts are stated. The question to be answered by the CT investigation should be included (e.g., "coronary artery disease?"). Also relevant are the patient's symptoms (such as angina, dyspnea, fatigue), risk factors

for coronary artery disease, history of previous revascularization therapies, and results of prior ischemia testing.

11.2.3   Technical Approach and Image Quality

The report should state the detector collimation, the acquisition method (retrospective [ECG gating] or prospective [ECG triggering]), the amount and type of contrast agent used, and the doses of nitroglycerin or beta blocker given. One may also add which coronary artery reconstruction phase was used for analysis because doing so will facilitate comparison with future examinations. However, this kind of information may also be stored elsewhere (e.g., in the radiology-information and/or picture archiving and communication system) instead of in the clinical report. It should be stated in the report whether nondiagnostic (not evaluable) coronary artery segments and/or artifacts were present that may have limited the interpretation.

11.2.4   Description of Findings

If one is comparing two studies, this is the best place in a report to mention to which examination the current findings are being compared (e.g., "compared to the prior cardiac CT of December 15, 2009"). The coronary artery dominance type (right, left, codominant) should be mentioned. If stenoses or plaques are present, it is critical to provide the location (ostial, near side-branch) and/or segment name or number (**Fig. 11.3**). Also, the estimated percent diameter stenosis (**Fig. 11.8**) should be given. As the characteristics of coronary stenoses may determine the success rate of percutaneous coronary interventions, it may be helpful to provide details regarding the length of a stenosis and its eccentricity as well as the presence of calcification or thrombus (**Fig. 11.29**). Further characteristics (e.g., plaque volume, Hounsfield units) may be given as well (Chap. 14).

Other cardiac findings such as global and regional cardiac function (Chap. 15) should be reported if imaging data have been acquired over the entire cardiac cycle. Further cardiac evaluation include evaluation of the myocardial tissue, cardiac chambers, and pericardium. Myocardial perfusion defects or other structural myocardial abnormalities, thrombi, and valve-leaflet or annulus calcifications are described if present (Chap. 16).

Cardiac and coronary artery evaluation is performed on a small reconstruction field of view using small slice thickness (0.5–0.9 mm) with overlap for optimal spatial

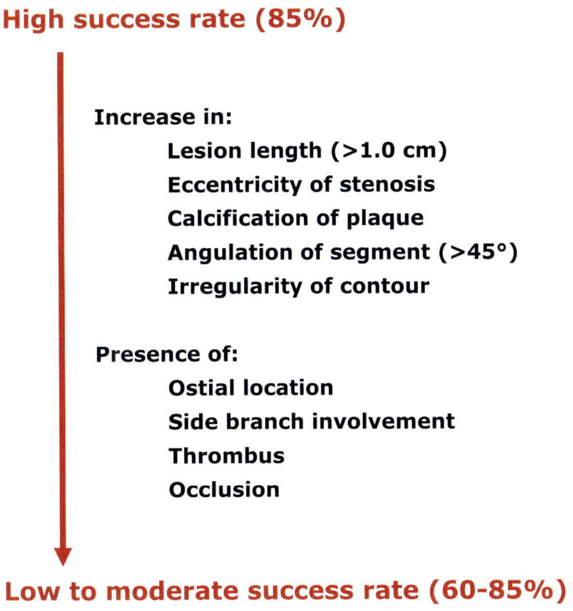

High success rate (85%)

Increase in:
   Lesion length (>1.0 cm)
   Eccentricity of stenosis
   Calcification of plaque
   Angulation of segment (>45°)
   Irregularity of contour

Presence of:
   Ostial location
   Side branch involvement
   Thrombus
   Occlusion

Low to moderate success rate (60-85%)

◘ **Fig. 11.29** Influence of different coronary artery stenosis characteristics on the success rate of percutaneous coronary interventions (Based on and modified from data provided in Ryan et al. J Am Coll Cardiol 1988 and Smith et al. JACT 2001). Success rates may be as low as 60% in patients with very long coronary lesions (>3.0 cm), lesions with severe angulation (>90°), or occlusions existing for more than 3 months. Other important characteristics that can be nicely evaluated with coronary CT are the eccentricity of the stenosis, degree of calcification, and presence of ostial or bifurcation lesions

resolution. However, these small reconstruction field of views cover only about one-third of the total chest volume, whereas about two-thirds of the chest volume has been exposed, which can be covered in the maximum field of view. The maximum field of view should always be evaluated for extracardiac findings. Extracardiac abnormalities in the lungs, bones, chest wall, mediastinum, etc. should be reported. Extracardiac findings are frequently encountered and may explain the patient's chest pain and/or dyspnea, e.g., in the case of incidentally found large diaphragmatic hernia, pulmonary embolism, or emphysema.

11.2.5 Overall Impression and Recommendations

The major findings regarding coronary artery stenoses (e.g., "2-vessel coronary artery disease with significant stenoses in …"), ventricular function, and relevant cardiac and extracardiac findings should be summarized and the differential diagnoses listed. If the relevance of

stenoses appears uncertain, one may recommend which test is indicated next (e.g., nuclear or any other ischemia test to further analyze a borderline stenosis). However, only further investigations that promise to be truly helpful are worth listing here. In case of extracardiac findings, it can be stated whether or not these findings might explain the patient's complaints.

Recommended Reading

1   Arnoldi E, Gebregziabher M, Schoepf UJ et al (2009) Automated computer-aided stenosis detection at coronary CT angiography: initial experience. Eur Radiol

2   Austen WG, Edwards JE, Frye RL et al (1975) A reporting system on patients evaluated for coronary artery disease. Report of the Ad Hoc Committee for Grading of Coronary Artery Disease, Council on Cardiovascular Surgery, American Heart Association. Circulation 51:5–40

3   Bonow RO, Carabello B, de Leon AC et al (1998) ACC/AHA guidelines for the management of patients with valvular heart disease. executive summary. A report of the American College of Cardiology/American Heart Association Task Force on Practice Guidelines (Committee on Management of Patients With Valvular Heart Disease). J Heart Valve Dis 7:672–707

4   Califf RM, Mark DB, Harrell FE Jr et al (1988) Importance of clinical measures of ischemia in the prognosis of patients with documented coronary artery disease. J Am Coll Cardiol 11: 20–26

5   Chin S, Ong T, Chan W et al (2006) 64 row multi-detector computed tomography coronary image from a centre with early experience: first illustration of learning curve. J Geriatric Cardiol 3:29–34

6   Coakley FV, Liberman L, Panicek DM (2003) Style guidelines for radiology reporting: a manner of speaking. AJR Am J Roentgenol 180:327–328

7   de Roos A, Kroft LJ, Bax JJ, Geleijns J (2007) Applications of multislice computed tomography in coronary artery disease. J Magn Reson Imaging 26:14–22

8   Dewey M, Müller M, Eddicks S et al (2006) Evaluation of global and regional left ventricular function with 16-slice computed tomography, biplane cineventriculography, and two-dimensional transthoracic echocardiography: comparison with magnetic resonance imaging. J Am Coll Cardiol 48:2034–2044

9   Dewey M, Schnapauff D, Laule M et al (2004) Multislice CT coronary angiography: evaluation of an automatic vessel detection tool. Fortschr Röntgenstr 176:478–483

10   Eagle KA, Guyton RA, Davidoff R et al (2004) ACC/AHA 2004 guideline update for coronary artery bypass graft surgery: a report of the American College of Cardiology/American Heart Association Task Force on Practice Guidelines (Committee to Update the 1999 Guidelines for Coronary Artery Bypass Graft Surgery). Circulation 110:e340–e437

11   Feuchtner GM, Dichtl W, Friedrich GJ et al (2006) Multislice computed tomography for detection of patients with aortic valve stenosis and quantification of severity. J Am Coll Cardiol 47:1410–1417

12   Feuchtner GM, Dichtl W, Schachner T et al (2006) Diagnostic performance of MDCT for detecting aortic valve regurgitation. AJR Am J Roentgenol 186:1676–1681

13 Friedman PJ (1983) Radiologic reporting: the hierarchy of terms. AJR Am J Roentgenol 140:402–403

14 Gibbons RJ, Abrams J, Chatterjee K et al (2003) ACC/AHA 2002 guideline update for the management of patients with chronic stable angina–summary article: a report of the American College of Cardiology/American Heart Association Task Force on Practice Guidelines (Committee on the Management of Patients With Chronic Stable Angina). Circulation 107:149–158

15 Hall FM (2000) Language of the radiology report: primer for residents and wayward radiologists. AJR Am J Roentgenol 175: 1239–1242

16 Hamon M, Morello R, Riddell JW (2007) Coronary arteries: diagnostic performance of 16- versus 64-section spiral CT compared with invasive coronary angiography–meta-analysis. Radiology 245: 720–731

17 Herzog C, Ay M, Engelmann K et al (2001) Visualization techniques in multislice CT-coronary angiography of the heart. Correlations of axial, multiplanar, three-dimensional and virtual endoscopic imaging with the invasive diagnosis. Rofo 173:341–349

18 Hoe JW, Toh KH (2007) A practical guide to reading CT coronary angiograms–how to avoid mistakes when assessing for coronary stenoses. Int J Cardiovasc Imaging 23:617–633

19 Hoffmann H, Dübel HP, Laube H, Hamm B, Dewey M (2007) Triage of patients with suspected coronary artery disease using multislice computed tomography. Acad Radiol 14:901–909

20 Jacobs JE, Boxt LM, Desjardins B, Fishman EK, Larson PA, Schoepf J (2006) ACR practice guideline for the performance and interpretation of cardiac computed tomography (CT). J Am Coll Radiol 3:677–685

21 Juergens KU, Fischbach R (2006) Left ventricular function studied with MDCT. Eur Radiol 16:342–357

22 Kelle S, Hug J, Kohler U, Fleck E, Nagel E (2005) Potential intrinsic error of noninvasive coronary angiography. J Cardiovasc Magn Reson 7:401–407

23 Koonce J, Schoepf JU, Nguyen SA, Northam MC, Ravenel JG (2009) Extra-cardiac findings at cardiac CT: experience with 1,764 patients. Eur Radiol 19:570–576

24 Kroft LJ, de Roos A, Geleijns J (2007) Artifacts in ECG-synchronized MDCT coronary angiography. AJR Am J Roentgenol 189:581–591

25 Kushner DC, Lucey LL (2005) Diagnostic radiology reporting and communication: the ACR guideline. J Am Coll Radiol 2:15–21

26 Leber AW, Becker A, Knez A et al (2006) Accuracy of 64-slice computed tomography to classify and quantify plaque volumes in the proximal coronary system: a comparative study using intravascular ultrasound. J Am Coll Cardiol 47:672–677

27 Libby P (2007) Braunwald's heart disease: a textbook of cardiovascular medicine. Saunders, An Imprint of Elsevier

28 MacMahon H, Austin JH, Gamsu G et al (2005) Guidelines for management of small pulmonary nodules detected on CT scans: a statement from the Fleischner Society. Radiology 237:395–400

29 Raff GL, Abidov A, Achenbach S et al (2009) SCCT guidelines for the interpretation and reporting of coronary computed tomographic angiography. J Cardiovasc Comput Tomogr 3:122–136

30 Ryan TJ, Faxon DP, Gunnar RM et al (1988) Guidelines for percutaneous transluminal coronary angioplasty. A report of the American College of Cardiology/American Heart Association Task Force on Assessment of Diagnostic and Therapeutic Cardiovascular Procedures (Subcommittee on Percutaneous Transluminal Coronary Angioplasty). Circulation 78:486–502

31 Schnapauff D, Zimmermann E, Dewey M (2008) Technical and clinical aspects of coronary computed tomography angiography. Semin Ultrasound CT MR 29:167–175

32 Smith SC Jr, Dove JT, Jacobs AK et al (2001) ACC/AHA guidelines of percutaneous coronary interventions (revision of the 1993 PTCA guidelines)--executive summary. A report of the American College of Cardiology/American Heart Association Task Force on Practice Guidelines (committee to revise the 1993 guidelines for percutaneous transluminal coronary angioplasty). J Am Coll Cardiol 37:2215–2239

33 Stillman AE, Rubin GD, Teague SD, White RD, Woodard PK, Larson PA (2008) Structured reporting: coronary CT angiography: a white paper from the American College of Radiology and the North American Society for Cardiovascular Imaging. J Am Coll Radiol 5:796–800

34 Vogel-Claussen J, Pannu H, Spevak PJ, Fishman EK, Bluemke DA (2006) Cardiac valve assessment with MR imaging and 64-section multi-detector row CT. Radiographics 26:1769–1784

35 Vogl TJ, Abolmaali ND, Diebold T et al (2002) Techniques for the detection of coronary atherosclerosis: multi-detector row CT coronary angiography. Radiology 223:212–220

The ACR practice guideline for the performance and interpretation of cardiac CT (Jacobs et al.) can be accessed at:

http://www.acr.org/SecondaryMainMenuCategories/quality_safety/ guidelines/dx/cardio/ct_cardiac.aspx

The ACR practice guideline for communication of diagnostic imaging findings (Kushner et al.) can be accessed at:

http://www.acr.org/SecondaryMainMenuCategories/quality_safety/ guidelines/dx/comm_diag_rad.aspx

The SCCT guidelines for the interpretation and reporting of coronary computed tomographic angiography (Raff et al.) can be accessed at:

http://www.scct.org/documents/SCCTGuidelinesforI&RofCCTA.pdf

Coronary Artery Bypass Grafts

E. Martuscelli

Abstract

This chapter provides practical information for optimizing scanning of coronary artery bypass grafts and reading the images.

12.1   Introduction

In patients who underwent coronary artery bypass grafting, recurrence of symptoms can be due to graft failure or progression of atherosclerosis in the native vessels. Conventional coronary angiography has so far been considered the reference standard for visualization of both native vessels and bypass grafts. With its inherent advantages and good diagnostic accuracy, noninvasive coronary angiography using CT is considered a viable alternative in symptomatic patients after coronary artery bypass grafting (Chap. 6).

CT was first proposed for noninvasive imaging of coronary artery venous bypass grafts by Brundage et al. in 1980. At that time the detection of flow-limiting stenoses was not possible. CT technology has since greatly improved (Chap. 8), which has important implications for the diagnostic evaluation of venous and arterial coronary bypass grafts since they are ideal vessels for visualization by CT because of their greater diameter, their reduced motion, and their relative freedom from calcification.

However, applicability of CT to all comers is limited by premature atrial or ventricular contractions, which can reduce image quality when occurring during scanning. Moreover, in patients with coronary artery bypass grafts, the investigation of the native vessels can pose a challenge because of the often times severe coronary calcifications present.

12.2   Vade Mecum of Coronary Surgery

There are two main approaches for performing coronary artery bypass grafting: (1) traditional on-pump surgery, the most common form of revascularization, which usually involves median sternotomy, a single period of aortic cross-clamping, intermittent infusion of cold cardioplegia, and use of cardiopulmonary bypass; (2) minimally invasive coronary artery bypass grafting. This includes 4 subtypes: (a) port access coronary artery bypass grafting performed with femoral-femoral cardiopulmonary bypass and cardioplegic arrest; (b) port access approach using a totally endoscopic robotically assisted technique with coronary artery bypass grafting in cardiac arrest; (c) off-pump surgery, performed using median sternotomy without cardiopulmonary bypass, stabilizing the target vessel by specific devices; and (d) minimally invasive direct coronary artery bypass grafting via left anterior thoracotomy without a cardiopulmonary bypass.

Depending on the approach used for revascularization, the surgeon can utilize different types of arterial and venous grafts, which the physician performing the scan needs to be familiar with (**Table 12.1**). Despite the more complex harvesting procedure, arterial grafts are commonly used because of a better patency rate than venous coronary artery bypass grafts.

M. Dewey, *Cardiac CT*,
DOI: 10.1007/978-3-642-14022-8_15, © Springer-Verlag Berlin Heidelberg 2011

◻ **Table 12.1** Arterial and venous grafts in coronary surgery

Graft	Preparation	Direction
LIMA	Pedicled	LAD/Dia/OM
	Skeletonized	LAD/Dia/OM
	Free graft	LAD/Dia/OM
RIMA	Pedicled	LAD/Dia/OM/proximal RCA
	Skeletonized	LAD/Dia/OM/proximal RCA
	Free graft	LAD/Dia/OM/proximal RCA
RA	Free graft	Any vessel
GEA	Skeletonized	PDA
	Free graft	Distal LAD (prolonging LIMA)
GSV	Free graft	Any vessel

Dia diagonals; *GEA* gastroepiploic artery; *GSV* great saphenous vein; *LAD* left anterior descending artery; *LIMA* left internal mammary artery; *OM* obtuse marginals; *PDA* posterior descending coronary artery; *RA* radial artery; *RCA* right coronary artery; *RIMA* right internal mammary artery

The left internal mammary artery is usually anastomosed to the left descending coronary artery, diagonals, and/or obtuse marginal branches both as a single graft (**Fig. 12.1**) or in a sequential arrangement. The right internal mammary artery is usually anastomosed to the left anterior descending coronary artery crossing the midline (**Fig. 12.2A**), to the proximal right coronary artery, to obtuse marginal branches or diagonals, via the transverse sinus (behind the aorta) (**Fig. 12.2B**), or to obtuse branches or diagonals (**Fig. 12.3**).

The great saphenous vein is usually directly anastomosed to the aorta to revascularize any coronary artery both in a single graft (**Figs. 12.4** and **12.5**) or in a sequential arrangement (**Fig. 12.6**). The radial artery is also used as free graft to all coronary arteries as a single graft (**Fig. 12.4C**) or in sequential arrangement. It is more frequently attached in a Y-configuration to left or right internal mammary grafts and less commonly to the aorta. The gastroepiploic artery is only rarely used to revascularize the posterior descending coronary artery; sometimes it is used as a free graft to extend a left internal mammary graft anastomosed to the very distal part of left anterior descending coronary artery (**Fig. 12.7**).

12.3   Technical Considerations

12.3.1   CT Scanner

CT of coronary artery bypass grafts requires a larger scan range (12.5–22.0 cm) and consequently a longer breath-hold. Due to the limited coverage of 4-row CT a very long, impractical breath-hold of over 50 s was required. 16-row CT slightly improved the situation, but it took the advent of 64-row systems to make CT of coronary artery bypasses a practical approach with a short breath-hold duration (12–15 s) and thin-slice imaging. Moreover, apart from enhancing diagnostic accuracy, 64-row scanners improved the applicability of the method in other ways as well. The latest generation of scanners with a very large detector coverage (320-row; Chap. 10a) or very fast table feed (Chap. 10b) promise a further reduction in radiation exposure and improvement in image quality. For clinical routine, at least 64 rows are recommended for follow-up of patients after coronary surgery.

12.3.2   Scan Range and Direction

The scan range depends on both the modality of grafting. Patients who have received a mammary artery bypass graft should be scanned starting at the subclavian arteries (about at the middle of the clavicle, Chap. 9). The scan usually ends at the inferior border of the heart with the exception of patients with a gastroepiploic artery graft, in whom the scan has to include the upper abdomen. Using 64-row CT the scan direction is usually craniocaudal.

12.3.3   Contrast Agent

Bolus tracking should be preferred for more consistent results and more homogeneous contrast in the coronary arteries (Chap. 9). An amount of approximately 60–100 ml of contrast agent followed by a saline flush is sufficient for bypass imaging using 64-row CT.

12.3.4   Acquisition Protocols

In case of a slow and stable heart rate (<65 beats per min), prospective ECG triggering is recommended because it can reduce the radiation dose by up to about 80–90% compared to retrospective spiral scanning.

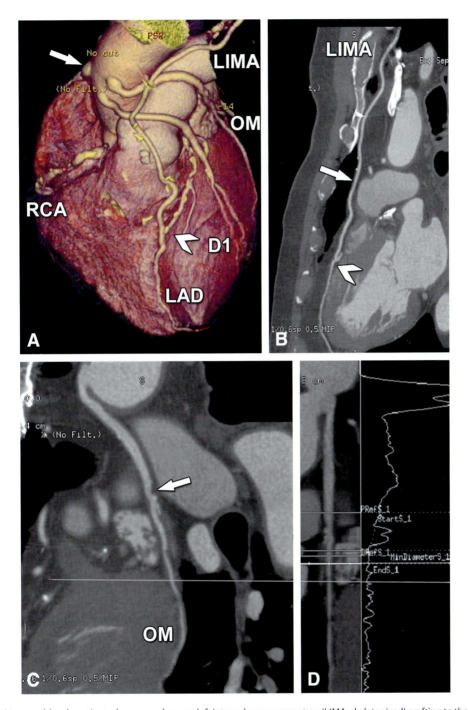

Fig. 12.1 64-year-old male patient who was underwent left internal mammary artery (LIMA, skeletonized) grafting to the left descending coronary artery and vein grafts to the right coronary artery (RCA), the diagonal branch (D1), and to the obtuse marginal branch (OM, **Panel A,** three-dimensional reconstruction) 14 years ago. CT was performed because of an inferior myocardial perfusion defect on single-photon emission computed tomography. The skeletonized LIMA graft is patent (*arrow* in **Panel B,** curved multiplanar reformation) with a normal distal anastomosis (*arrowhead* in **Panels A** and **B**) but the vein graft to the RCA is occluded (*arrow* in **Panel A**). The venous graft to the OM branch shows luminal narrowing (*arrow* in **Panel C,** curved multiplanar reformation), which was estimated to be not significant by quantitative analysis (14% diameter stenosis in **Panel D,** lumen stripe reformation)

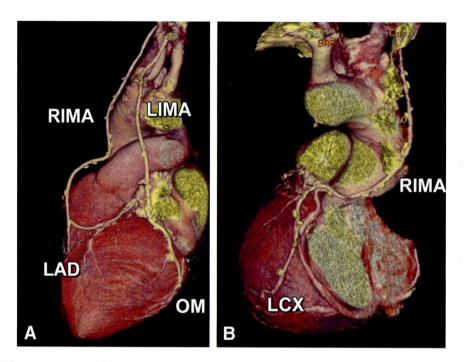

◘ **Fig. 12.2** Different examples of left and right internal mammary artery grafts. **Panel A** shows three-dimensional reconstructions of the CT in a 68-year-old female patient who underwent left internal mammary artery (LIMA, skeletonized) grafting to an obtuse marginal branch (OM) and right internal mammary artery (RIMA, also skeletonized) to the left anterior descending coronary artery (LAD) 6 years ago. The CT was performed because of atypical angina and shows that both arteries are patent (volume-rendered three-dimensional reconstruction). **Panel B** shows a RIMA (skeletonized) anastomosed to the left circumflex coronary artery (LCX) across the transverse sinus behind the aorta in a 58-year-old male patient who was operated on 8 years ago. CT was performed because of an inconclusive stress test. The grafts were patent in both patients

Since coronary artery bypass patients often have more irregular heart rates than patients scanned for suspected coronary artery disease, it may be wise to use some padding resulting in a somewhat lower radiation dose reduction (60–80%). The drawbacks of prospective acquisition are a lack of flexibility in reconstructing image data across the cardiac cycle and the impossibility to undertake functional analysis unless single-beat prospective triggering with tube current modulation is used. Retrospective ECG gating should be preferred in case of heart rate instability. Adjusting the tube current to body mass is a useful measure to reduce effective dose also in CT bypass imaging. For specific recommendations for scanners from different vendors see Chap. 10.

12.3.5 Reconstruction and Reading

Reconstruction of coronary artery bypass acquisitions is similar to standard coronary CT angiography protocols. Slice thickness and the reconstruction field of view should be as small as possible. Halfscan reconstruction is usually adequate in low heart rates (<65 beats per min), and dual-source CT and/or multisegment reconstruction are beneficial in higher heart rates. Sharp kernels (e.g., as used for stent imaging, see Chap. 13) may be used in heavily calcified vessels, which are common in patients after bypass grafting.

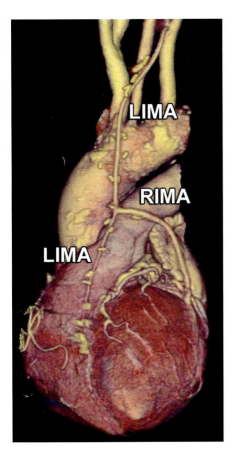

Fig. 12.3 66-year-old female who was operated on 7 years ago by left internal mammary artery (LIMA) to the left descending coronary artery, a right internal mammary artery (RIMA) used as free graft in Y configuration with the LIMA to revascularize an obtuse marginal branch. CT was carried out because of an inconclusive stress test. The grafts are patent without significant stenoses

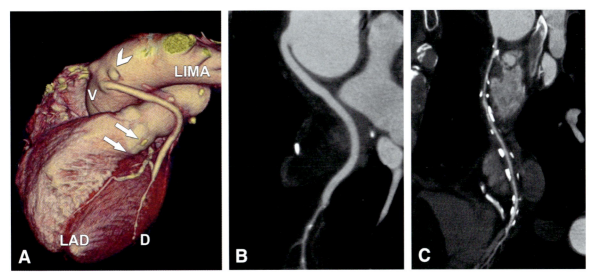

Fig. 12.4 63-year-old male patient who was underwent left internal mammary artery (LIMA) to the left descending coronary artery (LAD), two single vein (V) grafts to the obtuse marginal branch and diagonal (D) branch (**Panels A and B**) as well as radial artery (free graft) to the descending posterior coronary artery (**Panel C**) 10 years ago. CT was performed because of a positive perfusion stress test (lateral wall). The venous graft to the marginal branch (*arrowhead*) and the LIMA (*arrows*) is occluded (**Panel A,** volume rendering) whereas the venous graft to the D branch is patent (**Panel B,** curved multiplanar reformation). The assessability of the radial artery free graft is slightly impaired by the presence of the typical large number of metallic clips (**Panel C,** curved multiplanar reformation)

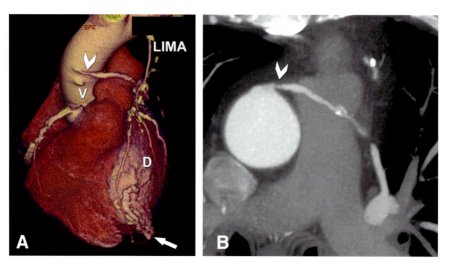

■ **Fig. 12.5** 65-year-old male patient who underwent left aneurysmectomy (*arrow*), left internal mammary artery (LIMA, pedicled) to the first diagonal branch (D), and a vein graft to the first and second obtuse marginal branches (**Panel A**) 5 years ago. CT was performed because of recurrence of atypical angina. The LIMA graft is patent but the vein graft to the first OM is occluded (V) and the one to the second obtuse marginal branch is severely stenosed (*arrowhead* in **Panels A** and **B**); the latter was found to be unsuitable for revascularization

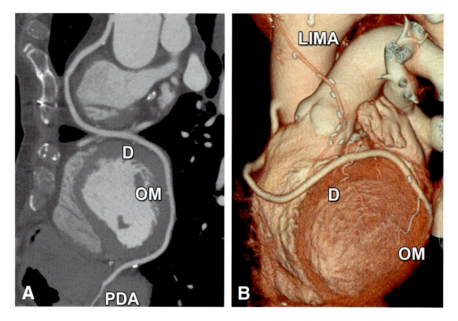

■ **Fig. 12.6** 68-year-old male patient who underwent venous circular (jump) grafting to the diagonal branch (D in **Panel A**, curved multiplanar reformation), obtuse marginal branch (OM), and the posterior descending coronary artery (PDA) 12 years ago. The left anterior descending coronary artery was revascularized by the left internal mammary artery (LIMA in **Panel B**). CT was carried out because of atypical angina and showed the venous circular graft to be patent

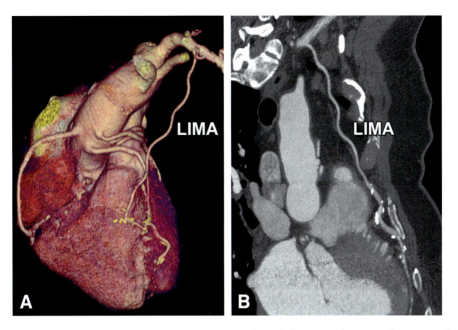

List 12.1 suggests a structured approach to reading coronary bypass CT datasets.

Three-dimensional volume rendering is particularly useful in patients who underwent surgical revascularization because it allows a quick overview of arterial and venous grafts and a quick evaluation of their anatomical condition. Significant stenoses are usually searched for by scrolling through axial images (with and without maximum-intensity projection). This should be supplemented by oblique multiplanar reformations and curved multiplanar reformations, which allows quantification of percent diameter stenosis on cross-sections along the vessel.

List 12.1. Systematic approach to reading coronary artery bypass CT

1. Volume-rendered images for a rapid overview of graft anatomy
2. Graft evaluation by axial scrolling and multiplanar reconstructions
3. Evaluation of graft anastomoses and run-off
4. Evaluation of native vessels
5. Anatomy of the thoracic aorta and left ventricle (diastolic dimensions)
6. Left ventricular and valve function in case of retrospective gating (Chaps. 15 and 16)

12.4 Diagnostic Accuracy of CT

Diagnostic accuracy and evaluability depend on the technical characteristics of the scanner available with a continuous improvement of performance from 4-row to 64-row (or more) scanners.

Four-row CT provided an anisotropic resolution, often times did not depict the distal anastomosis, and 38% of the patent grafts could not be evaluated because of respiratory/motion/metallic clip artifacts. The advent of 16-row CT improved assessment of occlusion/significant stenosis; however, about 20% were judged not assessable because of artifacts (**Table 12.2**).

Table 12.2 Meta-analysis of diagnostic performance of 16- and 64-row CT for detection of coronary artery bypass obstruction (stenosis and occlusion)

Scanner	Graft assessability	Sensitivity	Specificity	Positive predictive value	Negative predictive value
16-row	78%	96.9% (94.2–98.6%)	96.4% (94.8–97.6%)	91.3% (87.6–94.2)	98.8% (97.7–99.4%)
64-row	100%	98.1% (96.0–99.3%)	96.9% (95.3–98.1%)	94.1% (91.0–96.3%)	99.1% (98.0–99.7)

Adapted from Hamon et al. Radiology 2008

Numbers in parentheses are 95% confidence intervals

Sixty-four-row CT improved the depiction of the distal anastomosis and showed excellent diagnostic results (**Table 12.2**) in the evaluation of arterial and venous grafts without excluding grafts from analysis. However, the investigation of native vessels showed somewhat mixed results with about 10% of coronary segments being nondiagnostic, mostly because of severe calcifications. In evaluable native vessel segments, sensitivity and specificity are significantly lower than in patients with suspected coronary artery disease. Thus, image quality is important in coronary artery bypass patients to allow a comprehensive assessment of the grafts and the native vessels.

Recommended Reading

1   Achenbach S, Marwan M, Ropers D et al (2010) Coronary CT angiography with a consistent dose below 1 mSv using prospectively electrocardiogram-triggered high-pitch acquisition. Eur Heart J 31:340–346

2   Brundage BH, Lipton MJ, Herfkens RJ et al (1980) Detection of patent artery bypass grafts by CT. Circulation 61:826–831

3   Dewey M, Zimmermann E, Deissenrieder F et al (2009) Non invasive coronary angiography by 320 row CT with lower radiation exposure and maintained diagnostic accuracy. Circulation 120:867–875

4   Hamon M, Lepage O, Malagutti P et al (2008) Diagnostic performance of 16 and 64 section spiral CT for coronary artery bypass grafts assessment. Radiology 247:679–686

5   Hermann F, Martinoff S, Meyer T et al (2008) Reduction of radiation estimates in cardiac 64-slice CT angiography in patients after coronary by artery bypass graft surgery. Invest Radiol 43:253–260

6   Martuscelli E, Romagnoli A, D'Eliseo A et al (2004) Evaluation of venous and arterial conduit patency by 16-slice spiral CT. Circulation 110:3234–3238

7   Nazeri I, Shahabi P, Tehrai M, Sharif-Kashani B, Nazeri A (2009) Assessment of patients after aortocoronary bypass grafting using 64-slice computed tomography. Am J Cardiol 103:667–673

8   Ropers D, Ulzheimer S, Orlov B et al (2001) Investigation of aorto-coronary artery bypass grafts by multislice spiral CT with electrocardiographic – gated image reconstruction. Am J Cardiol 88:792–795

9   Ropers D, Pohle FK, Kuetter A et al (2006) Diagnostic accuracy of non invasive coronary angiography in patients after bypass surgery using 64-slice spiral CT with 330-ms gantry rotation. Circulation 114:2334–2341

10 Steigner M, Otero H, Mitsouras D et al (2009) Narrowing the phase window width in prospectively ECG gated single heart beat 320-detector row coronary CT angiography. Int J Cardiovasc Imaging 25:85–90

12

Coronary Artery Stents

K. Anders

Abstract

This chapter details the demands on coronary artery stent CT angiography and the typical challenges when reading these datasets.

13.1 Clinical Background

In most patients with relevant coronary artery disease (CAD), interventional treatment comprises placement of a coronary artery stent rather than angioplasty alone. Stent material, coating, drug-eluting properties, and anticoagulant drugs influence re-endothelialization rates, recurrent intimal hyperplasia, in-stent restenosis, and thrombosis. Conventional bare-metal stents have a clinically symptomatic restenosis rate of about 20–30%. Initial results for drug-eluting stents first published in 2002 and 2003 (sirolimus- and paclitaxel-eluting stents) were very favorable with significantly decreased restenosis rates at short- and mid-term follow-up (up to 1 year). However, more recent literature suggests that – possibly due to vessel wall inflammation in the vicinity of drug-eluting stents and reduced re-endothelialization – late in-stent thrombosis rates may be increased.

Multislice CT angiography has been contemplated as a noninvasive follow-up tool for detecting in-stent restenosis or occlusion in patients with coronary stents. The increasing number of stent implantations performed every year heightens our chances of having to report on stents in cardiac CT examinations performed for some other reason.

13.2 Challenges

Coronary stent sizes vary with the diameter of the artery treated and usually range between 2.5 and 5 mm. Depending on the skills of the interventionalist involved, they might be found nearly anywhere within the coronary tree, including coronary artery bifurcations, rather distal segments, and bypass grafts. As most coronary segments take an oblique course relative to the scan axis, isotropic datasets with the best possible spatial resolution in any direction are desirable.

Most current stents are made of metal struts with a strut thickness between approximately 0.07 and 0.15 mm; mesh design can show considerable differences (e.g., sinusoidal ring, slotted tube, or multicell design), with different metal-to-surface ratios causing different degrees of attenuation. **Fig. 13.1** shows an overview of stents used and their different appearances in ex-vivo CT scans. Drug-eluting stents are additionally covered with a polymer, storing the drug to be released to the vessel wall within 6–8 weeks following implantation.

M. Dewey, *Cardiac CT*,
DOI: 10.1007/978-3-642-14022-8_16, © Springer-Verlag Berlin Heidelberg 2011

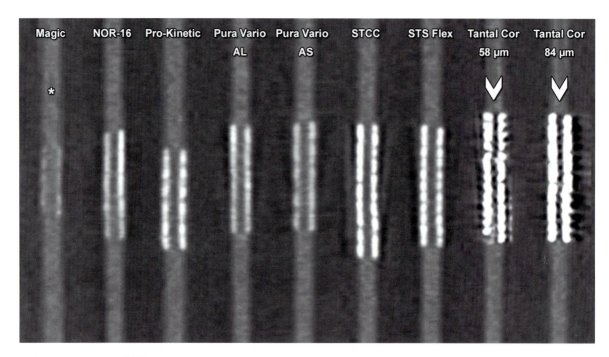

⬛ Fig. 13.1 Overview of different coronary stents using ex-vivo CT. Stent lumen visibility and artifacts differ greatly for the currently available coronary artery stents. This is mainly due to differences in material, strut size, and design. The visibility of the lumen of the Magic stent (*asterisk*), which is made of magnesium (plus less than 5% of zirconium, yttrium, and rare earth metals each), is far superior to that of tantalum-coated stents (strut thickness of 58 and 84 μm) with pronounced artificial lumen narrowing (*arrowheads*). Modified and used with permission from Maintz et al. Eur Radiol 2009

In CT, any kind of metal will cause typical artifacts resulting from the pronounced attenuation due to its very high density. The severity of metal artifacts in the final image is determined by spatial resolution on the one hand and the use of noise filters and special reconstruction algorithms on the other. Residual motion artifacts due to high heart rates, irregular beats, or paradoxical ventricular motion patterns – conditions likely to be met in patients with manifest CAD – enhance the artifacts caused by the metal stents. Furthermore, decreased cardiac output, also common in patients with CAD, influences individual contrast dynamics.

13.3   Beam Hardening, Blooming, and Artificial Lumen Narrowing

13.3.1   Beam Hardening

Beam hardening refers to a shift in the X-ray spectrum to higher energy photons caused by absorption of lower energy photons within very dense structures such as metallic material. It may lead to a virtual loss of

CT density in surrounding soft tissue (i.e., it may look "darker" than it should and black streaks may occur). This is because higher energy photons are less sensitive to soft tissue and iodine attenuation. **Fig. 13.2** shows beam hardening with corresponding tissue or filling defects caused by high density contrast agent or metal. Dedicated image reconstruction algorithms (see below) may correct or even overcorrect for this effect and may thus eventually even exaggerate soft tissue densities.

13.3.2   Blooming and Artificial Lumen Narrowing

So-called blooming of stent struts is an apparent increase in strut size in x-, y-, and z-direction and is mainly caused by partial volume effects. Its magnitude is influenced by the reconstruction algorithm used for image computation. Whenever a voxel includes two different densities (e.g., parts of stent struts as well as lumen), the average density of the two will be displayed. As CT density values of metal are extremely high, those average values will always be way above those of body tissue and – in the window-level settings used in CT angiography – will rather resemble those

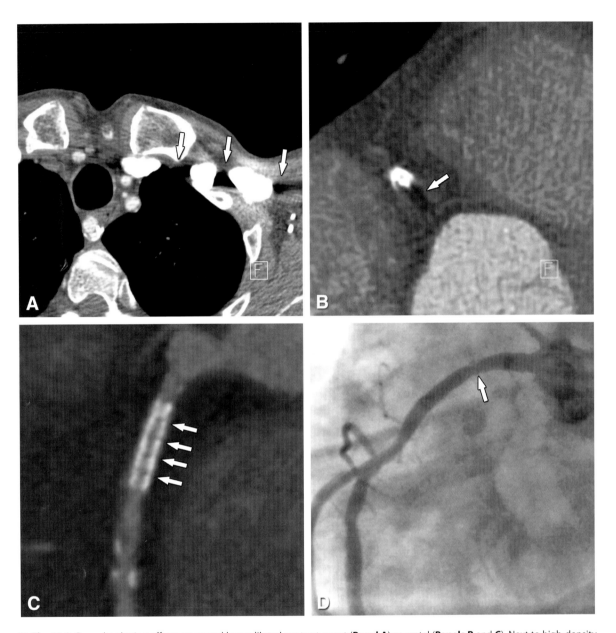

◘ **Fig. 13.2** Beam-hardening effects as caused by undiluted contrast agent (**Panel A**) or metal (**Panels B** and **C**). Next to high-density inflowing contrast agent, the relative increase in X-ray energy decreases the visualization of low-density soft tissue, causing black streaks and artificial tissue defects (*arrows* in **Panel A**). The same effect can be witnessed in surrounding tissue next to coronary stents (*arrow* in **Panel B**). Within the stent, beam hardening artifacts depend on the individual stent structure and may look like repeated dark spots inside the stent lumen (*arrows* in **Panel C**). They preclude rule-out of in-stent restenosis in this 56-year-old male patient, which thus had to be excluded by conventional coronary angiography. The corresponding angiogram in **Panel D** shows only mild focal waisting (*arrow*) but no relevant stenosis

of the stent struts. Thus the better spatial resolution gets, which means the smaller the voxels are, the fewer partial volume effects will be seen. However, even state-of-the-art high-end CT scanners do not provide a spatial resolution equivalent to current stent strut size (0.07–0.15 mm). One of the most bothersome effects of blooming is artificial lumen narrowing. The in-stent lumen is systematically underestimated in CT: artificial narrowing ranges from 20% to 100% depending on stent material. When using current 64-row CT with smaller slice thickness and dedicated reconstruction kernels, artificial narrowing is reduced (**Fig. 13.3**) but still considerable at about 30–40%.

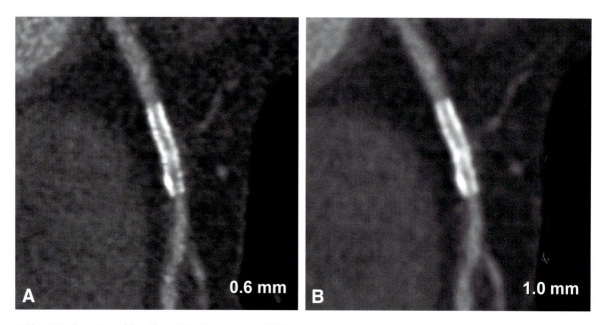

□ **Fig. 13.3** Illustration of the effect of slice thickness on visibility of in-stent lumina. Curved multiplanar reformations of a 3.0-mm stent in the right coronary artery using a slice thickness of 0.6-mm (**Panel A**) and 1.0 mm (**Panel B**). The improved resolution shows greater detail, but also increases noise (**Panel A**), whereas there is pronounced blooming and reduced lumen visibility with thicker slices (**Panel B**). Both datasets were reconstructed at a slice increment equal to two thirds of the slice thickness (0.4 and 0.7 mm) with an intermediate sharp reconstruction kernel and are displayed with identical window-level settings (1500/300)

13.4 Data Acquisition and Image Reconstruction

13.4.1 Temporal Resolution

Considering the general challenges of cardiac CT (motion) and the special challenges of imaging coronary artery stents (metal artifacts enhanced by motion), individualized contrast timing and premedication (e.g., beta blocker and nitroglycerin) as well as a fast gantry rotation speed and the use of the scanner´s best possible temporal resolution are important. Please be reminded that a scanner´s temporal resolution is best at the center of the scan field since the influence of the fan angle increases in off-center positions. So try to ensure optimal positioning of the heart by adjusting table height and patient position on the table accordingly (Chap. 9).

13.4.2 Spatial Resolution: Scanning

The scanner's detector size (e.g., 0.5 mm) determines the thinnest possible reconstructed slice thickness and thus spatial resolution in Z-direction. Coronary artery stent imaging demands submillimeter collimation. Yet, smaller detector elements will result in images with higher noise. Unfortunately, increased image noise degrades the depiction of fine details. Thus, the X-ray input needs to be increased when the smallest possible detector collimation is to be used, especially in larger individuals.

13.4.3 Spatial Resolution: Image Reconstruction

The reconstruction field of view determines pixel size within the axial image. For coronary stent evaluation, the field of view should be just large enough to contain the entire heart, but small enough to take advantage of its 512 × 512 matrix (Chap. 9). Of course, a second reconstruction with a larger field of view to cover possible noncoronary findings is also needed.

The reconstruction algorithms used for image calculation from raw data can manipulate the original data in several ways. They can smoothen the overall image impression by stretching the transition between different tissues/densities over several voxels or emphasize tissue

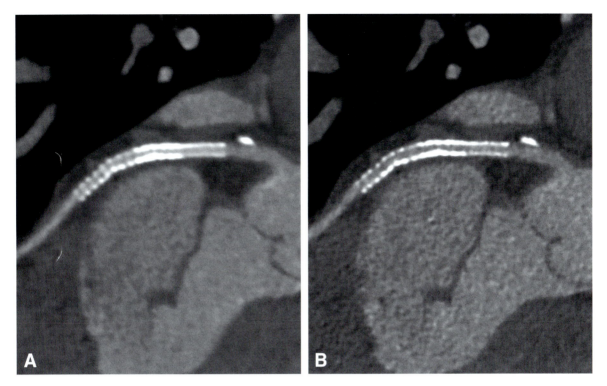

Fig. 13.4 Effect of reconstruction kernels on stent visibility. Curved multiplanar reformations (0.75 mm slice thickness) of a 3-mm stent in the left circumflex coronary artery using soft (**Panel A**) and intermediate sharp reconstruction kernels (**Panel B**). There is a smooth impression, but reduced stent lumen visibility using the soft kernel (**Panel A**) compared to the grainy appearance (higher image noise) of the sharper kernel in **Panel B**, which however allows better in-stent lumen assessment. Identical window-level settings (1500/300) were used

differences by sharpening the delineation of neighboring CT attenuation values. Unless confounded by additional filtering, smoothing algorithms will decrease and edge-enhancing filters will enhance background image noise. The different image impressions resulting from use of a soft vs. intermediate reconstruction kernel with identical window-level settings are shown in **Fig. 13.4**. The recommended reconstruction kernels for the evaluation of coronary artery stents are frequently identical to those used in the presence of heavy coronary calcifications. **Table 13.1** gives an overview of the reconstruction algorithms recommended for coronary artery stent imaging.

In addition, reconstruction algorithms may contain corrections for local artifacts such as beam hardening or weakening in the vicinity of high-density material. An increase in Hounsfield unit (HU) values within the stent lumen compared to lumen attenuation proximal and distal to the stented segment may result from both limited spatial resolution and overcorrection of the algorithm

◘ **Table 13.1** Vendor-specific reconstructions kernels for coronary CT angiography

CT vendor	Reconstruction kernel recommended for routine coronary CT angiography	Reconstruction kernel recommended for calcium/coronary stents
GE	SOFT	Detail (DTL), Bone C2
Philips	CA	CD (calcium: CC)
Siemens	B26f (B30f)	B46f
Toshiba	Cardiac CTA (FC 3)	Cardiac stent (FC 5)

used. False-high in-stent densities can be reduced by using dedicated sharp reconstruction algorithms for coronary stent visualization (**Fig. 13.5**).

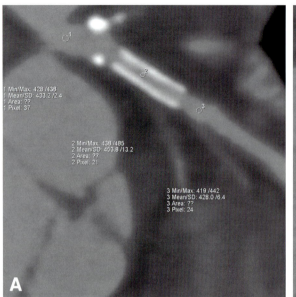
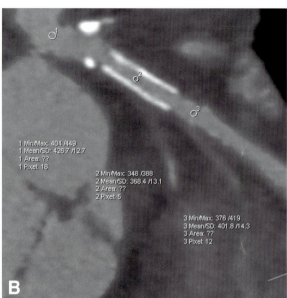

■ Fig. 13.5 Decrease of false-high in-stent HU values (**Panel A**) when using sharp reconstruction kernels (**Panel B**). A decrease in partial volume effects and different filtering techniques included in recommended reconstruction kernels lead to different in-stent HU values in the same LAD stent reconstructed with a soft (B26f) (**Panel A**) vs. a sharp (B46f) (**Panel B**) reconstruction kernel. Whereas in **Panel A**, in-stent values exceed those measured before and after the stent (mean of about 454 HU versus 433 and 428 HU), in-stent HU values in **Panel B** are not higher but slightly lower than those in the adjacent nonstented vessel (about 368 HU versus 427 and 402 HU). Of course, standard deviation as a surrogate of image noise shows higher values in **Panel B**

13.5   CT Wish List

The evaluation of the small coronary in-stent lumen, which may contain low-density soft tissue, e.g., neointima or plaque, demands higher spatial resolution because it is surrounded by high-density stent struts leading to artificial lumen narrowing. Also, datasets without motion artifacts and with optimal contrast are required. However, whenever wishes have to be put into practice, some trade-offs arise. At present, it is impossible to provide all of the above at once. **Table 13.2** gives an overview of the wish list and the issues involved.

13.6   Reading and Interpretation

A systematic approach to reading cardiac CT as described in Chap. 11 should also be used for evaluating coronary stents. Interactive multiplanar reading and curved multiplanar reformation using thin-slice isotropic datasets are recommended for evaluation of the stent lumen. Maximum-intensity projections or three-dimensional reconstructions merely provide an overview of stent locations while lumen information is always obscured by the dense stent struts on these images.. Attention should be paid to the window-level settings in reading stents. In

Table 13.2 CT wish list for coronary CT angiography of stented arteries

What do we want?	Why don't we get it?	What is the remedy?
No blooming and no artificial lumen narrowing	Slice thickness and matrix are subject to technical limitations. We cannot go thinner than current detector elements. Noise reduction decreases visibility of details	Use the thinnest detector collimation available, and try to adapt X-ray input and image reconstruction (see kernels in **Table 13.1**) in order to get diagnostic images
No image noise	There is always image noise in CT – even when scanning just air (electronic noise); and in humans, the amount of photons cannot be deliberately increased. The demand for detailed images requires noisy reconstruction algorithms	As much X-ray as is required should be used. Noise in the final image is also determined by the reconstruction algorithm used, and here, unfortunately, noise and detail increase or decrease conjointly
Optimal vessel contrast	Circulation time, cardiac output, blood volume, and distribution determine contrast, but are not always easy to predict or control	We can get close to optimal contrast by using individual contrast timing and weight- or BMI-adapted flow rates (see Chap. 9)
Motion-free images	Heart rate acceleration during breath-hold, involuntary expiration, extrasystolic beats, and ECG misregistration cause motion artifacts	Thorough patient preparation (beta blockers), breath-hold instruction, and prescan ECG check will help (see Chap. 7)

order to not obscure vessel wall calcifications and overestimate vessel dimensions in case of high attenuation, standard mediastinal or abdominal settings (e.g., window/level 350/50 or 400/50) cannot be used. A CT angiography window-level preset (usually around 600/200) can be adapted for stents, depending on individual vessel contrast and calcium load. Whereas earlier studies used a 700/200 or 1000/200 window-level setting, recent recommendations derived from phantom studies advise to go up to 1500/300 for stent reading. **Fig. 13.6** demonstrates the great influence of window-level settings on the visibility of the stent lumen.

Any in-stent finding should be confirmed by excluding motion artifacts, e.g., by comparison with the same stent in another cardiac phase. Unfortunately, low attenuation in-stent findings sometimes cannot be differentiated from beam hardening artifacts caused by the individual stent structure, calcium in the vessel wall next to the stent struts, radiopaque stent markers, or overlapping struts. If the presence of artifacts cannot be ruled out, the in-stent lumen becomes nondiagnostic and conventional coronary angiography has to be performed (see **Fig. 13.7**). Interestingly, the presence of contrast agent within a distal vessel segment does not rule out in-stent stenosis or even occlusion because of possible collaterals. **Fig. 13.8** shows a true-negative as well as a true-positive coronary stent seen with CT.

13

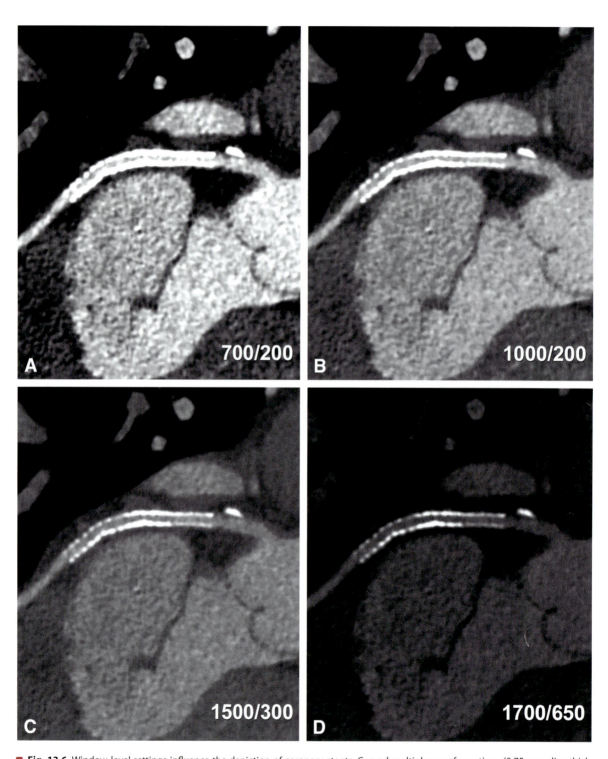

■ **Fig. 13.6** Window-level settings influence the depiction of coronary stents. Curved multiplanar reformations (0.75-mm slice thickness) of the same stent as shown in **Fig. 13.4** displayed with different window-level settings: in **Panel A** with 700/200, which is often used for CT angiography and nicely displays contrast-filled vessels, but enhances stent blooming. In **Panel B** with 1000/200, the increase in window width reduces blooming, but is still insufficient to adequately visualize the in-stent lumen. In **Panel C** with 1500/300, which is a reasonable trade-off, blooming is greatly reduced while vessel contrast is maintained. In **Panel D** with 1700/650, window values are shifted closer towards "bone-window"-like settings. Here, blooming becomes less significant but vessel contrast and the ability to depict noncalcified plaque decreases considerably. All images were reconstructed with a sharp kernel

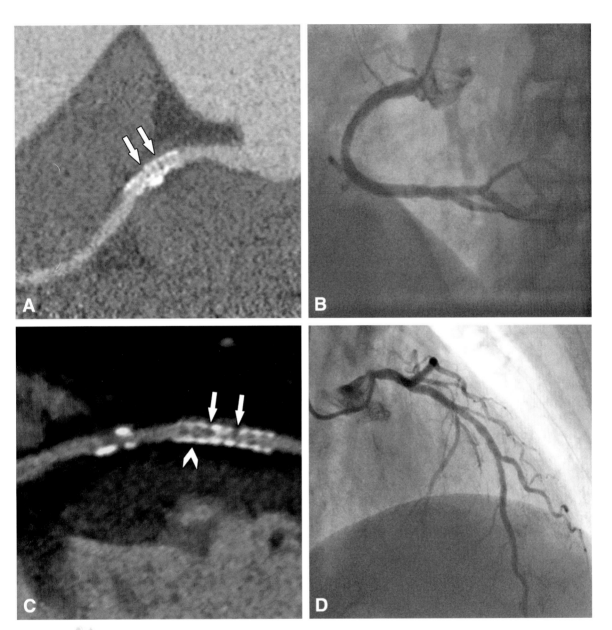

Fig. 13.7 Examples of nondiagnostic coronary artery stents. **Panel A** shows a proximal 3.5-mm stent in the right coronary artery in a 67-year-old female patient presenting with worsening shortness of breath. In this case multiple black streaks, most likely artifacts caused by the stent struts, cross the lumen, making it uninterpretable (*arrows* in **Panel A**). Thus, conventional coronary angiography had to be performed to rule out significant in-stent restenosis (**Panel B**). In a 56-year-old male patient presenting with exercise-induced chest pain but with inconclusive stress ECG changes, blurry streaks (*arrows*) as well as reduced attenuation in the proximal third of the stent (*arrowhead*) preclude ruling out significant stenosis in a 3-mm stent in the mid left anterior descending coronary artery (**Panel C**). No significant stenosis is present in the corresponding conventional coronary angiogram (**Panel D**). Images courtesy of S. Achenbach

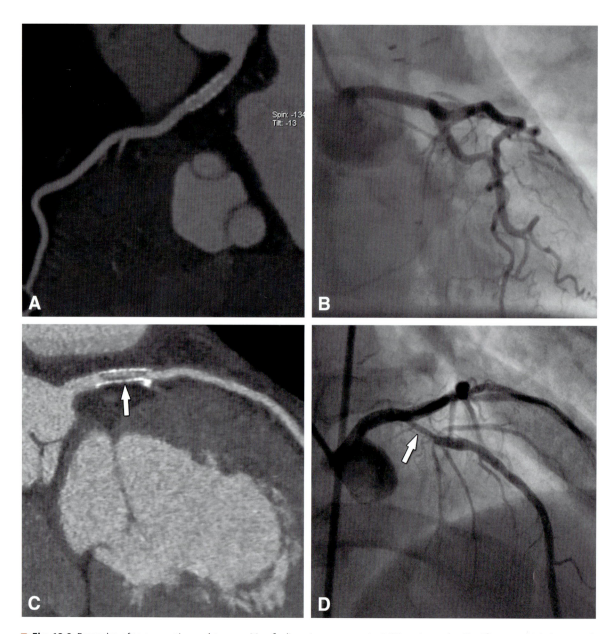

◘ Fig. 13.8 Examples of true-negative and true-positive findings in coronary stent CT angiography. Significant stenosis is correctly ruled out (**Panel A**) using a curved multiplanar reformation along the left main and left anterior descending coronary artery in a 62-year-old female patient presenting with atypical angina pectoris. Absence of significant left main in-stent stenosis is confirmed on conventional coronary angiography (**Panel B**). True-positive significant in-stent restenosis in a proximal left anterior descending coronary artery stent in a 60-year-old male patient presenting with typical angina (**Panel C**). This curved multiplanar reformation along this proximal left anterior descending coronary artery stent with filling defects is suggestive of relevant in-stent stenosis (*arrow*). The corresponding conventional coronary angiogram in **Panel D** confirms this diagnosis (*arrow*, 65% diameter stenosis on quantitative coronary angiography). Conventional angiograms courtesy of S. Achenbach

13

13.7 Clinical Results and Recommendations

Four-row CT was shown to be inappropriate for the visualization of the coronary stent lumen due to pronounced artificial lumen narrowing (60–100%). Evaluation was mostly limited to determining patency vs. occlusion. Whereas 16- and 64-row in-vitro data suggested improved visualization of coronary artery stent lumen, clinical results remained very heterogeneous. In several single-center clinical trials, between 13% and 51% (16-row) and 0–40% (64-row) of all stents had to be excluded from analysis due to artifacts. The reported sensitivity values of 16- and 64-row CT ranged from 54% to 92% and 75–100%, respectively, with a negative predictive value of up to 97–99%. Meta-analyses summarizing clinical trials using 16-, 40- and 64-row CT confirmed the improved diagnostic accuracy, but clearly emphasized its limitations in unselected patients and its shortcomings in stents <3 mm. Thus, coronary CT angiography for in-stent lesion evaluation is regarded as inappropriate in asymptomatic individuals, whereas the benefit remains uncertain in symptomatic patients. Further and larger studies will have to determine whether current recommendations need to be revised. **List 13.1** summarizes current exclusion criteria.

List 13.1. Coronary stent CT angiography should not be performed

1. Asymptomatic patients (if not part of an approved study protocol)
2. Arrhythmic patients
3. Patients with elevated heart rate and contraindications to beta blockers (see Chap. 7)
4. Stents with a diameter of below 3.0–3.5 mm
5. Tantalum stents or gold–coated stents (all sizes)

13.8 Outlook

13.8.1 Scanners

Further improvements in spatial resolution would help to reduce partial volume effects in coronary stent visualization. Flat-panel detector CT improves lumen visibility in ex-vivo coronary stents. However, inherent to flat-panel detector use with its smaller detector elements is a pronounced increase in image noise, which would have to be compensated for by raising X-ray input. Furthermore, currently available flat-panel scanners have a rather long gantry rotation time and comparably slow data read-out and are not suited for in-vivo cardiac examinations in clinical routine but might become a valuable alternative in the future.

13.8.2 Stents

Replacement of the metal struts by some low-density = low-attenuating material could be a different promising approach. Another alternative would be the use of biodegradable stents, dissolving within 4–6 months, leaving only the original vessel wall to be evaluated. The PROGRESS-AMS trial evaluated clinical results up to 1 year following coronary implantation of a biodegradable magnesium stent in de novo 50–99% coronary artery stenoses; according to intravascular ultrasound follow-up, stent struts were fully absorbed within the first 4 months and are also not visible in CT. However, the re-stenosis rate was relatively high with an overall target lesion revascularization rate of 45% at 1 year. Polymer drug-eluting stents as described in the ABSORB study (everolimus-eluting poly-L-lactid acid stent) are fully absorbed after 2 years with no target lesion revascularization required in the study cohort. Apart from radiopaque markers at the stent entry and exit, they seem to be virtually invisible in conventional coronary angiography and are thus compatible with follow-up coronary CT angiography.

At present, both flat-panel CT and novel (absorbable) stents are not available for everyday clinical practice.

Recommended Reading

1   Beohar N, Davidson CJ, Kip KE et al (2007) Outcomes and complications associated with off-label and untested use of drug-eluting stents. JAMA 297:1992–2000

2   Cademartiri F, Schuijf JD, Pugliese F et al (2007) Usefulness of 64-slice multislice computed tomography coronary angiography to assess in-stent restenosis. J Am Coll Cardiol 49:2204–10

3   Ehara M, Kawai M, Surmely JF et al (2007) Diagnostic accuracy of coronary in-stent restenosis using 64-slice computed tomography: comparison with invasive coronary angiography. J Am Coll Cardiol 49:951–9

4   Erbel R, Di Mario C, Bartunek J et al (2007) PROGRESS-AMS (Clinical Performance and Angiographic Results of Coronary Stenting with Absorbable Metal Stents) Investigators. Temporary scaffolding of coronary arteries with bioabsorbable magnesium stents: a prospective, non-randomised multicentre trial. Lancet 369:1869–75

5   Hamon M, Champ-Rigot L, Morello R, Riddell JW, Hamon M (2008) Diagnostic accuracy of in-stent coronary restenosis detection with multislice spiral computed tomography: a meta-analysis. Eur Radiol 18:217–25

6   Kumbhani DJ, Ingelmo CP, Schoenhagen P et al (2009) Meta-analysis of diagnostic efficacy of 64-slice computed tomography in the evaluation of coronary in-stent restenosis. Review Am J Cardiol 103:1675–81

7   Lell MM, Panknin C, Saleh R et al (2007) Evaluation of coronary stents and stenoses at different heart rates with dual source spiral CT (DSCT). Invest Radiol 42:536–41

8   Mahnken AH, Buecker A, Wildberger JE et al (2004) Coronary artery stents in multislice computed tomography: in vitro artifact evaluation. Invest Radiol 39:27–33

9   Mahnken AH, Seyfarth T, Flohr T et al (2005) Flat-panel detector computed tomography for the assessment of coronary artery stents: phantom study in comparison with 16-slice spiral computed tomography. Invest Radiol 40:8–13

10 Maintz D, Seifarth H, Raupach R et al (2006) 64-slice multidetector coronary CT angiography: in vitro evaluation of 68 different stents. Eur Radiol 16:818–826

11 Maintz D, Burg MC, Seifarth H et al (2009) Update on multidetector coronary CT angiography of coronary stents: in vitro evaluation of 29 different stent types with dual-source CT. Eur Radiol 19:42–9

12 Morice MC, Serruys PW, Sousa JE et al (2002) RAVEL Study Group. Randomized Study with the Sirolimus-Coated Bx Velocity Balloon-Expandable Stent in the Treatment of Patients with de Novo Native Coronary Artery Lesions.A randomized comparison of a sirolimus-eluting stent with a standard stent for coronary revascularization. N Engl J Med 346:1773–80

13 Moses JW, Leon MB, Popma JJ et al (2003) SIRIUS Investigators. Sirolimus-eluting stents versus standard stents in patients with stenosis in a native coronary artery. N Engl J Med 349:1315–23

14 Oncel D, Oncel G, Tastan A, Tamci B (2008) Evaluation of coronary stent patency and in-stent restenosis with dual-source CT coronary angiography without heart rate control. AJR Am J Roentgenol 191:56–63

15 Rixe J, Achenbach S, Ropers D et al (2006) Assessment of coronary artery stent restenosis by 64-slice multi-detector computed tomography. Eur Heart J 27:2567–72

16 Schepis T, Koepfli P, Leschka S et al (2007) Coronary artery stent geometry and in-stent contrast attenuation with 64-slice computed tomography. Eur Radiol 17:1464–73

17 Schlosser T, Scheuermann T, Ulzheimer S et al (2007) In vitro evaluation of coronary stents and in-stent stenosis using a dynamic cardiac phantom and a 64-detector row CT scanner. Clin Res Cardiol 96:883–90

18 Schuijf JD, Pundziute G, Jukema JW et al (2007) Evaluation of patients with previous coronary stent implantation with 64-section CT. Radiology 245:416–23

19 Seifarth H, Ozgun M, Raupach R et al (2006) 64- Versus 16-slice CT angiography for coronary artery stent assessment: in vitro experience. Invest Radiol 41:22–7

20 Serruys PW, Ormiston JA, Onuma Y et al (2009) A bioabsorbable everolimus-eluting coronary stent system (ABSORB): 2-year outcomes and results from multiple imaging methods. Lancet 373:897–910

21 Sun Z, Davidson R, Lin CH (2009) Multi-detector row CT angiography in the assessment of coronary in-stent restenosis: a systematic review. Eur J Radiol 69:489–95

22 Vanhoenacker PK, Decramer I, Bladt O et al (2008) Multidetector computed tomography angiography for assessment of in-stent restenosis: meta-analysis of diagnostic performance. Review BMC Med Imaging 8:14

23 Vermeersch P, Agostoni P, Verheye S et al (2006) Randomized double-blind comparison of sirolimus-eluting stent versus bare-metal stent implantation in diseased saphenous vein grafts: six-month angiographic, intravascular ultrasound, and clinical follow-up of the RRISC Trial. J Am Coll Cardiol 48:2423–31

24 Vermeersch P, Agostoni P, Verheye S et al (2007) DELAYED RRISC (Death and Events at Long-term follow-up AnalYsis: Extended Duration of the Reduction of Restenosis In Saphenous vein grafts with Cypher stent) Investigators Increased late mortality after sirolimus-eluting stents versus bare-metal stents in diseased saphenous vein grafts: results from the randomized DELAYED RRISC Trial. J Am Coll Cardiol 50:261–7

25 Win HK, Caldera AE, Maresh K et al (2007) EVENT Registry Investigators. Clinical outcomes and stent thrombosis following off-label use of drug-eluting stents. JAMA 297:2001–9

13

Coronary Artery Plaques

P. Schoenhagen, H. Niinuma, T. Gerber, and M. Dewey

Abstract

This chapter describes the rationale, clinical approach, and incremental value of plaque analysis as a component of coronary CT angiography performed in patients with suspected luminal stenosis.

14.1 Plaque Imaging

Plaque imaging describes the identification and characterization of atherosclerotic changes of the vessel wall. Plaque imaging *research* contributes to the understanding of disease progression/regression and the development of novel antiatherosclerotic treatment strategies. *Clinical* plaque imaging is performed to identify disease characteristics associated with a high risk for future cardiovascular events with the goal of reducing the risk through appropriate preventive strategies. In this context, two related imaging and treatment approaches are conceivable: (1) the focal identification of individual unstable, vulnerable plaques with potential subsequent local/interventional treatment and (2) the systemic assessment of the total plaque burden and activity with subsequent systemic/pharmacological treatment.

The local identification of the most vulnerable plaques is a concept derived from invasive imaging in the catheterization laboratory, for example intravascular ultrasound (IVUS) and optical coherence tomography. Theoretically, such lesions could be treated locally ("plaque sealing") before causing clinical events. However, none of the current invasive or noninvasive imaging modalities can reliably identify such lesions, in part because the proposed imaging criteria of instability are not very specific and are also found in non-culprit lesions. Moreover, we have no evidence at present that local treatment of such lesions is associated with clinical benefit.

A clinically more important goal of plaque imaging is to identify systemic vulnerability by assessing plaque burden, composition, and activity in the entire coronary tree. The experience with IVUS, noninvasive carotid intima-media thickness measurement using ultrasound, and coronary artery calcium scoring with CT demonstrates that overall plaque burden is a predictor of future cardiovascular events, independent of the severity of luminal stenosis. Similarly, there is recent, emerging data from coronary CT angiography in patients with suspected obstructive CAD, suggesting that both the extent and characteristics of plaque can predict the risk of future cardiovascular events. This information is particularly important in the evaluation of symptomatic, intermediate-risk populations because in many of these patients coronary CT angiography will show (nonobstructive) atherosclerotic changes in the absence of significant stenosis. Clinical management in these patients is focused on optimally reducing the long-term risk. However, there is currently no definitive evidence-based data demonstrating that choosing a

M. Dewey, *Cardiac CT*,
DOI: 10.1007/978-3-642-14022-8_17, © Springer-Verlag Berlin Heidelberg 2011

particularly aggressive management strategy on the basis of nonobstructive plaque will improve outcome. For this reason and because coronary CT angiography carries potential risks related to radiation exposure and contrast administration, it is currently not recommended for the identification of plaque in the context of screening or primary prevention in asymptomatic individuals.

14.2 Plaque Identification, Characterization, and Quantification

14.2.1 Plaque Identification

Coronary atherosclerotic plaque starts accumulating long before the development of luminal stenosis. The early stages of coronary atherosclerotic plaque accumulation are typically associated with expansion of the vessel wall (positive remodeling Glagov et al. N Engl J Med 1987). The resulting enlargement of the vessel cross-section typically prevents development of luminal narrowing until the plaque area exceeds 40% of the vessel area. Because coronary CT angiography allows simultaneous assessment of luminal dimensions/stenosis and the vessel wall/plaque, it can identify these early disease stages, which are not well reflected by coronary angiography. Plaque identification with CT is possible with two types of acquisition/scanning protocols: (1) calcium scoring (no contrast agent, low radiation) and (2) contrast-enhanced angiography (IV contrast, higher radiation).

There is extensive evidence-based data in support of calcium scoring, in particular in asymptomatic, intermediate-risk populations, documenting that the amount of calcium predicts the risk of future events. The identification of noncalcified plaque and overall plaque burden is more complex and requires outlining the lumen with contrast. Preclinical CT plaque imaging of ex-vivo arteries after static filling or perfusion of the lumen with contrast and in-vivo imaging of animal models with subsequent histologic verification have been performed for validation of plaque imaging. Plaque imaging using standard clinical contrast-enhanced CT protocols has been validated against IVUS. These studies have demonstrated reliable identification of calcified and noncalcified plaque (**Table 14.1**).

14.2.2 Plaque Characterization

Characterization of plaque components based on tissue attenuation described by Hounsfield units (HU) allows

◘ **Table 14.1** Accuracy of plaque detection with CT in comparison to IVUS

Study	Scanner generation	N	Sensitivity %	Specificity %
Achenbach et al. Circulation 2004	16-row	22	94	86
Leber et al. JACC 2004	16-row	58	85	92
Leber et al. JACC 2006	64-row	20	92	94
Sun et al. AJR 2008	64-row	26	96	90
Petranovic et al. JCCT 2009	64-row	11	96	89

differentiation into broad groups of noncalcified, mixed, and calcified plaque types (**Figs. 14.1–14.4**). Comparison of the plaque types differentiated by CT with IVUS plaque characterization has revealed a correlation between IVUS echodensity and HU values but significant overlap of attenuation values between the different noncalcified plaque types, in particular between lipid-rich and fibrous plaque components (**Table 14.2**). In addition, recent CT studies suggest that the attenuation of plaques may be influenced by contrast density in the lumen and by contrast enhancement of the vessel wall itself, the latter presumably related to the vasa vasorum (**List 14.1**). It should also be noted that IVUS echodensity has limited value as a reference standard because it correlates only modestly with histology.

> **List 14.1. Confounders of plaque analysis**
>
> 1. Plaque HU and lumen density
> 2. Plaque/Wall enhancement with contrast

14.2.3 Plaque Quantification

Even more complex than the qualitative identification and characterization of plaque and plaque components is the reliable quantification of overall plaque burden and its components. The simple approach of classifying all voxels above a defined HU threshold (e.g., 130 HU for calcium

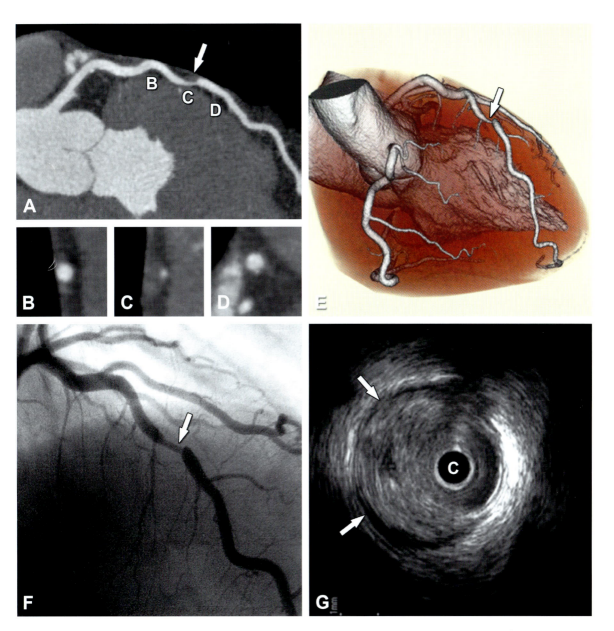

□ **Fig. 14.1** Noncalcified plaque (*arrow*) in the proximal left anterior descending coronary artery associated with significant luminal stenosis in a 65-year-old male patient. **Panel A** shows a curved multiplanar reformation (with cross-sections along the vessel in **Panels B–D** and **Panel E** is a volume-rendered three-dimensional reconstruction of CT. **Panel F** is the conventional coronary angiography of this plaque, which resulted in a 70% diameter stenosis, while **Panel G** is the intravascular ultrasound confirming the eccentric noncalcified plaque (*arrows*). C intravascular ultrasound catheter

scoring) along the course of a coronary artery as calcium is not sufficient for this purpose. In contrast-enhanced scans, there is overlap of the density values of noncalcified and calcified plaque with soft-tissue surrounding the artery and the contrast-enhanced lumen, respectively. Therefore it is necessary to first outline the lumen/vessel wall and vessel wall/adventia borders before, in a second step, the vessel wall and plaque contained between these borders can be characterized based on HU. The first step allows quantification of plaque area or volume, the second step allows characterization of plaque components and quantification (**Fig. 14.5**).

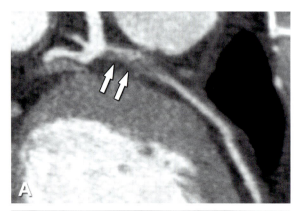

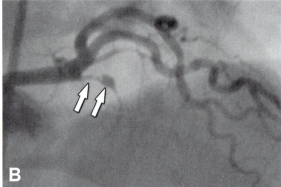

◘ **Fig. 14.2** Noncalcified plaque (*arrows*) of the proximal left anterior descending coronary artery associated with (subtotal) occlusion in a 48-year-old male patient presenting with a vague history of recent episodes of chest pain. **Panel A** shows a curved multiplanar reformation of CT. **Panel B** shows the corresponding conventional coronary angiogram

14

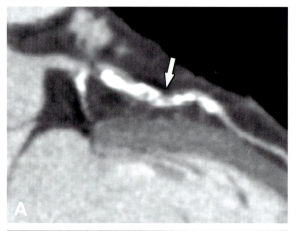

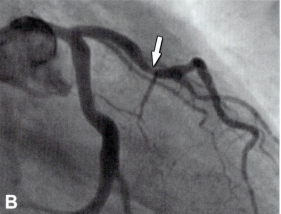

◘ **Fig. 14.4** Densely calcified plaque in the proximal and mid left anterior descending coronary artery (*arrow*) in a 65-year-old female patient presenting with chronic angina pectoris. **Panel A** shows a curved multiplanar reformation while the corresponding conventional coronary angiogram (**Panel B**) shows a hazy stenotic lesion (diameter stenosis of 75%) in the mid part of the calcified plaque. Importantly, the densely calcified plaques in the proximal and distal segment show no evidence of a significant angiographic stenosis

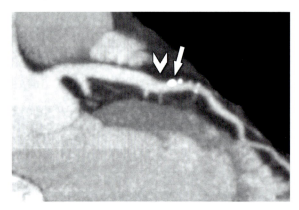

◘ **Fig. 14.3** Mixed plaque with calcified (*arrow*) and noncalcified components (*arrowhead*) in the mid left anterior descending coronary artery associated with mild luminal narrowing in a 55-year-old female patient presenting with atypical angina pectoris. The image shown here is a maximum-intensity projection along the vessel

◻ **Table 14.2** Plaque characterization by CT in comparison to IVUS

Study	Lipid-rich (HU)	Fibrous (HU)	Calcified (HU)
Schroeder et al. JACC 2001	14 ± 26	91 ± 21	419 ± 194
Leber et al. JACC 2004	49 ± 22	91 ± 22	391 ± 156
Becker et al. Eur Radiol 2006	47 ± 9	104 ± 28	
Carrascosa et al. AJC 2006	72 ± 32	116 ± 36	383 ± 186
Pohle et al. Atherosclerosis 2007	58 ± 43	121 ± 34	
Motoyama et al. JACC 2007	11 ± 12	78 ± 21	516 ± 198
Sun et al. AJR 2008	79 ± 34	90 ± 27	772 ± 251
Petranovic et al. JCCT 2009	100 ± 28	77 ± 39	608 ± 217

HU densities are given as mean ± standard deviation. There is considerable overlap between the HU measurements in lipid-rich and fibrous plaques. The reference standard classification into lipid-rich, fibrous, and calcified is based on IVUS criteria

◻ **Table 14.3** Interobserver variability of plaque quantification

Study	Segments	Interobserver variability
Leber et al. JACC 2006	All	37%
Pflederer et al. Roefo 2008	Proximal LAD Proximal LCX Proximal RCA	17% 29% 32%
Petranovic et al. JCCT 2009	All	30%

Clinical experience with CT in comparison to histology and IVUS for quantification of coronary artery plaque is limited. Limitations are the lower spatial resolution (>0.4 mm for each voxel edge) and difficulties in defining intimal and adventitial borders. As a result, the interobserver variability of plaque volume quantification with CT angiography is relatively high (**Table 14.3**).

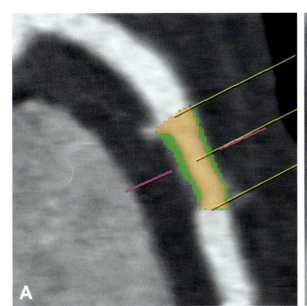
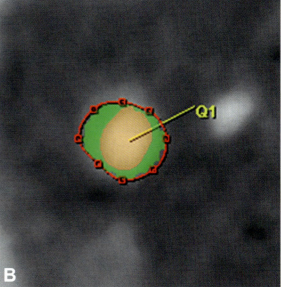

◻ **Fig. 14.5** Noncalcified plaque without significant diameter loss in the left anterior descending coronary artery in a 42-year-old male patient presenting with atypical angina pectoris. **Panel A** is a curved multiplanar reformation and **Panel B** is a corresponding cross-section. The semiautomated analysis of this noncalcified plaque is shown as a color overlay with the plaque colored in green and the lumen in orange, while a red line traces the endothelial-adventitial border

The assessment of arterial remodeling is an important aspect of plaque quantification. Remodeling describes characteristic changes in vessels dimensions associated with plaque accumulation and is related to plaque stability. Remodeling is described by comparing the vessel size at the lesion and an adjacent reference site. The remodeling index is a quantitative measure calculated by dividing the vessel area (external elastic membrane area) at the lesion and adjacent normal reference site. Values higher than 1 or 1.05 indicate positive (expansive) remodeling. Based on IVUS data, positive remodeling is associated with an increased risk of future coronary events. While remodeling can be assessed with CT, clinical experience is still limited (**Table 14.4**).

Quantification of plaque burden and remodeling will eventually allow serial noninvasive examination of coronary anatomy and plaque burden in pharmacological studies, similar to other imaging modalities, such as IVUS, if the concerns of cumulative radiation exposure and of reproducibility can be addressed by future technical developments. **Figure 14.6** shows the clinical steps of plaque identification and quantification.

14.3 Retrospective Analysis of Composition of Individual Lesions: Relationship to Clinical Presentation

The above-described validation of plaque imaging with CT has allowed retrospective evaluation of lesion criteria and their relationship to clinical presentation. Based on existing knowledge from histologic post-mortem studies, criteria of vulnerable lesions (thin-cap fibroatheroma) include: (1) large overall plaque burden, (2) a necrotic core, separated from the lumen by a thin fibrous cap (<65 μm), (3) positive arterial remodeling, and (4) presence of cell populations associated with inflammatory response.

Corresponding in-vivo imaging findings have been described with invasive modalities. In gray-scale IVUS studies, low echodensity, positive remodeling, and small "spotty" calcifications have been identified as high-risk criteria for culprit lesions in patients with acute coronary events. Based on further analysis with IVUS radiofrequency analysis, the IVUS-derived thin cap fibroatheroma is defined as a plaque with significant plaque burden, a confluent necrotic core >10–20% of the total plaque volume, amount of calcium >10% with a speckled appearance, and no imaging evidence of a fibrous cap (i.e., thin cap is below spatial resolution). IVUS assessment of these criteria typically serves as the gold standard for the evaluation with CT. However, it should be considered that IVUS identification of lesion vulnerability is a limited gold standard with moderate correlation to histology.

CT allows identification of low-density plaques, pattern and extent of calcification, and remodeling. In populations with intermediate risk for CAD examined with CT, noncalcified coronary plaque is found in about 30% of patients, often together with adjacent coronary calcifications. The prevalence of noncalcified plaques as the only manifestation of CAD is less than 10%. In patients with acute coronary syndromes, culprit lesions on coronary CT angiography are to a large proportion noncalcified or mixed plaques, and less frequent densely calcified (**Table 14.5**). Mixed plaque identified with CT appears to correspond with IVUS-derived thin cap fibroatheroma. However, differentiation of noncalcified plaque components based on HU is limited, and there is overlap of the above high-risk criteria between stable and unstable lesions (Kitagawa et al. JACC Cardiovasc Imaging 2009). Therefore, the value of focal identification of "vulnerable lesions" is limited and should currently not be used to justify prospective clinical management.

■ **Table 14.4** Assessment of arterial remodeling

Study	Scanner	n	Definition[a]
Schoenhagen et al. Coronary Artery Disease 2003	16-row	14	Qualitative assessment
Achenbach et al. JACC 2004	16-row	44	Quantitative remodeling index
Imazeki et al. Circ J 2004	4-row	31 with ACS 26 with SA	Quantitative remodeling index
Motoyama et al. JACC 2007; 2009	16- and 64-row	38 with ACS 33 with SA	Quantitative remodeling index
Meijs et al. Am J Cardiol 2009	64-row	50 with UAP 64 with SA	Quantitative remodeling index[b]

[a] Remodeling is assessed by comparison between lesion and reference vessel diameter

[b] This study found no significant difference in remodeling index between UAP and SA patients but significantly more UAP patients had noncalcified plaques.

ACS acute coronary syndrome; *SA* stable angina pectoris; *UAP* unstable angina pectoris

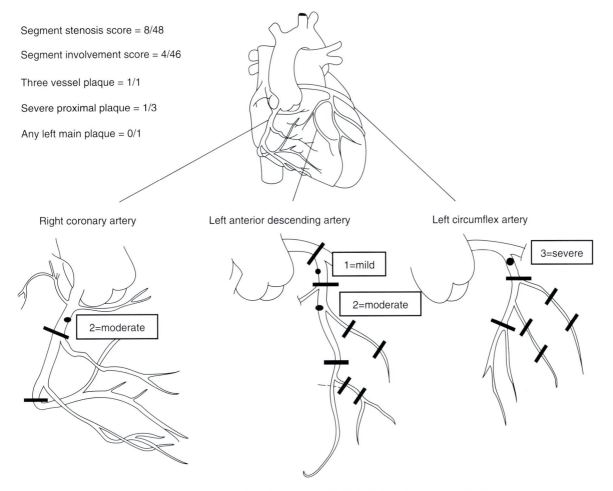

Segment stenosis score = 8/48

Segment involvement score = 4/46

Three vessel plaque = 1/1

Severe proximal plaque = 1/3

Any left main plaque = 0/1

Right coronary artery   Left anterior descending artery   Left circumflex artery

1=mild

2=moderate

3=severe

2=moderate

2=moderate

☐ **Fig. 14.6** Semiquantitative grading system, based on the angiographic Duke index, of atherosclerotic disease burden in a patient with mild narrowing in the proximal LAD, moderate narrowing in the mid LAD, severe narrowing in the proximal LCX, and moderate narrowing in the proximal RCA. Modified from Min et al. J Am Coll Cardiol 2007 with permission from Elsevier

☐ **Table 14.5** Characteristics of unstable plaques

Criteria	Suggested definition
Low density, noncalcified plaque	HU < 20–40
Positive arterial remodeling	Remodeling index >1.05
Spotty calcification	Calcium < 3 mm

14.4   Prospective Prognostic Value of Plaque Burden and Composition

The most important goal of atherosclerosis imaging is to prospectively identify an increased risk of cardiovascular events based on plaque burden and characteristics.

CT calcium scoring has demonstrated an incremental predictive value for future coronary events over "traditional" multivariate risk assessment models in selected asymptomatic, intermediate-risk populations. In symptomatic patient populations with clinical indications for coronary CT angiography, there is emerging prospective data demonstrating that presence of plaque and plaque composition predict future events (**Table 14.6**).

These papers categorize both severity and distribution of luminal stenosis and presence of nonobstructive atherosclerotic plaque. In the largest study by Min et al., 1,127 patients were assessed for presence and severity of luminal stenosis and plaque burden using a number of scores based on presence of plaque, moderate stenosis (50% luminal diameter stenosis), or severe stenosis (70% stenosis) in all coronary segments. In multivariate analysis, CT

◘ Table 14.6 Prognostic value of plaque burden and composition

Study	n	Follow-up length	Score details	Endpoint
Min et al. JACC 2007	1,127	15 months	Luminal stenosis and plaque	All-cause mortality
Carrigan et al. EHJ 2009	227	28 months	Luminal stenosis and plaque	Composite: cardiac mortality, MI, revascularization
Motoyama et al. JACC 2009	1,059	27 months	Remodeling, low-attenuation	ACS
van Werkhoven et al. EHJ 2009	432	670 days	Luminal stenosis and plaque versus calcium score	Composite: all-cause mortality, MI, unstable angina

ACS acute coronary syndrome; *MI* myocardial infarction

angiography scores measuring plaque/stenosis severity, global plaque extent, plaque distribution, presence of left main or left anterior descending artery plaque, and three-vessel plaque were all independently predictive of all-cause mortality. However, while presence and distribution of plaque was examined, plaque composition was not part of this analysis. The impact of high-risk characteristics of plaque composition was examined in a recent study analyzing 10,037 coronary segments in 1,059 patients (Motoyama et al. J Am Coll Cardiol 2007). Low-attenuation plaque and positive vessel remodeling independently predicted subsequent development of acute coronary syndrome with a hazard ratio of 22.8 (95% confidence interval, 6.9–75.2). Another study examined whether CT angiography has an incremental prognostic value to calcium scoring in 432 patients (van Werkhoven et al. Eur Heart J 2009). After multivariate correction for calcium score, presence of ≥50% stenosis, number of diseased segments, obstructed segments, and noncalcified plaques were independent predictors with an incremental prognostic value to calcium score.

In conclusion, emerging data supports the prognostic value of comprehensive assessment of atherosclerotic coronary disease burden for all-cause mortality as a component of coronary CT angiography.

14.5   Clinical Recommendations

The data reviewed demonstrates that plaque imaging is feasible as part of routine coronary CT angiography and provides incremental information to the assessment of luminal narrowing in symptomatic intermediate-risk populations. It is becoming increasingly obvious that CT, while limited in comparison to conventional angiography for the quantification of stenoses, allows imaging "beyond luminography" with potential impact on further clinical management. Additional studies and eventual

multicenter trials are required to elucidate the clinical impact of both focal identification of the most vulnerable lesions and, more importantly, overall atherosclerotic disease burden. However, there is currently no evidence that the increased risk indicated by the presence of certain forms of subclinical plaque can be mitigated by commencing or modifying medical therapy. Based on the emerging literature, preliminary clinical recommendations can be proposed (**Tables 14.7** and **14.8**).

14.6   Future of Plaque Imaging

Rapid technical development of CT scanners and scanner software and the accumulating data from preclinical and clinical studies have greatly improved our understanding of the potential and the limitations of plaque imaging by cardiac CT. **List 14.2** summarizes some of the more recent developments.

List 14.2. Future of plaque imaging

1. Better detector material (e.g., K-edge imaging based on photon-counting detectors)
2. Dual-energy for plaque characterization
3. Wider Z-coverage
4. Improved temporal resolution
5. Prospective triggering
6. Fast pitch
7. Improved reconstruction algorithm, e.g., iterative reconstruction
8. Volumetric analysis (with semiautomated software tools)
9. Clinical scoring systems (**Table 14.8**)
10. Contrast agents with specific binding (e.g., to intercellular adhesion molecules or cellular markers of inflammatory response)

▪ Table 14.7 Clinical approach and recommendations

Approach	Recommendations
Indication	– Plaque imaging alone is currently not an indication for CT angiography. In other words, screening of asymptomatic patient cannot be recommended (Chaps. 6 and 21). – The indication for CT is based on the need to exclude luminal stenosis in symptomatic patients with intermediate pretest probability (Chaps. 5 and 6). – In patients in whom coronary CT angiography is clinically indicated, analyzing plaque burden for its prognostic value may be performed, but the implications for clinical management are not well established.
Data acquisition	– The data acquisition protocol should be determined by the primary indication for CT – Standard coronary CT angiography scanning protocols should not be modified solely for the purpose of facilitating plaque imaging, especially if the modification will increase radiation dose to the patient
Data analysis –technique	– General approach as described in Chap. 11 – Multiplanar reformations, maximum–intensity projections, and curved multiplanar reformations – Window-level setting: beginning at 155%/65% of HU mean luminal intensity (Leber et al. JACC 2006) then adjusting to optimize differentiation between vessel wall and surrounding soft tissue
Data analysis –clinical aspects	– Identification of obstructive and nonobstructive plaque in all visualized coronary segments – Classification into noncalcified and calcified plaque – Summarize plaque burden with semiquantitative scores (Table 14.8)
High-risk plaque criteria	– Spotty calcification, mixed, and noncalcified plaque components – Low–attenuation plaque components – Positive (expansive) remodeling
Atherosclerosis research	– Manual and semiautomated quantitative and volumetric analysis – Dedicated plaque characterization beyond HU, including functional analysis with molecular imaging of plaque for cellular or humoral markers of inflammation

▪ Table 14.8 Approaches to clinical scores of overall disease burden

Approach	Description	Study
Vessel stenosis/involvement score	Major epicardial vessels (LM, LAD, LCX, RCA) with moderate (> 50%) or severe (>70%) luminal diameter narrowing	Min et al.
Segment involvement score	Presence of plaque irrespective of the degree of luminal stenosis within each segment Yields a total score ranging from 0 to 16	Min et al. Carrigan et al.
Segment stenosis score	Grade of luminal diameter stenosis (0 = none, 1 = <50%, 2 = ≥50%, 3 = >70%) in each coronary segment Yields a total score ranging from 0 to 48.	Min et al. Carrigan et al.
Vulnerability score	Low-density plaque and arterial remodeling in each segment	Motoyama et al.

Recommended Reading

1   Achenbach S, Moselewski F, Ropers D et al (2004) Detection of calcified and noncalcified coronary atherosclerotic plaque by contrast-enhanced, submillimeter multidetector spiral computed tomography: a segment-based comparison with intravascular ultrasound. Circulation 109:14–17

2   Achenbach S, Ropers D, Hoffmann U et al (2004) Assessment of coronary remodeling in stenotic and nonstenotic coronary atherosclerotic lesions by multidetector spiral computed tomography. J Am Coll Cardiol 43:842–847

3   Barreto M, Schoenhagen P, Nair A et al (2008) Potential of dual-energy computed tomography to characterize atherosclerotic plaque: ex vivo assessment of human coronary arteries in comparison to histology. J Cardiovasc Comput Tomogr 2:234–242

4   Cademartiri F, Mollet NR, Runza G et al (2005) Influence of intracoronary attenuation on coronary plaque measurements using multislice computed tomography: observations in an ex vivo model of coronary computed tomography angiography. Eur Radiol 15:1426–1431

5   Carrigan TP, Nair D, Schoenhagen P et al (2009) Prognostic utility of 64-slice computed tomography in patients with suspected but no documented coronary artery disease. Eur Heart J 30:362–371

6   Cheruvu PK, Finn AV, Gardner C et al (2007) Frequency and distribution of thin-cap fibroatheroma and ruptured plaques in human coronary arteries: a pathologic study. J Am Coll Cardiol 50:940–949

7   Glagov S, Weisenberg E, Zarins CK, Stankunavicius R, Kolettis GJ (1987) Compensatory enlargement of human coronary arteries. N Engl J Med 316:1371–1375

8   Greenland P, Bonow RO, Brundage BH et al (2007) ACCF/AHA 2007 clinical expert consensus document on coronary artery calcium scoring by computed tomography in global cardiovascular risk assessment and in evaluation of patients with chest pain. J Am Coll Cardiol 49:378–402

9   Halliburton SS, Schoenhagen P, Nair A et al (2006) Contrast enhancement of coronary atherosclerotic plaque: a high-resolution, multidetector-row computed tomography study of pressure-perfused, human ex-vivo coronary arteries. Coron Artery Dis 17:553–560

10 Hendel RC, Patel MR, Kramer CM et al (2006) ACCF/ACR/SCCT/SCMR/ASNC/NASCI/SCAI/SIR 2006 appropriateness criteria for cardiac computed tomography and cardiac magnetic resonance imaging. J Am Coll Cardiol 48:1475–1497

11 Imazeki T, Sato Y, Inoue F et al (2004) Evaluation of coronary artery remodeling in patients with acute coronary syndrome and stable angina by multislice computed tomography. Circ J 68:1045–1050

12 Kitagawa T, Yamamoto H, Horiguchi J et al (2009) Characterization of noncalcified coronary plaques and identification of culprit lesions in patients with acute coronary syndrome by 64-slice computed tomography. JACC Cardiovasc Imaging 2:153–160

13 Leber AW, Becker A, Knez A et al (2006) Accuracy of 64-slice computed tomography to classify and quantify plaque volumes in the proximal coronary system: a comparative study using intravascular ultrasound. J Am Coll Cardiol 47:672–677

14 Meijboom WB, Van Mieghem CA, van Pelt N et al (2008) Comprehensive assessment of coronary artery stenoses: computed tomography coronary angiography versus conventional coronary angiography and correlation with fractional flow reserve in patients with stable angina. J Am Coll Cardiol 52:636–643

15 Meijs MF, Meijboom WB, Bots ML et al (2009) Comparison of frequency of calcified versus non-calcified coronary lesions by computed tomographic angiography in patients with stable versus unstable angina pectoris. Am J Cardiol 104:305–311

16 Min JK, Shaw LJ, Devereux RB et al (2007) Prognostic value of multidetector coronary computed tomographic angiography for prediction of all-cause mortality. J Am Coll Cardiol 50:1161–1170

17 Motoyama S, Kondo T, Sarai M et al (2007) Multislice computed tomographic characteristics of coronary lesions in acute coronary syndromes. J Am Coll Cardiol 50:319–326

18 Motoyama S, Sarai M, Harigaya H et al (2009) Computed tomographic angiography characteristics of atherosclerotic plaques subsequently resulting in acute coronary syndrome. J Am Coll Cardiol 54:49–57

19 Nair A, Kuban BD, Tuzcu EM, Schoenhagen P, Nissen SE, Vince DG (2002) Coronary plaque classification with intravascular ultrasound radiofrequency data analysis. Circulation 106:2200–2206

20 Rodriguez-Granillo GA, García-García HM, Mc Fadden EP et al (2005) In vivo intravascular ultrasound-derived thin cap fibroatheroma detection using ultrasound radiofrequency data analysis. J Am Coll Cardiol 46:2038–2042

21 Schoenhagen P, Tuzcu EM, Stillman AE et al (2003) Non-invasive assessment of plaque morphology and remodeling in mildly stenotic coronary segments: comparison of 16-slice computed tomography and intravascular ultrasound. Coron Artery Dis 14:459–462

22 Schoenhagen P, Ziada KM, Kapadia SR, Crowe TD, Nissen SE, Tuzcu EM (2000) Extent and direction of arterial remodeling in stable versus unstable coronary syndromes. Circulation 101:598–603

23 Schroeder S, Kopp AF, Baumbach A et al (2001) Noninvasive detection and evaluation of atherosclerotic coronary plaques with multislice computed tomography. J Am Coll Cardiol 37:1430–1435

24 Springer I, Dewey M (2009) Comparison of multislice computed tomography with intravascular ultrasound for detection and characterization of coronary artery plaques: a systematic review. Eur J Radiol 71:275–282

25 Sun J, Zhang Z, Lu B et al (2008) Identification and quantification of coronary atherosclerotic plaques: a comparison of 64-MDCT and intravascular ultrasound. Am J Roentgenol 190:748–754

26 van Werkhoven JM, Schuijf JD, Gaemperli O et al (2009) Incremental prognostic value of multi-slice computed tomography coronary angiography over coronary artery calcium scoring in patients with suspected coronary artery disease. Eur Heart J 30: 2622–2629

Cardiac Function

F. Wolf and G. Feuchtner

Abstract

In this chapter, clinical indications, examination techniques, and postprocessing methods for evaluation of cardiac function with CT are presented.

15.1   Performance of CT for Assessment of Cardiac Function

Global left ventricular function is an important parameter for defining clinical management of patients in the routine setting. Cardiac computed tomography (CT) enables evaluation of global left ventricular function and shows good agreement with magnetic resonance imaging (MRI), the gold standard (see Chap. 20). The agreement of CT with MRI is better than that of both cine-ventriculography and echocardiography with MRI. Evaluation of right ventricular function is feasible by CT, and initial study results are promising. Still, the complex geometry of the right ventricle makes its segmentation more difficult.

If a retrospectively gated CT scan is performed and images are reconstructed at 5% (or 10% at most) steps during the cardiac cycle, cardiac function can be analyzed as part of coronary CT angiography. The analysis can be performed on commercially available three-dimensional postprocessing workstations using automated or semiautomated software tools.

Regional left ventricular dysfunction occurs in various underlying diseases, e.g., ischemic heart disease (**Fig. 15.1**). A convenient approach for assessing regional left ventricular function is to evaluate wall motion abnormalities on cardiac short- and long-axis views (four-chamber, three-chamber, and two-chamber views) in the four-dimensional cine-mode. Datasets allowing four-dimensional cine viewing need to be acquired using retrospective ECG gating with image reconstruction at 5% or 10% intervals throughout the cardiac cycle. Regional wall motion abnormalities and global left ventricular function can be evaluated from the same datasets.

In normal ventricles, left ventricular free wall thickness increases by more than 40% during systole (normokinetic myocardium) with a slightly smaller increase in the thickness of the ventricular septum. In patients with ischemic or nonischemic heart disease, wall motion abnormalities can be observed. Hypokinesia is defined as a systolic wall thickening of less than 30%, and akinesia as wall thickening of less than 10%. Dyskinesia is defined as outward myocardial motion during systole, usually in association with systolic wall thinning, and aneurysms

M. Dewey, *Cardiac CT*,
DOI: 10.1007/978-3-642-14022-8_18, © Springer-Verlag Berlin Heidelberg 2011

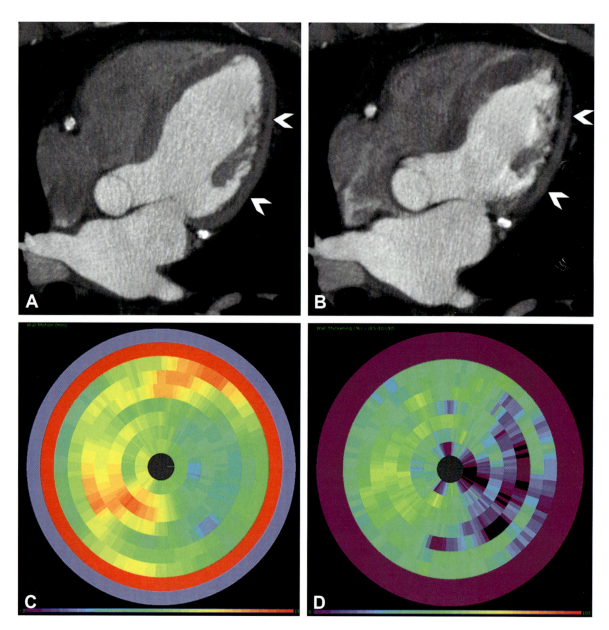

🔲 **Fig. 15.1** Fifty-nine-year-old patient with regional akinesia after a large infarct in the lateral wall of the left ventricle. Note thinning of the lateral wall (*arrowheads*) during end-diastole (**Panel A**, four-chamber view) and end-systole (**Panel B**, four-chamber view). **Panel C** shows the colored bull's eye plot of wall motion in mm and **Panel D** shows wall thickening in percent

are defined as distinct areas of abnormal left ventricular diastolic contour.

Wall motion abnormalities are systematically evaluated and reported using the 17-segment model of the AHA (see Chap. 3). Each segment can be assigned a score on the basis of its contractility as assessed visually (normal = 1, hypokinesia = 2, akinesia = 3, dyskinesia = 4, and aneurysm = 5). A wall motion score index can be calculated to semiquantitatively describe the extent of regional wall motion abnormalities:

Wall motion score index = sum of wall motion scores / number of segments.

Normally contracting left ventricular myocardium has a wall motion score index of 1 (17/17 = 1). The evaluation of wall motion abnormalities can be performed automatically or semiautomatically on dedicated cardiac CT workstations (see Sect. 15.5).

To summarize, although recent technical developments have improved the capabilities of CT, temporal resolution is still lower than that of cardiac MRI. Hence MRI should be preferred as first-line imaging modality in clinical practice. However, if retrospective ECG-gated datasets are available for coronary CT angiography, comprehensive evaluation of regional wall motion abnormalities or global left ventricular function may have added value.

15.2 Clinical Use of Cardiac CT

Current cardiac CT should not be used as first-line imaging modality for evaluation of left ventricular function because it involves radiation exposure. Cardiac MRI or echocardiography should be preferred for primary evaluation of right and left ventricular function. MRI is regarded as the gold standard method with the highest reproducibility.

Cardiac CT has the advantage that the datasets acquired for coronary CT angiography using retrospective ECG gating can also be used for evaluating cardiac function. No additional injection of contrast agent or exposure to further radiation is necessary. Because of the importance of global as well as regional cardiac function for a patient's individual prognosis and further clinical management, we thus strongly encourage to perform cardiac function analysis in all patients undergoing coronary CT angiography if datasets are acquired with conventional retrospective ECG gating.

15.3 Adjustment of CT Examination Protocols for Evaluation of Cardiac Function

15.3.1 Contrast Bolus Design

For evaluation of cardiac function, it is recommended to adjust the contrast agent injection protocol. Homogeneous enhancement of the right ventricle is desirable for better delineation of the interventricular septum. If a single bolus is injected for arterial phase at high flow rate (~5 ml/s), followed by a saline chaser, as commonly used for coronary CT angiography, most of the contrast agent will have left the right ventricle by the time the scan is taken. Hence, the interventricular septum and the right ventricle will not be delineated. If contrast bolus timing

is suboptimal, e.g., if the injection time is too long, and/or if the bolus volume is too large, the right ventricle will appear inhomogeneous and show streak artifacts hampering image quality.

As mentioned before in Chap. 9, whenever assessment of cardiac function is required, biphasic injection of the contrast agent or injection of a mixture of contrast agent and saline have shown to improve image quality by providing low but homogeneous contrast attenuation of the right chambers. Streak artifacts, resulting from persisting flow of contrast agent, impair segmentation of the right chambers using fully automated software tools and degrade image quality of the right coronary artery. Therefore, the attenuation of the right chambers should be as homogeneous as possible.

Vrachliotis et al. describe a biphasic injection protocol including a first phase bolus of contrast at high flow rate (100 ml at 5 ml/s) and a second phase at decreased flow (30 ml at 3 ml/s), resulting in an overall contrast agent volume of 130 ml. This protocol allows triple rule-out because it ensures rather homogenous enhancement in the coronary, aortic, and pulmonary vasculature as well as in the right ventricle using 64-row CT.

15.3.2 ECG-Gating Techniques

Retrospective ECG gating is required for assessment of cardiac function, which permits the acquisition of multiphase datasets over the entire cardiac cycle. ECG-dependent tube current modulation can be applied, resulting in diagnostic images in most cases despite higher image noise during systole.

Prospectively EGG-triggered datasets ("step-and-shoot") preclude evaluation of cardiac function if the padding window is placed at end-diastole.

The recently introduced prospective ECG-triggered adaptive sequential scan mode, with additional tube current modulation throughout the cardiac cycle enables estimation of cardiac function parameters and may provide a reasonable alternative in patients with stable heart rates.

15.3.3 Image Reconstruction

Reconstruction of the multiphase dataset covering the entire cardiac cycle should be performed in 5% or 10% steps from 0% to 90% of the RR interval. For detailed information on how to generate multiphase datasets on the different scanners, please see Chap. 10.

We recommend reconstructing a slice width of 1 mm (overlap, 70%) to ensure highest spatial resolution and highest accuracy of measurements; however, one needs to keep in mind that multiphase datasets produce large amounts of images. If one experiences difficulties in uploading large datasets, slice thickness may be increase to 1.5–2 mm to reduce the number of images.

Most of the commercially available workstations provide tools for automated detection of the maximum end-systolic and end-diastolic volumes. Using these tools, it is generally possible to automatically identify systole and diastole and reduce data volume and analysis time.

15.4   Definition of Cardiac Function Parameters

A large number of cardiac function parameters exist. **Table 15.1** presents clinically relevant parameters, which can be calculated with all commercially available postprocessing workstations equipped with cardiac software packages. **Table 15.2** lists other important cardiac parameters, which can be evaluated depending on the ECG-gating technique (retrospective or prospective ECG gating) and the specific workstation used.

▣ Table 15.1 Clinically relevant cardiac function parameters

Parameter	Unit	Description
End-diastolic volume (EDV)	ml	Largest volume of the left ventricle during any cardiac phase. An increase in venous return to the heart increases the EDV, which stretches the muscle fibers and increases the preload. This leads to an increase in ventricular contraction in order to eject the additional blood, resulting in a higher SV
End-systolic volume (ESV)	ml	Smallest volume of the left ventricle during any cardiac phase
Stroke volume (SV)	ml/stroke	Blood volume ejected during systole ($SV = EDV - ESV$)
Ejection fraction (EF)	%	Percentage of blood in the left ventricle ejected during systole ($EF = SV/EDV \times 100\%$)
Cardiac output (CO)	l/min	Blood volume ejected from the heart per minute ($CO = $ heart rate $\times SV/1{,}000$). CO is regulated principally by the oxygen demand of the body cells and is increased during infection and sepsis and decreased in cardiomyopathy and heart failure

▣ Table 15.2 Parameter unit description

Parameter	Unit	Description
Myocardial volume (MV)	Ml	Volume of myocardium of the left ventricle (inclusion or exclusion of the papillary muscles depending on the workstation)
Myocardial mass (MM)	G	$MM = MV \times 1.05$ g/ml (1.05 g/ml = specific mass of the myocardium)
Myocardial mass index (MMI)	g/kg	MMI = MM (g)/body weight (kg)
Body surface area (BSA)	m²	$BSA = 0.007184 \times$ body height $^{0.725}$ (cm) $\times$ body weight $^{0.425}$ (kg)
Stroke index (SI)	(ml/beat)/m²	SI = SV/BSA
Cardiac index (CI)	(l/min)/m²	CI = CO/BSA
Wall motion (WM)	mm	Maximum motion of the outer (epicardial) contours between systole and diastole
Wall thickening (WT)	%	WT = (ES wall thickness – ED wall thickness)/ED wall thickness $\times 100\%$

15.5 Analysis of Cardiac Function on Different Commercial Workstations

Cardiac software packages from all major CT vendors and dedicated cardiac workstations allow evaluation of cardiac function. Most workstations have automated or semiautomated tools to facilitate and accelerate function analysis. All vendors have tools to evaluate left ventricular function; some of them also developed tools to evaluate right ventricular function.

15.5.1 Vital Images (Vitrea Workstation)

After loading a multiphase dataset (**Fig. 15.2**), this software tool fully automatically identifies the cardiac axes, the endo- and epicardial contours as well as end-systole and end-diastole of the left ventricle. The cardiac axes as well as the endo- and epicardial contours should be checked in all phases to avoid false measurements of function parameters. If necessary, these parameters including the mitral valve plane can be adjusted

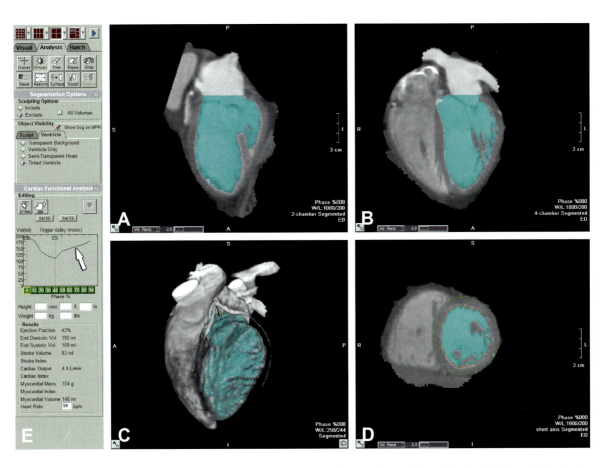

■ **Fig. 15.2** Fully automated cardiac function analysis software (Vitrea, Vital Images) in a patient with reduced left ventricular ejection fraction (43%). Images are presented in two-chamber view (**Panel A**), four-chamber view (**Panel B**), three-dimensional display (**Panel C**), and short-axis view (**Panel D**). The blood pool of the left ventricle is marked in blue. The papillary muscles are excluded. The epicardial contours are indicated with green lines, the endocardial contours with red lines (**Panel D**). **Panel E** shows a volume curve of the left ventricle (*arrow*) over the cardiac cycle. End-diastole (ED, 0% of RR interval) and end-systole (ES, 40% of RR interval) are automatically recognized and marked. Moreover, results of the function analysis are shown. If the patient's weight and height and the heart rate are given, the software calculates stroke index, cardiac index, cardiac output, and myocardial index. Figure courtesy of Vital Images

manually. For evaluation of function parameters such as ejection fraction or stroke volume, the papillary muscles are excluded, whereas for the evaluation of myocardial mass, the papillary muscles are included. Regional wall motion analysis using this tool is shown in **Fig. 15.3**.

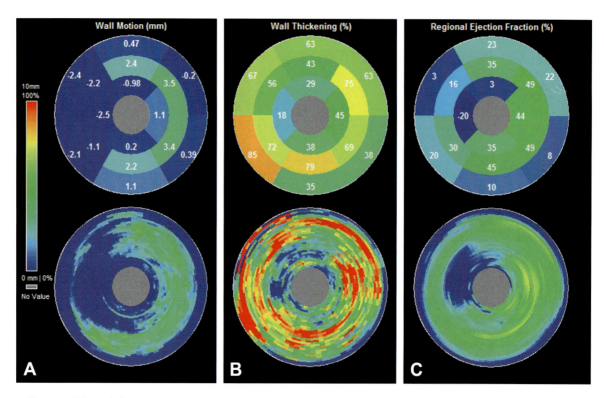

Fig. 15.3 Color-coded map (Vitrea, Vital Images) of the left ventricle using the 17-segment model of the American Heart Association (AHA) obtained with automated cardiac function analysis software (Vitrea, Vital Images). Wall motion is shown in mm (**Panel A**), while wall thickening and the regional ejection fraction are presented as percentages (**Panels B** and **C**). Images show that all three parameters are reduced in the anteroseptal segments in the apical third of the left ventricle in a patient with high-grade LAD stenosis. Figure courtesy of Vital Images

15.5.2 Siemens (syngo.via™, Cardio-vascular Engine)

After loading a multiphase dataset, automatic recognition of the left heart epi- and endocardial and the right heart endocardial contours is performed (**Fig. 15.4**). All contours can be adjusted manually, if necessary. Despite the use of maximal tube current modulation (**Fig. 15.5**) (MinDose™), endocardial and epicardial boarder contour tracking is feasible. Cardiac function results are presented for the left and right ventricle including a time-volume curve (**Fig. 15.4E**) and bull's eye plots for wall motion, wall thickening, and wall thickness (**Fig. 15.6B**). Hypoattenuated myocardium (e.g., myocardial infarction) is segmented based on Hounsfield units (**Fig. 15.6C**).

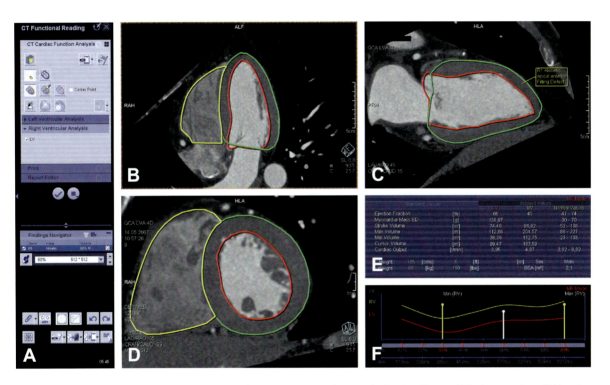

Fig. 15.4 Cardiac function analysis software (**Panel A**, syngo.via™, Cardio-Vascular Engine, Siemens). The inner endocardial borders of the left (*red*) and right (*yellow*) ventricle including the papillary muscles are traced automatically. Left ventricular function parameters are shown in four-chamber (**Panel B**), two-chamber (**Panel C**), and short-axis-view (**Panel D**). Cardiac function parameters are presented for the left and right ventricle and compared with the normal values (**Panel E**). **Panel F** shows a time-volume curve for the left (*red*) and right (*yellow*) ventricle. Figure courtesy of Siemens

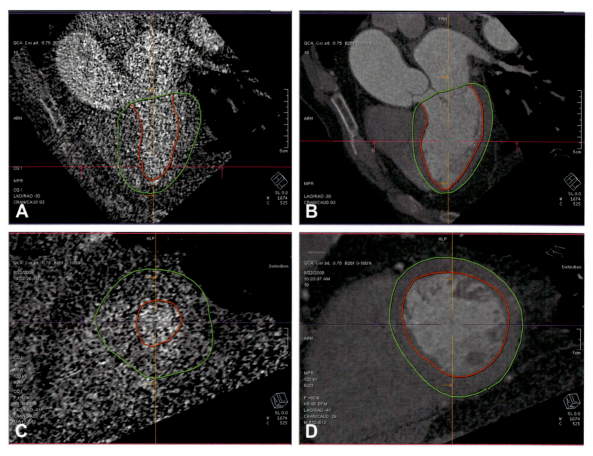

◘ Fig. 15.5 Recently introduced software (syngo.via™, Cardio-Vascular Engine, Siemens) allows endo- and epicardial contour tracking despite high image noise during systole (**Panels A** and **C**) through the use of MinDose™ (Siemens). Note full tube current is applied during end-diastole (**Panels B** and **D**) only. Contour tracking results may be corrected manually if necessary. Figure courtesy of Siemens

15

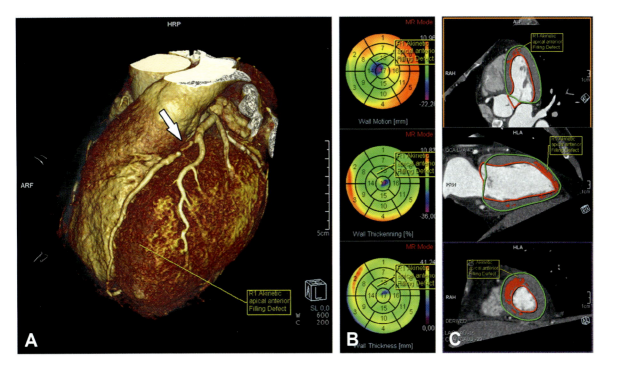

▫ Fig. 15.6 Assessment of myocardial infarction using syngo.via™, Cardio-Vascular Engine (Siemens). This patient is the same as in **Fig. 15.4** and had a 90% LAD stenosis (*arrow* in **Panel A**), which matched with an anteroseptal perfusion defect (*colored red* in **Panel C**). The perfusion defect, defined as hypoattenuating region, is segmented automatically based on Hounsfield unit ratio. **Panel B** shows the corresponding wall motion deficit (segments 13, 14, and 17 in the bull's eye plot). Figure courtesy of Siemens

15.5.3   Philips (Brilliance Workspace, Comprehensive Cardiac)

At least two (end-systole and end-diastole) or more datasets (e.g., 0–90% in 10% steps) can be uploaded into the comprehensive cardiac tool. Cardiac function analysis works fully automated, and endo- and epicardial borders as well as cardiac axes and the position of the mitral valve can be adjusted manually if necessary. Function analysis can be performed using the conventional short-axis method (**Fig. 15.7**). Alternatively, the user can select the fully automated method allowing segmentation of all four cardiac chambers (**Figs. 15.8 and 15.9**)

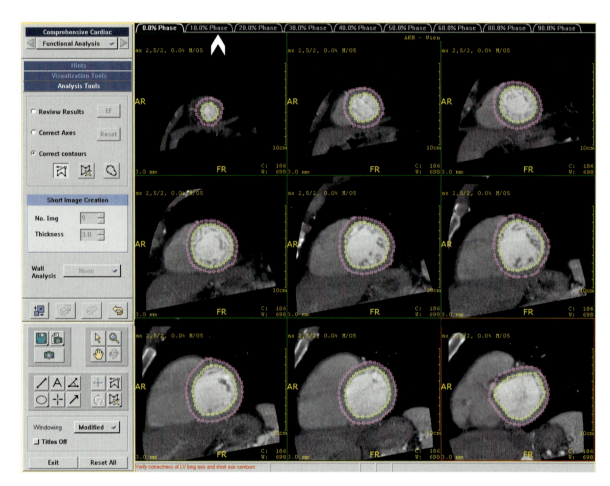

◘ Fig. 15.7 Conventional cardiac function analysis tool (Comprehensive Cardiac, Philips) in a patient with normal left ventricular function. Multiple datasets (0–90%, at 10% steps) can be evaluated by clicking on the different phase cards (*arrowhead*). Endo- and epicardial contours of the left ventricle can be adjusted manually if necessary. Left ventricular function parameters are calculated using Simpson's method

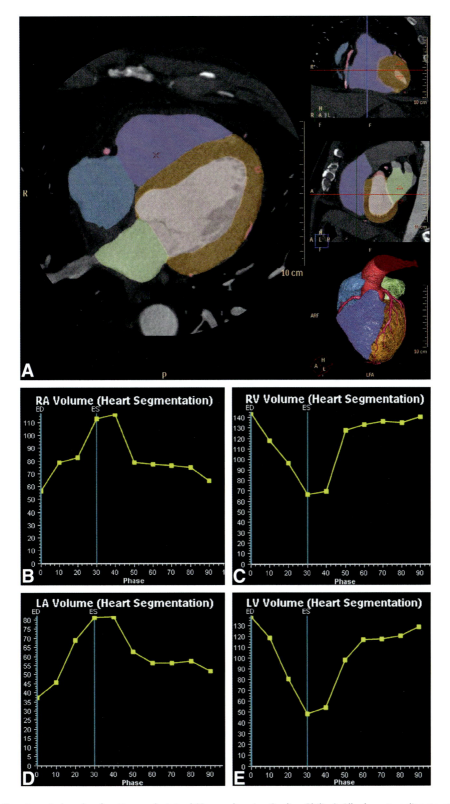

■ **Fig. 15.8** Fully automated cardiac function analysis tool (Comprehensive Cardiac, Philips). All relevant cardiac structures are recognized and color-coded (**Panel A**). Volume-over-time curves for all four cardiac chambers (*LA* left atrium; *LV* left ventricle; *RA* right atrium; *RV* right ventricle) can be generated (**Panels B–E**)

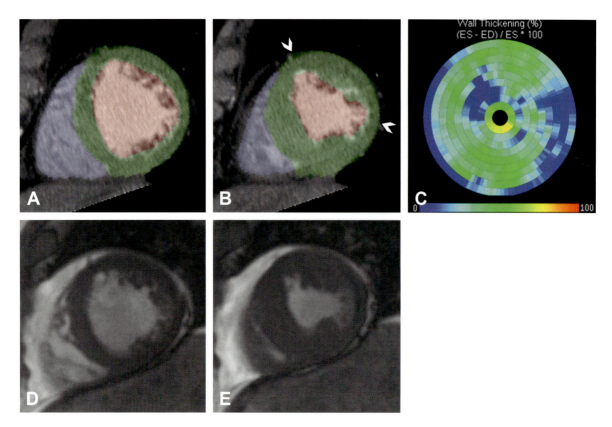

🔴 **Fig 15.9** Cardiac function analysis in a patient 2 years after myocardial infarction using a fully automated tool (Comprehensive Cardiac, Philips). **Panels A** and **B** show end-diastolic and end-systolic short-axis views, respectively. There is a small area of hypokinesia anteriorly and a larger area of akinesia inferolaterally (*arrowheads* in **Panel B**). **Panel C** presents a color-coded bull's eye plot of the CT examination showing the reduced wall thickening (*dark-blue areas*). **Panel D** shows end-diastolic and **Panel E** end-systolic short-axis images obtained in the same patient with MRI

15.5.4   GE (Advantage Workstation)

A three-dimensional model of the left ventricle at end-systole and end-diastole is segmented (**Fig. 15.10**). All function parameters are calculated and shown for each chamber. Automated endocardial (**Fig. 15.10**) and epicardial contour tracking (**Fig. 15.11**) of the left ventricle is feasible. The program allows measurement of left ventricular wall thickness and wall motion in the bull's eye view (**Fig. 15.11**).

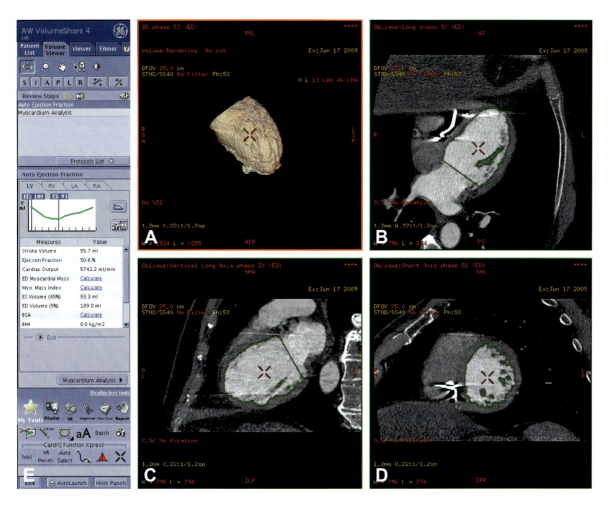

■ **Fig. 15.10** Fully automated global left ventricular function evaluation tool (Advantage Workstation, GE) shown in a patient with normal function and a pacemaker lead in the right ventricle (artifacts). The data are shown as a three-dimensional model (**Panel A**), four-chamber view (**Panel B**), two-chamber view (**Panel C**), and a short-axis view (**Panel D**). The endocardial contours are traced in green color. **Panel E** shows a volume-over-time curve and the numerical results of the left ventricle analysis. Figure courtesy of E. Martuscelli

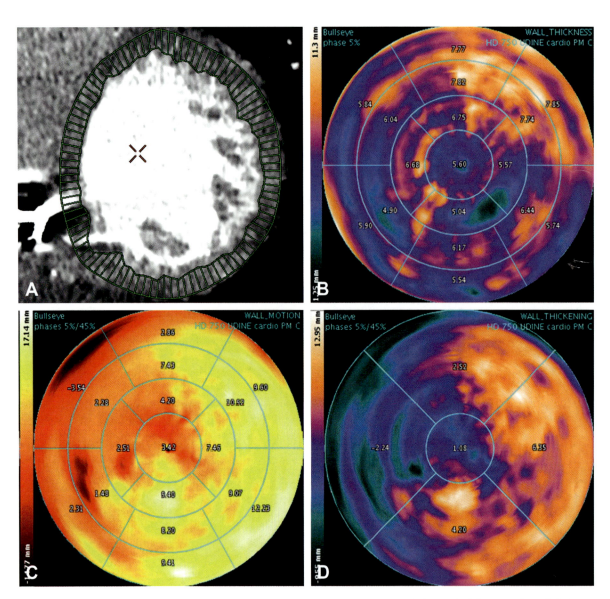

15

▣ **Fig. 15.11** By using "myocardium analysis" tool (Advantage Workstation, GE), the myocardial mass, the left ventricular wall thickness, wall motion, and systolic wall thickening can be measured. Epi- and endocardial contours are recognized automatically and can be adjusted manually if necessary (**Panel A**). Results are presented in the bull's eye view for left ventricular wall thickness (**Panel B**), left ventricular wall motion (**Panel C**), and systolic wall thickening (**Panel D**). Figure courtesy of E. Martuscelli

15.5.5 Terarecon (Aquarius iNtuition)

The cardiac function tool from Terarecon allows uploading datasets with multiple cardiac phases. Epi- and endocardial contours of the left ventricle are recognized automatically and can be adjusted manually (**Fig. 15.12**). The software recognizes end-systole and end-diastole.

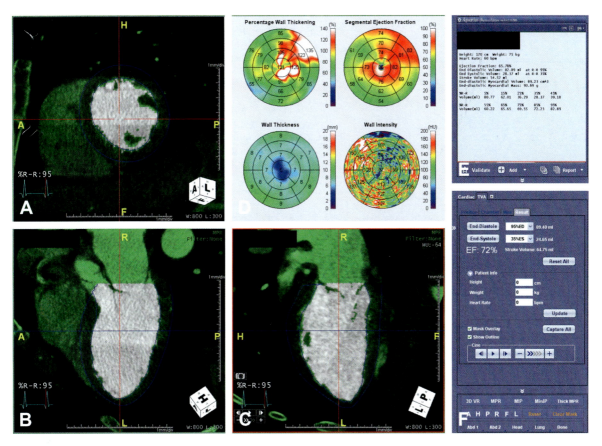

☐ **Fig. 15.12** Left ventricular function analysis with the software tool from Terarecon (Aquarius iNtuition). Epi- and endocardial contours of the left ventricle are recognized, the myocardium is colored in green and shown as short-axis view (**Panel A**) and long-axis views (**Panels B** and **C**). Results are presented numerically (**Panels E** and **F**) and also in the bull's eye view (**Panel D**). In addition to the standard values – percentage wall thickening, segmental ejection fraction and wall thickness – the wall intensity is also evaluated, which represents the segmental Hounsfield units of the left ventricle myocardium. Figure courtesy of Terarecon

Recommended Reading

1   Bansal D, Singh RM, Sarkar M et al (2008) Assessment of left ventricular function: comparison of cardiac multidetector-row computed tomography with two-dimension standard echocardiography for assessment of left ventricular function. Int J Cardiovasc Imaging 24:317–325

2   Cury RC, Nieman K, Shapiro MD et al (2008) Comprehensive assessment of myocardial perfusion defects, regional wall motion, and left ventricular function by using 64-section multidetector CT. Radiology 248:466–475

3   Dewey M, Müller M, Eddicks S et al (2006) Evaluation of global and regional left ventricular function with 16-slice computed tomography, biplane cineventriculography, and two-dimensional transthoracic echocardiography: comparison with magnetic resonance imaging. J Am Coll Cardiol 48:2034–2044

4   Dewey M, Müller M, Teige F et al (2006) Multisegment and halfscan reconstruction of 16-slice computed tomography for assessment of regional and global left ventricular myocardial function. Invest Radiol 41:400–409

5   Dewey M, Müller M, Teige F, Hamm B (2006) Evaluation of a semi-automatic software tool for left ventricular function analysis with 16-slice computed tomography. Eur Radiol 16:25–31

6   Fischbach R, Juergens KU, Ozgun M et al (2007) Assessment of regional left ventricular function with multidetector-row computed tomography versus magnetic resonance imaging. Eur Radiol 17:1009–1017

7   Gilard M, Pennec PY, Cornily JC et al (2006) Multi-slice computer tomography of left ventricular function with automated analysis software in comparison with conventional ventriculography. Eur J Radiol 59:270–275

8   Jensen CJ, Jochims M, Hunold P et al (2010) Assessment of left ventricular function and mass in dual-source computed tomography coronary angiography influence of beta-blockers on left ventricular function: comparison to magnetic resonance imaging. Eur J Radiol. 74:484-91

9   Juergens KU, Seifarth H, Range F et al (2008) Automated threshold-based 3D segmentation versus short-axis planimetry for assessment of global left ventricular function with dual-source MDCT. Am J Roentgenol 190:308–314

10   Kerl JM, Ravenel JG, Nguyen SA et al (2008) Right heart: split-bolus injection of diluted contrast medium for visualization at coronary CT angiography. Radiology 247:356–364

11   Kristensen TS, Kofoed KF, Møller DV et al (2009) Quantitative assessment of left ventricular systolic wall thickening using multi-detector computed tomography. Eur J Radiol 72:92–97

12   Mühlenbruch G, Das M, Hohl C et al (2006) Global left ventricular function in cardiac CT. Evaluation of an automated 3D region-growing segmentation algorithm. Eur Radiol 16:1117–1123

13   Müller M, Teige F, Schnapauff D, Hamm B, Dewey M (2009) Evaluation of right ventricular function with multidetector computed tomography: comparison with magnetic resonance imaging and analysis of inter- and intraobserver variability. Eur Radiol 19:278–289

14   Remy-Jardin M, Delhaye D, Teisseire A, Hossein-Foucher C, Duhamel A, Remy J (2006) MDCT of right ventricular function: impact of methodologic approach in estimation of right ventricular ejection fraction, part 2. Am J Roentgenol 187:1605–1609

15   Schepis T, Gaemperli O, Koepfli P et al (2006) Comparison of 64-slice CT with gated SPECT for evaluation of left ventricular function. J Nucl Med 47:1288–1294

16   Stolzmann P, Scheffel H, Trindade PT et al (2008) Left ventricular and left atrial dimensions and volumes: comparison between dual-source CT and echocardiography. Invest Radiol 43:284–289

17   Stolzmann P, Scheffel H, Leschka S et al (2008) Reference values for quantitative left ventricular and left atrial measurements in cardiac computed tomography. Eur Radiol 18.1625–1634

18   van der Vleuten PA, de Jonge GJ et al (2009) Evaluation of global left ventricular function assessment by dual-source computed tomography compared with MRI. Eur Radiol 19:271–277

19   Vrachliotis TG, Bis KG, Haidary A et al (2007) Atypical chest pain: coronary, aortic, and pulmonary vasculature enhancement at biphasic single-injection 64-section CT angiography. Radiology 243:368–376

15

Cardiac Valves

G. Feuchtner

Abstract

This chapter reviews the current role of cardiac CT in valve imaging and outlines potential clinical applications and future developments.

16.1   Reading and Reporting

Through improvements in temporal resolution and the use of ECG gating during the entire cardiac cycle, four-dimensional cine imaging of cardiac valve function (**Fig. 16.1**) by computed tomography (CT) is feasible. The main advantage of cardiac CT is that the cardiac valves can be evaluated from the CT datasets acquired for assessment of the coronary arteries and left ventricular function.

The standard views for evaluation of the aortic valve and the mitral valve are summarized in **Table 16.1**. Please see also Chaps. 3 and 11 for details on anatomy and image interpretation.

16.2   CT Examination Technique

For evaluation of valvular morphology, at least one cardiac phase is necessary (e.g., for imaging of the bicuspid valve, the end-diastolic phase is sufficient). Hence, low-dose techniques such as prospective ECG gating can be used for evaluation of morphology. Also, aortic regurgitation can be assessed on static end-diastolic phases.

For evaluation of valvular function, CT data need to be acquired during the entire cardiac cycle. To date, retrospective ECG gating is the mode of first choice. ECG tube current modulation (with ~20% tube current reduction during systole) can be applied in the conventional mode, but leads to an increase in image noise, which can reach nondiagnostic levels, especially in morbidly obese patients. Special care needs to be taken when adjusting scan parameters for tube current modulation in obese patients (e.g., by tube current or tube voltage elevation). Very recently introduced prospective scan modes using dual-source and wide-area detector CT allow expansion of the scan window during the entire cardiac cycle, hence evaluation of cardiac function has become feasible.

A biphasic contrast agent injection protocol is advantageous over a monophasic injection for optimal timing of the contrast bolus to ensure right ventricular enhancement and adequate evaluation of all four cardiac valves and cardiac regional and global function. If only the aortic and mitral valves need to be assessed, a monophasic bolus injection as commonly applied for coronary CT angiography is appropriate.

M. Dewey, *Cardiac CT*,
DOI: 10.1007/978-3-642-14022-8_19, © Springer-Verlag Berlin Heidelberg 2011

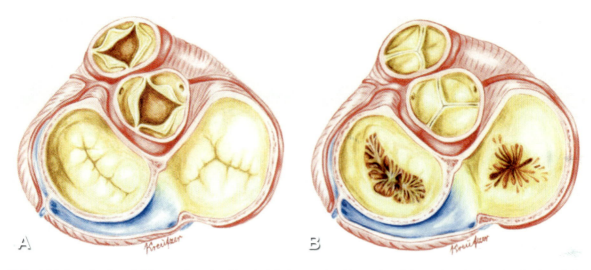

☐ **Fig. 16.1** Posterior view of all four cardiac valves (drawing) during systole with opening of the aortic and pulmonic valve (**Panel A**) as well as during early diastole (**Panel B**). Also shown are the left and right coronary artery arising from the left and right sinus of Valsalva, respectively, the posterior noncoronary sinus of Valsalva, and the great cardiac vein with the coronary sinus opening into the right atrium

☐ **Table 16.1** Standard views for cardiac valve evaluation

Aortic valve	Mitral valve
Left coronal oblique (**Figs. 16.2A, 16.3B**, and **16.9A and B**)	Two-chamber view (**Fig. 16.9C**)
Three-chamber view (**Figs. 16.3C, 16.5A,** and **16.8A,** and **16.10C,** and **D**)	
Cross-sectional LVOT (**Figs. 16.2C, 16.3A, 16.4,** and **16.5B**)	Short-axis LV at the level of the mitral annulus (**Fig. 16.6B**)

LVOT left ventricular outflow tract; *LV* left ventricle

16.3   Valvular Heart Disease

16.3.1   Aortic Stenosis

Degenerative aortic stenosis is very common with a prevalence of 2–5% in the elderly population >65 years. The pathomechanisms are similar to those in coronary heart disease, involving a degenerative process leading to aortic valve calcification and developing slowly during a lifetime. Rheumatic disease can cause aortic stenosis as well.

Transthoracic echocardiography is the clinical reference modality to establish the diagnosis of aortic stenosis, based on measurement of transvalvular pressure gradients and calculation of the aortic valve orifice area using the Doppler-velocity time integral (continuity equation). This formula has some limitations and its accuracy for hemodynamic estimation of the effective aortic valve orifice is limited, e.g., in the presence of low-flow, low-pressure gradient aortic stenosis, or in case of reduced cardiac output. In addition, other factors such as eccentricity of left ventricular outflow tract (LVOT) influence these measurements. In contrast, the anatomic (= geometric) aortic valve area obtained directly from cross-sectional imaging techniques such as cardiac CT (**Fig. 16.2**) or magnetic resonance imaging (MRI) is not affected by external factors and flow phenomena. Several studies, with more than 300 patients enrolled, showed a high correlation of CT with transthoracic echocardiography. The size of the aortic valve area is used to classify the severity of aortic stenosis as mild, moderate, and severe (**Table 16.2**). Images should be reconstructed at early/mid systole, which is the time point of maximal aortic valve opening. The

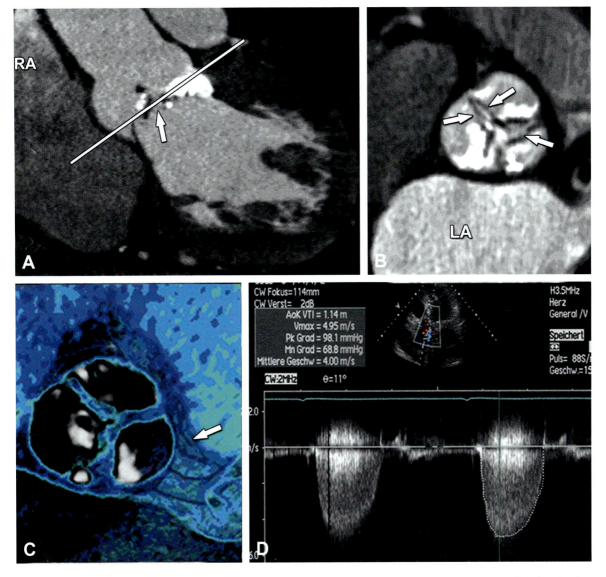

Fig. 16.2 Tricuspid aortic valve with severe calcification and stenosis. Left coronal oblique view of aortic root (**Panel A**). The white line in **Panel A** indicates the position of the cross-sectional image of the aortic root (**Panel B**) which allows measurement of the inner aortic valve orifice area (delineated with *arrows*). The calcifications are also nicely shown in a three-dimensional volume rendering (**Panel C**) with the *arrow* pointing at the left coronary ostium. Transthoracic echocardiography (**Panel D**) shows increased velocity of 4 m/s and transvalvular pressure gradient (PK Grad = peak gradient; Mn Grad = mean gradient) over the aortic valve. *RA* right atrium; *LA* left atrium

views for evaluation of the aortic valve are shown in **Fig. 16.3** and listed in **Table 16.1**. Multiplanar reformations should be applied.

There may be two useful clinical applications for measurement of the aortic valve area: first, in patients referred for coronary CT angiography, if valve calcification is present, the aortic valve area may be measure because these patients may have aortic stenosis or just non-stenotic valve calcification. Second, patients who require a second imaging modality for accurate sizing of the aortic valve area, e.g., in case of pending cardiac surgery,

Table 16.2 Staging of aortic stenosis (AS)

Classification	Staging	AVA
AS I	Mild	>1.5 cm²
AS II	Moderate	1.0–1.5 cm²
AS III	Severe	<1.0 cm²
	Severe critical	<0.7 cm²

AVA aortic valve area

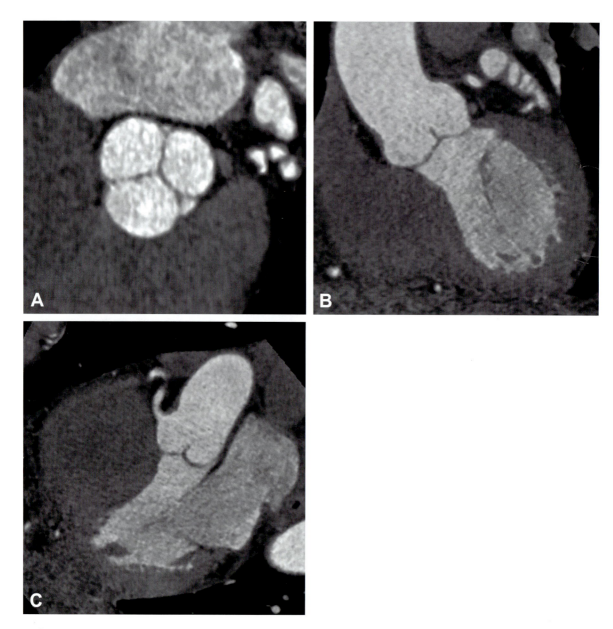

▫ **Fig. 16.3** Three standard views of the aortic valve. Cross-sectional axial oblique (**Panel A**), left coronal oblique (**Panel B**), and three-chamber view (**Panel C**) reconstructed with double-oblique multiplanar reformations

and/or if echocardiography has inherent limitations such as in low-flow low-gradient aortic stenosis. In these patients, CT can also yield information about the presence of coronary artery disease, left ventricular function, and the size of the aortic annulus. Left ventricular function is a valuable predictor of outcome in severe aortic stenosis. Accurate sizing of aortic root dimensions is required especially before minimally invasive aortic valve replacement or percutaneous transcatheter valve implantation.

16.3.2 Bicuspid Aortic Valve

CT can also identify bicuspid or tricuspid valve morphology (**Fig. 16.4**). The aortic valve can be congenitally bicuspid (without or with fused raphe) or develop a secondary degenerative bicuspid shape due to calcification and adhesions. This information is of interest in clinical practice for cardiac surgeons to define the surgical approach (valve replacement versus possible surgical reconstruction) or to define further patient management.

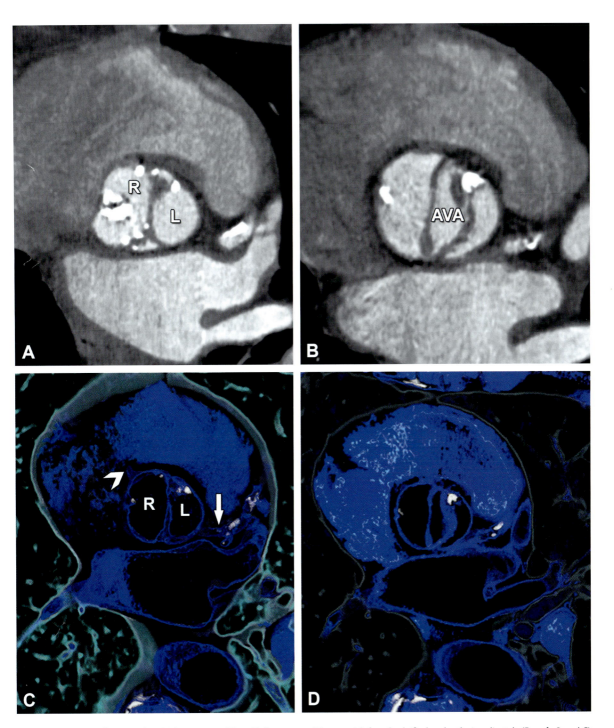

Fig. 16.4 Bicuspid aortic valve. Right coronary (R) and left coronary (L) cusp with fused calcified raphe during diastole (**Panels A** and **C**). During mid-systole (**Panels B** and **D**), the inner aortic valve orifice area (AVA) can be visualized and quantified (**Panel B**). Note the characteristic "fish-mouth" opening of the bicuspid valve (**Panels B** and **D**). Postprocessing with multiplanar reformations (**Panels A** and **B**) and black-blood volume rendering (**Panels C** and **D**). Volume rendering enables imaging of aortic root morphology and the origin of coronary ostia (**Panel C**) with the left (*arrow*) and the right coronary artery (*arrowhead*)

Congenital bicuspid valves are prone to developing dysfunction (regurgitation or stenosis), hence those patients may need to be followed up closer.

16.3.3   Aortic Valve Calcification

CT allows quantification of aortic valve calcifications by using the same commercially available software as for coronary artery calcium scores. The aortic valve calcium score provides independent prognostic information in patients with asymptomatic aortic stenosis. Moreover, an aortic valve calcium score cut-off of 1,100 Agatston units is associated with a high likelihood of aortic stenosis. Thus all patients referred for nonenhanced coronary calcium scoring, in whom aortic valve calcification is an incidental finding, should be referred for transthoracic echocardiography for further evaluation.

16.3.4   Aortic Regurgitation

The onset of aortic regurgitation is either acute or chronic. Whilst acute aortic regurgitation is seen in fulminant infective endocarditis or ascending aortic dissection involving the valve, chronic aortic regurgitation can develop on the basis of several underlying diseases, the most common being aortic root dilatation and aneurysm formation (**Fig. 16.5**) as well as degenerative or rheumatic disease.

In patients with aortic regurgitation, cardiac CT allows visualization of the anatomic regurgitant orifice area. This area can be seen as central valvular leakage area, reflecting an incomplete co-adaption of cusps (**Fig. 16.5**), by selecting end-diastolic CT datasets, which are usually reconstructed for coronary CT angiography. The regurgitant orifice area is a reliable diagnostic criterion for identifying aortic regurgitation. Several studies demonstrated the ability of CT to detect moderate and severe aortic regurgitation. Mild aortic regurgitation can be missed in the presence of dense valvular calcification or in patients with bicuspid valves. Contradictory data are available regarding the accuracy of CT in grading the severity of aortic regurgitation. One study mostly including patients with prevailing aortic root dilatation and rather mildly calcified valves, found a good performance of CT in differentiating moderate (cut-off: regurgitant orifice area >25 mm^2) and severe aortic regurgitation (cut-off: regurgitant orifice area >75 mm^2). Other studies recruited mainly patients with degenerative valve disease and observed a limited accuracy of CT in distinguishing the degrees of aortic regurgitation based on the regurgitant orifice area. Besides measurement of the regurgitant orifice area, newly introduced software modules enable right and left ventricular volume segmentation, hence they may provide a quantification tool for functional calculation of the aortic regurgitation fraction and volume, based on right and left stroke volume mismatch.

Preoperative triage is an important clinical application of cardiac CT in patients with aortic regurgitation. CT allows differentiation between bicuspid and tricuspid valve morphology and offers the advantage of simultaneous, accurate sizing of the aortic root and the ascending aorta as well as the evaluation of coronary arteries and left ventricular function within one scan.

The aortic valve should be evaluated in all patients undergoing CT angiography for possible concomitant underlying aortic regurgitation, in particular if no recent echocardiography exam was performed. In case of a visible regurgitation on CT, the patients should be further evaluated with echocardiography.

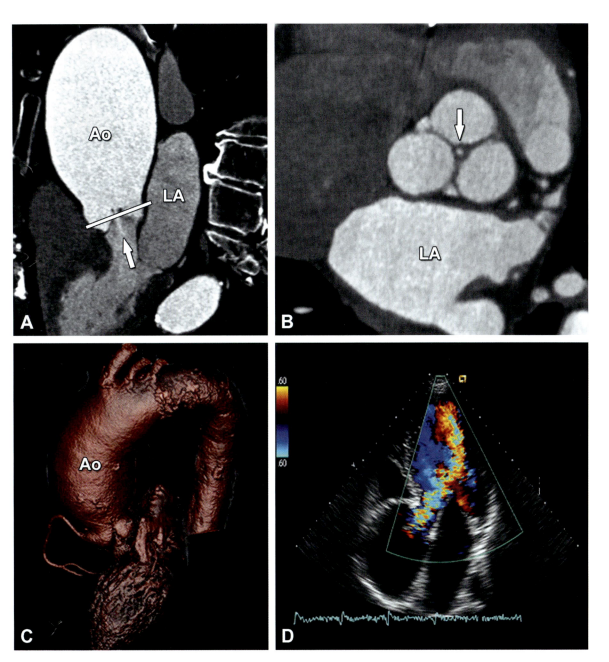

Fig. 16.5 Aortic regurgitation due to ascending aortic (Ao) aneurysm. The three-chamber view (**Panel A**) shows incomplete closure of the aortic leaflets during diastole with a regurgitant jet downstream into the left ventricular outflow tract (*arrow*). The white line in **Panel A** indicates the position of the cross-section through the aortic root (**Panel B**). This cross-section shows central valvular leakage (*arrow*, aortic regurgitant orifice area). The ascending aortic aneurysm is shown in a three-dimensional volume rendering in (**Panel C**) and the corresponding echocardiography (**Panel D**) shows a Doppler regurgitation jet ("vena contracts") towards the left atrium. *LA* left atrium

16.3.5   Mitral Stenosis

The prevailing etiology of mitral stenosis is rheumatic disease, leading to leaflet thickening and structural degeneration of the valve apparatus including the chordae and causing obstruction of left ventricular inflow. Echocardiography is the imaging method of choice for grading mitral stenosis. Evaluation encompasses a combination of transvalvular pressure gradients, pulmonary artery systolic pressure, and an assessment of the mitral valve orifice area for differentiating between mild, moderate, and severe stages of disease. Mitral valve stenosis is regarded as significant if the mitral orifice area is less than 1 cm²/m² body surface area. Only one study has assessed the value of CT in mitral stenosis, showing good correlation of planimetric measurement of the mitral valve orifice area (**Fig. 16.6**) with those obtained from transesophageal echocardiography. Doming of mitral leaflets (**Fig. 16.6A**) is a further very typical imaging finding in mitral stenosis.

Left atrial dilatation, subsequently inducing atrial fibrillation, is common in advanced mitral stenosis. Hence, left atrial appendage thrombus, is a typical result.

Importantly, cardiac CT allows accurate exclusion of left atrial thrombus. Care needs to be taken when filling defects are seen in the left atrial appendage, since these may represent either spontaneous echo contrast or artificial lack of contrast agent due to incomplete filling. A transesophageal echocardiography exam or a late-phase CT is required in case of uncertainty.

16.3.6   Mitral Regurgitation

The etiology of mitral regurgitation is variable. Mitral regurgitation may develop as a primary condition, such as in the course of rheumatic, degenerative or infectious disease, but also secondary to mitral annulus dilatation in ischemic or nonischemic cardiomyopathy. Another underlying disease is classic mitral valve prolapse.

One study employed the potential of CT to quantify the degree of mitral regurgitation and showed good correlation of planimetric measurement of the regurgitant orifice area at CT with both echocardiography and ventriculography. However, an overlap between the different

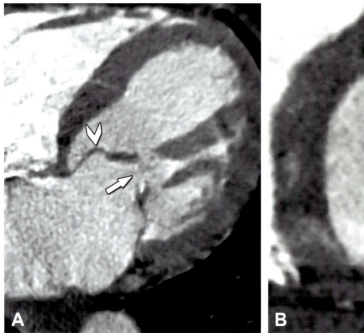
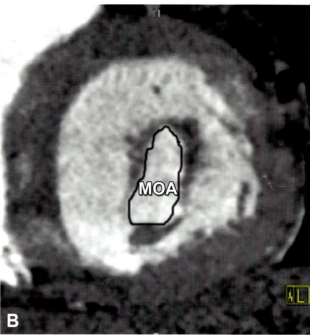

□ Fig. 16.6 Mitral stenosis with a four-chamber view (**Panel A**) showing the stenotic mitral valve orifice (*arrow*) and doming of anterior leaflet (*arrowhead*). The short-axis view of the left ventricle (**Panel B**) at the level of the mitral valve during diastole allows quantification of the mitral orifice area (MOA)

grades of mitral regurgitation as determined with CT was found. Thus, given few scientific data, accurate identification and quantification of the disease with CT seems not feasible at this time.

16.3.7   Mitral Annular Calcification

However, CT provides a valuable imaging modality for clarifying valvular morphology and masses that are unclear on echocardiography. Mitral annular calcification is a degenerative process, which typically shows slow circular progression from an initial U-shape or J-shape to O-shape in end-stage disease. On occasion, these calcifications appear mass-like with a mass effect, typically protruding into the adjacent myocardium from the base of the annulus (**Fig. 16.7**). A special subtype of mitral annular calcification is mitral caseous calcification, which typically presents as a central echolucent mass on echocardiography which can be difficult to distinguish from other tumors. With cardiac CT, the diagnosis of mitral annular calcification can be easily established or confirmed based on a prevailing calcific component (**Fig. 16.7B**).

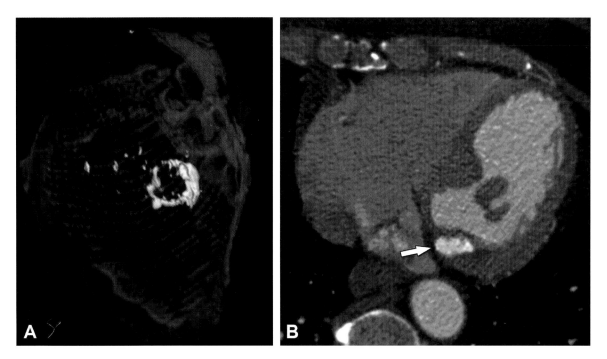

☐ **Fig. 16.7** Mitral annular calcification. Such an annulus calcification typically originates from the base of the annulus (U-shape) and progresses upstream in a circular fashion until involving the entire annulus, finally forming an O-shape (**Panel A**, three-dimensional reconstruction). Ovoid calcified mass (*arrow* in **Panel B**) at the base of the mitral annulus, which can mimic a fibrous mass on echocardiography. CT can help to clarify the exclusively calcific nature. Mitral annular calcification may serve as a marker for other cardiac structural abnormalities such as mitral regurgitation

16.3.8   Mitral Valve Prolapse

Mitral valve prolapse is defined as systolic displacement of mitral valve leaflets below the mitral annulus plane (**Fig. 16.8**). The prevalence is 2.3% in the general population. There are two types of prolapsed. The first, *billowing,* (bowing of the leaflet), typically develops in the course of myxomatous degeneration and thickening due to redundant leaflets with increased thickness (>2–5 mm). A mid-systolic click murmur is characteristic.

In contrast, a *flail leaflet* (=free leaflet edge prolapse) is a result of chordal rupture, e.g., in the presence of rheumatic disease, infective endocarditis, or rarely of trauma or myocardial infarction, which is not necessarily associated with concomitant leaflet thickening. In general, a mitral leaflet is regarded as thickened if it measures more than 2 mm during diastole.

Transthoracic echocardiography is the reference method to establish the diagnosis of mitral valve prolaps. Three-dimensional transesophageal echocardiography is used for detailed preoperative characterization of the extent of involvement if surgical mitral reconstruction is planned. A recent study has shown that CT allows accurate diagnosis of prolapse, if three-chamber and two-chamber views reconstructed during systole are used in combination. The criterion used for definite diagnosis of mitral valve prolapse is leaflet displacement of more than 2 mm below the mitral annulus. However, the saddle-shape of the mitral valve leads to overestimation of the extent of prolapse on four-chamber views on CT, similar to echocardiography.

16.3.9   Infective Endocarditis

Valvular involvement is most commonly found in infective endocarditits, however, the entire endocardium can become involved in inflammation. Notably, intracardiac devices such as prosthetic valves, pacemaker leads, or atrial septal defect occluders are prone to infections and subsequently, vegetations. Masses attached to those devices can represent either thrombi, pannus, or vegetations. A differentiation cannot be made based on imaging findings; laboratory parameters are needed as evidence of infection.

Imaging findings are the key to establishing the diagnosis of infective endocarditis according to the modified Duke criteria, besides clinical parameters such as

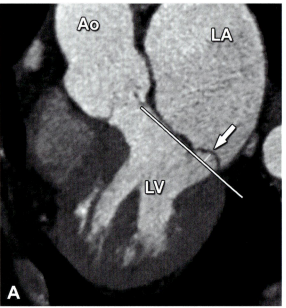
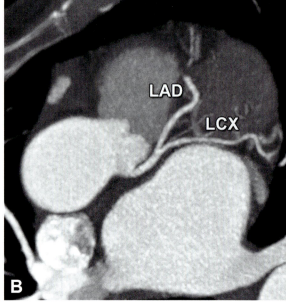

■ **Fig. 16.8** Mitral valve prolapse. Billowing (=bowing) of posterior leaflet (*arrow*) below the annulus plane (white line) on a three-chamber view (**Panel A**). Note myxomatous thickening of anterior leaflet without prolapse (**Panel A**). The mitral valve is closed during systole. In this patient, also coronary artery disease could be excluded (**Panel B**). Note normal left anterior descending coronary artery (LAD) and left circumflex coronary artery (LCX). *Ao* ascending aorta; *LA* left atrium; *LV* left ventricle positive blood culture and signs of infections (major/minor criteria). Transesophageal echocardiography is the current reference method to assess imaging findings. Further, exact morphological evaluation defines the management of patients: small (<1 cm) and nonmobile lesions, without paravalvular involvement, can be treated conventionally with medication while cardiac surgery is indicated for large and mobile lesions or paravalvular involvement.

Typical imaging findings are shown in **Fig. 16.9** and recommendations for image reformation are summarized in **Table 16.3**.

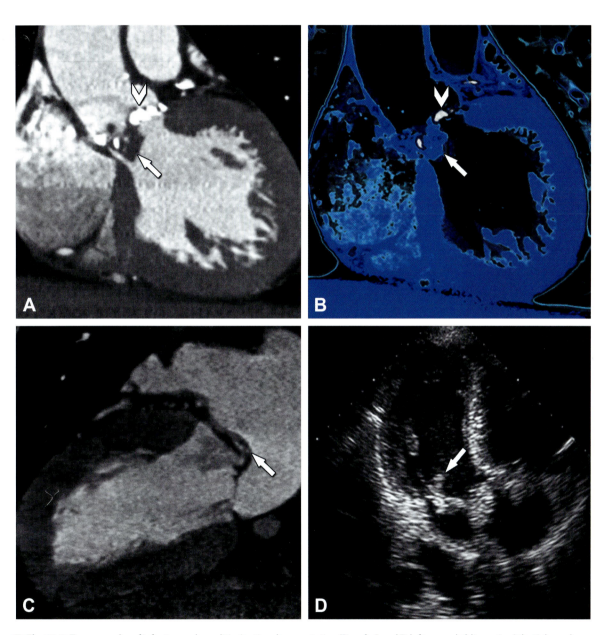

🔲 **Fig. 16.9** Two examples of infective endocarditis. Aortic valve vegetation (**Panels A** and **B**, left coronal oblique view) that is hypodense and prolapses into the left ventricular outflow tract (*arrow*). Note calcified spots on the aortic valve, which can be clearly distinguished from the vegetation (*arrowhead* in **Panels A** and **B**). Mitral leaflet perforation and vegetation in another patient (*arrow* in **Panel C**) with contrast agent between the split two layers of thickened leaflets in a two-chamber view. The corresponding echocardiography with the mitral valve vegetation (*arrow*) is shown in **Panel D**

> ▣ **Table 16.3** CT Imaging findings in infective endocarditis

	CT findings
Vegetations	Hypodense (~30HU) soft tissue masses Varying in size and shape, ranging from well-defined masses (typically round, ovoid, or pedunculated) to rather diffuse irregular leaflet thickening.
Cusp perforation	Discontinuation in cusps (= contrast agent between cusps)
Paravalvular involvement	
– abscess	Loss of perivascular/periaortic fatty tissue and diffuse infiltration (>0 HU, ca. 10–50 HU)
– aneurysm	Cavity filled with contrast agent
Valvular regurgitation	
– aortic	Incomplete closure of cusps during diastole
– mitral	Incomplete closure of cusps during systole
Fistula	Communication between chambers or extracardiac vascular system (e.g., aorta)
Dehiscence (prosthetic valve)	Displacement >5° above annulus plane

MPR multiplanar reformation; *VRT* volume rendering technique; *CH* chamber; *LV* left ventricle; *LVOT* left ventricular outflow tract; *SA* short axis

CT allows imaging of valvular abnormalities and extravalvular involvement in infective endocarditis. Its advantage is the differentiation between calcifying and soft-tissue masses, which can be difficult on echocardiography. Hence, CT can help to clarify uncertain echocardiography findings, in particular in patients with equivocal or contradicting clinical findings. Moreover, the main advantage of CT in those patients is comprehensive evaluation of coronary arteries before surgery. Thus, conventional coronary angiography, with the risk of embolization originating from valvular vegetations, may be avoided.

16.3.10 Prosthetic Valves

There are two different prosthetic valve types: mechanical and bioprosthetic valves. The St. Jude bileaflet mechanical valve (**Fig. 16.10**) is currently the most commonly implanted type. Cardiac CT allows dynamic four-dimensional cine imaging of leaflet motion. Thus, CT can assist echocardiography in defining the cause of prosthetic valve dysfunction such as broken metallic leaflets, or stuck valves. Masses attached to a prosthetic valve can represent either thrombus or pannus (=chronic organized thrombus) or vegetations in case of clinical signs of infection. Another type of dysfunction is dehiscence, a loose connection between the prosthesis and the annulus (**Table 16.3**). Paravalvular leakage and regurgitation can occur after prosthetic valve implantation, which may need intervention depending on severity of backflow. In contrast, bioprosthetic valves may tend to slowly develop structural degeneration over time, leading to leaflet thickening, calcification, and destruction of leaflets and the apparatus. Paravalvular leakage may occur as a result of a disconnection between the prosthesis and the annulus (=dehiscence or suture loosening).

The detection rate of mechanical aortic valve dysfunction is low with ~51% by echocardiography, since metal artifacts hamper image quality. CT has shown to be a promising and valuable imaging modality in patients with suspected prosthetic valve dysfunction. Initial data suggest that the diagnostic performance of CT may be better than that of echocardiography. Thus, CT may be considered as an additional modality in case of uncertain echocardiography findings in patients with suspected prosthetic valve dysfunction or infection.

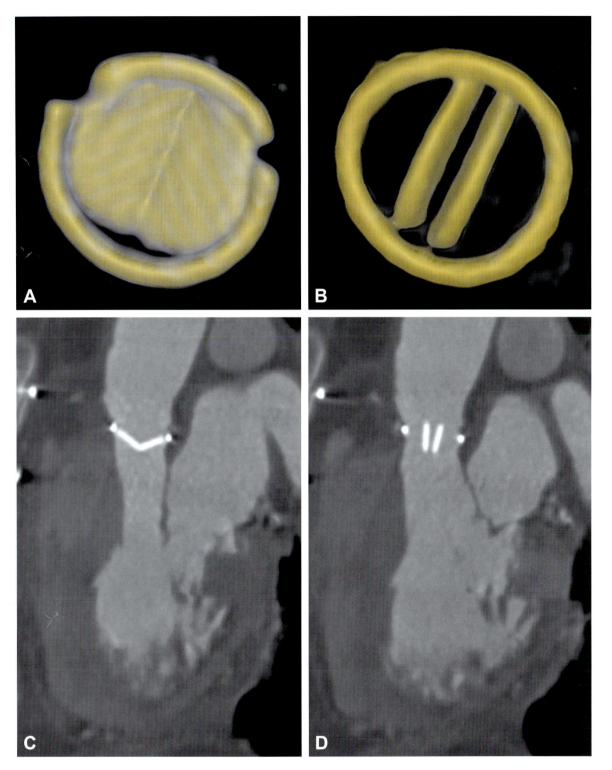

🔲 **Fig. 16.10** Mechanical aortic prosthetic valve (bileaflet type, St. Jude). Closed valve during end-diastole (**Panels A** and **C**) and opened valve during systole (**Panels B** and **D**). Data are displayed using volume rendering (**Panels A** and **B**) and multiplanar reformations in the three-chamber view (**Panels C** and **D**)

To summarize, aortic valve disease is currently considered the main use of CT in the context of valvular disease. New promising clinical applications of cardiac CT include infective endocarditis, prosthetic valves, and the implementation of CT for planning of minimally invasive surgical or transcatheter valvular interventions.

Recommended Reading

1   Alkadhi H, Desbiolles L, Husmann L et al (2007) Aortic regurgitation: assessment with 64-Section CT. Radiology 245:111–121

2   Alkahdi H, Bettex D, Wildermuth S et al (2005) Dynamic cine imaging of the mitral valve with 16-MDCT: a feasibility study. AJR Am J Roentgenol 185:636–646

3   Bonow RO, Carabello BA, Chatterjee K et al (2006) ACC/AHA 2006 guidelines for the management of patients with valvular heart disease. J Am Coll Cardiol 48:e1–e148

4   Bouvier E, Logeart D, Sablayrolles JL et al (2006) Diagnosis of aortic valvular stenosis by multislice cardiac computed tomography. Eur Heart J 27:3033–3038

5   Dewey M, Müller M, Eddicks S et al (2006) Evaluation of global and regional left ventricular function with 16-slice computed tomography, biplane cineventriculography, and two-dimensional transthoracic echocardiography: comparison with magnetic resonance imaging. J Am Coll Cardiol 48:2034–2044

6   Feuchtner GM (2009) The utility of computed tomography in the context of aortic valve disease. Int J Cardiovasc Imaging 25:611–614

7   Feuchtner GM, Dichtl W, Friedrich GJ et al (2006) Multislice computed tomography for detection of patients with aortic valve stenosis and quantification of severity. J Am Coll Cardiol 47: 1410–1417

8   Feuchtner GM, Dichtl W, Müller S et al (2008) 64-MDCT for diagnosis of aortic regurgitation in patients referred to CT coronary angiography. Am J Roentgenol 191:W1–W7

9   Feuchtner G, Alkadhi H, Karlo C et al (2010) Cardiac CT angiography for the diagnosis of mitral valve prolapse: comparison with echocardiography. Radiology 254:374–383

10 Feuchtner GM, Stolzmann P, Dichtl W et al (2009) Multislice computed tomography in infective endocarditis: comparison with transesophageal echocardiography and intraoperative findings. J Am Coll Cardiol 53:436–444

11 Kim YY, Klein AL, Halliburton SS et al (2007) Left atrial appendage filling defects identified by multidetector computed tomography in patients undergoing radiofrequency pulmonary vein antral isolation: a comparison with transesophageal echocardiography. Am Heart J 154:1199–1205

12 Konen E, Goitein O, Feinberg MS et al (2008) The role of ECG-gated MDCT in the evaluation of aortic and mitral mechanical valves: initial experience. Am J Roentgenol 191:26–31

13 Messika-Zeitoun D, Aubry MC, Detaint D et al (2004) Evaluation and clinical implications of aortic valve calcification measured by electron-beam computed tomography. Circulation 110:356–362

14 Messika-Zeitoun D, Serfaty JM, Laissy JP et al (2006) Assessment of the mitral valve area in patients with mitral stenosis by multislice computed tomography. J Am Coll Cardiol 48:411–413

15 Meijboom WB, Mollet NR, Van Mieghem CA et al (2006) Preoperative computed tomography coronary angiography to detect significant coronary artery disease in patients referred for cardiac valve surgery. J Am Coll Cardiol 48:1658–1665

16 Pouleur AC, le Polain de Waroux JB et al (2007) Aortic valve area assessment: multidetector CT compared with cine MR imaging and transthoracic and transesophageal echocardiography. Radiology 244:745–754

17 Tops LF, Wood DA, Delgado V et al (2008) Noninvasive evaluation of the aortic root with multislice computed tomography implications for transcatheter aortic valve replacement. JACC Cardiovasc Imaging 1:321–330

18 Shah RG, Novaro GM, Blandon RJ et al (2009) Aortic valve area: meta-analysis of diagnostic performance of multi-detector computed tomography for aortic valve area measurements as compared to transthoracic echocardiography. Int J Cardiovasc Imaging 25:601–609

19 Tsai IC, Lin YK, Chang Y et al (2009) Correctness of multi-detector-row computed tomography for diagnosing mechanical prosthetic heart valve disorders using operative findings as a gold standard. Eur Radiol 19:857–867

16

Coronary Artery Anomalies

P.G.C. Begemann, M. Grigoryev, G. Lund, G. Adam, and M. Dewey

Abstract

This chapter gives an overview of coronary anomalies and their development, the course of anomalous coronary arteries, and their classification and clinical importance.

17.1 Embryonic Development

The development of the coronary arteries is a self-organizing process in the subepicardial space, resulting in the formation of a vascular plexus, which connects to the aorta in later stages. This process comprises three major developmental steps: vasculogenesis, angiogenesis, and embryonic arteriogenesis (**Fig. 17.1**).

In the initial stage of embryonic development of the heart, the endocardium and myocardium are being nourished by the blood flowing through the lumen of the heart tube. By the beginning of the third week, as the walls of the developing heart become thicker, diffusion is no longer sufficient to supply the heart tube. At this stage endothelial precursor cells migrate into the myocardium and commence forming the primordial vascular structures (vasculogenesis). The initial channels formed within the epicardial covering are scattered throughout the myocardium, inducing an epicardial-to-endocardial vascular gradient, regulated among others by ventricular epicardial growth factor.

Similar to the first stage, the second stage of development – angiogenesis – also appears to be regulated by hypoxia. There is still no continuity between the separate vascular structures and there is no circulation of systemic blood within them. Later, the vessels coalesce to form the primary vascular plexus. The complex network of the subepicardial primary plexus expands along the dorsal and ventral interventricular sulcus, the atrioventricular sulcus, and then along the base of the truncus arteriosus throughout the myocardium. The vessels sprouting from the primary plexus form new septa and pillars within the vascular lumen, giving rise to the peritruncal ring of capillaries.

Only at the late stages of development will the vascular network gain access to the aortic root (arteriogenesis, **Fig. 17.2**). The vessels from the peritruncal ring sprout preferentially into the aorta, establishing multiple connections to the left and right aortic sinuses and much

M. Dewey, *Cardiac CT*,
DOI: 10.1007/978-3-642-14022-8_20, © Springer-Verlag Berlin Heidelberg 2011

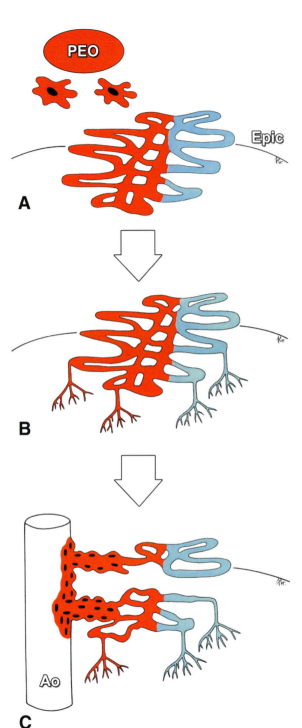

Fig. 17.1 Development of the coronary arteries. Vasculogenesis includes the in situ formation of a primitive capillary plexus in the subepicardial space from immature endothelial precursors partly originating from the proepicardial organ (PEO in **Panel A**). This is also the phase during which early differentiation into arterial (*red*) and venous (*blue*) endothelium occurs. Angiogenesis is initiated by the formation of a vascular network via transmyocardial sprouting from preexisting vessels and intussusception, i.e., formation of new pillars and septations within the vascular sprouts (**Panel B**). Subsequent embryonal arteriogenesis begins with the connection of the network to the aorta (Ao) and continues with extensive remodeling, formation of distinct vascular provinces, recruitment of smooth muscle cells, and vascular stabilization (**Panel C**). For details on arteriogenesis of the coronaries see **Fig. 17.2.** *Epic* epicardium. Modified from Y. von Kodolitsch et al. Zeitschrift für Kardiologie 2004

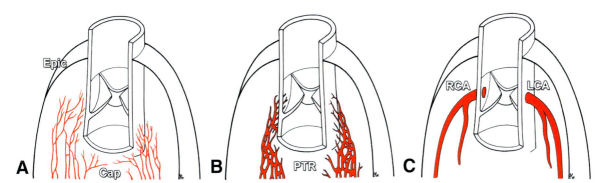

Fig. 17.2 Arteriogenesis of the coronary arteries. Multiple capillaries (Cap) form the primary vascular plexus beneath the epicardium (Epic in **Panel A**). Around the aorta and pulmonary trunk the capillaries coalesce to form a peritruncal ring (PTR in **Panel B**). Subsequently, multiple vessels extend towards the aorta and invade it. The peritruncal ring is reduced to the mainline coronary artery pattern with the right (RCA) and left coronary artery (LCA) attached to the aorta at the corresponding coronary sinuses (**Panel C**). Modified from Bernanke et al. Anat Rec 2002

fewer to the posterior (noncoronary) aortic sinus. The hemodynamic changes associated with this access to the aortic root appear to initiate the vascular maturation of the network and its aortic orifices. The migration of smooth muscle cells and pericytes from the epicardium and the aortic root to the primitive vascular structures and their coalescence with them are the next step of a vascular maturation. As a result, stable arteries are formed; they grow radially and the peritruncal ring with its numerous vessels undergoes partial regression (**Fig. 17.2**). Defects at any stage of this complex development can lead to coronary anomalies.

□ **Table 17.1** Modified classification of coronary anomalies according to Paolo Angelini

A. Anomalies of origin and course
1. Absent LM with split origin of LCA (**Fig. 17.4**).
2. Anomalous location (high, low, commissural) of coronary ostium within aortic root or near proper aortic sinus of Valsalva
3. Anomalous location of coronary ostium outside normal "coronary" aortic sinuses Right posterior aortic sinus, ascending aorta or aortic arch, left or right ventricle, pulmonary artery, etc.
4. Anomalous location of coronary ostium at improper sinus, including joint origin (**Fig. 17.3**, **Figs. 17.5–17.10**)
5. Single coronary artery
B. Anomalies of intrinsic coronary arterial anatomy
1. Congenital ostial stenosis or atresia, coronary ectasia or aneurysm, absence or hypoplasia of coronary artery etc. (**Fig. 17.12**)
2. Intramural (muscular bridge, Chap. 3) or subendocardial course or coronary crossing
3. Anomalous origin of PD, split LAD or RCA, or ectopic origin of first septal branch
C. Anomalies of coronary termination
1. Inadequate arteriolar/capillary ramifications
2. Fistulas from RCA or LCA (**Figs. 17.14** and **17.15**)
D. Anomalous anastomotic vessels

LM left main coronary artery; *LCA* left coronary artery; *LAD* left descending coronary artery; *RCA* right coronary artery; *LCX* left circumflex artery; *PD* posterior descending

The table and classification was modified from Angelini Circulation 2007

17.2   Classification

Many different classifications of coronary artery anomalies have been proposed to categorize the enormous number of variations in coronary artery anatomy. This section gives an overview to serve as a basis for an adequate description of coronary anomalies and to facilitate identification of potentially clinically important variants. Most classifications of coronary anomalies rely exclusively on the description of the anatomic variant. The approach favored here is based on the classification proposed by Paolo Angelini (Circulation 2007). Other classifications group anomalous coronary arteries according to their origin, course, or termination. Coronary artery anomalies can also be functionally divided into hemodynamically significant (malignant type) and hemodynamically nonsignificant (benign type). The malignant type consists of coronary artery variants that can cause ischemia and even sudden cardiac death.

According to Angelini, coronary anomalies can be anatomically divided into anomalies of origin and course, of intrinsic anatomy, of termination, and anomalous anastomotic vessels (**Table 17.1**). The origin and course of the anomalous coronary artery determine its possible clinical impact to the greatest extent. Instead of an origin from the proper sinus of Valsalva, coronary arteries can arise from the opposite sinus and take different pathways to reach the myocardial area they are supplying. On its course to the opposite site, the coronary artery can pass anterior to the pulmonary artery (**Fig. 17.3**), posterior to the aorta, or interarterially between the aorta and pulmonary trunk, or even intraseptally (subpulmonic course). Coronary anomalies also occur in association with congenital heart disease, for example with tetralogy of Fallot, transposition of the great arteries or pulmonary atresia (Chap. 18).

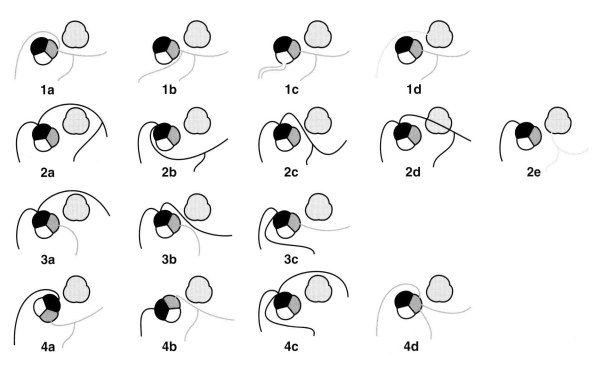

☐ **Fig. 17.3** Different courses of anomalously located coronary ostia at improper sinus with

1 showing anomalies of the right coronary artery (RCA) (a: anterior interarterial course, b: posterior course from left sinus of Valsalva, c: posterior course from the noncoronary sinus, d: anterior course from the pulmonary artery),

2 of the left main coronary artery (LM) (a: anterior course, b: posterior course, c: interarterial course, d: septal course, e: from the pulmonary artery (Bland–White–Garland syndrome)),

3 of the central branches of the left coronary artery (a: anterior course, b: interarterial course, c: posterior course), and

4 of both the right and left coronary arteries (a: orthotopic origins from clockwise rotated aortic bulb, b: orthotopic origins from counter-clockwise rotated aortic bulb, c: three origins from the right sinus, d: three origins from the left sinus). Aortic root: black: right sinus, grey: left sinus, white: noncoronary sinus. The pulmonary artery is shown completely in grey anterolateral to the aortic root. With permission from Schmitt et al. Eur Radiol 2005

17.3   Clinical Relevance

The prevalence of coronary anomalies is reported to be 0.3% up to 5.6%, depending on the literature source. In a large study of over 100,000 patients examined by conventional coronary angiography the prevalence of coronary anomalies was found to be around 1.3%. There is also evidence that prevalence varies according to geographic region.

17.3.1   Benign Coronary Anomalies

Coronary anomalies without compromise of blood flow to the myocardium or severe fistulas are considered benign. The simplest coronary anomaly is the absence of the left main coronary artery (split left coronary) with a separate origin of the left anterior descending and left circumflex coronary artery (**Fig. 17.4**). The most common course of a benign anomalous coronary artery is the prepulmonary (**Fig. 17.5**) and retroaortic path (**Fig. 17.6**).

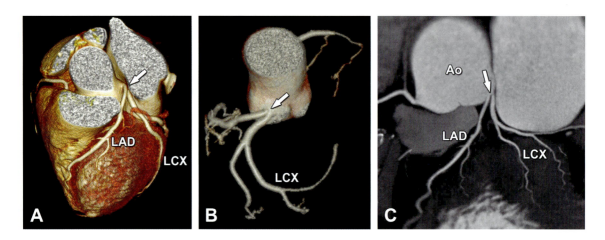

■ **Fig. 17.4** Absence of the left main coronary artery (so-called split left coronary artery). The left anterior descending coronary artery (LAD) and the left circumflex coronary artery (LCX) arise separately (*arrow*) from the left sinus of Valsalva of the aorta (Ao) in a 68-year-old woman who was referred to cardiac CT to exclude coronary artery disease based on atypical chest pain. **Panel A** shows a cranial view of a three-dimensional volume-rendered image. The separate ostia cannot be recognized definitely. Better evaluation is possible on a volume-rendered reconstruction of the coronary tree (**Panel B**) or a two-dimensional map view (**Panel C**)

17

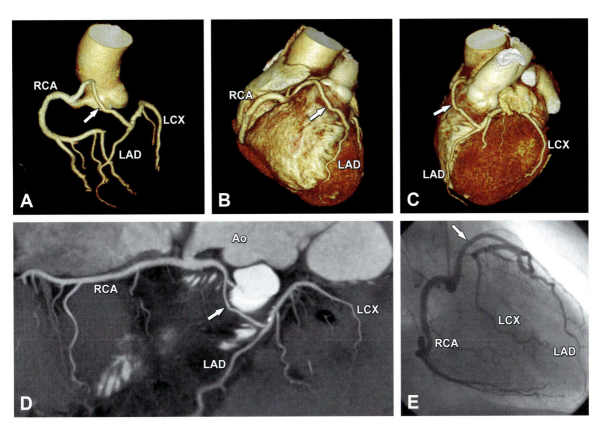

🔲 **Fig. 17.5** Prepulmonary benign course of the left coronary artery arising from the right coronary artery after a short common trunk, which originates from the right sinus of Valsalva. The anomalously coursing left coronary artery (*arrow* in **Panels A–D**) passes anterior to the pulmonary artery to the anterior interventricular sulcus, where it splits into left anterior descending coronary artery (LAD) and left circumflex coronary artery (LCX). Due to the prepulmonary course of the left coronary artery, this anomaly is considered benign. The CT of this 52-year-old male patient was performed to exclude coronary artery disease based on hypertension and atypical chest pain. Conventional coronary angiography also showed the coronary anomaly, but the course of the proximal part of the left coronary artery was unclear (**Panel E**), therefore, the patient was referred for CT. The patient was medically treated and the further clinical course was uneventful. **Panel A** shows a volume-rendered reconstruction of the coronary tree. **Panels B** and **C** are three-dimensional volume-rendered images from two different views showing the anterior course of the anomalous left coronary artery, while **Panel D** gives an overview on a two-dimensional map view. **Panel E** shows the corresponding invasive angiography. *Ao* aorta; *RCA* right coronary artery

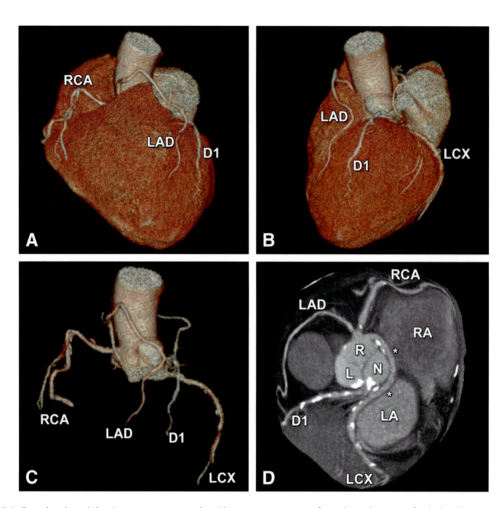

◻ **Fig. 17.6** Complex though benign coronary anomaly with two coronary ostia from the right sinus of Valsalva (R) and no coronary ostium on the left sinus of Valsalva (L). There are two separate vessels supplying the area of the left anterior descending, which were assumed to be the LAD and D1 (**Panels A–C**) according to their location (split LAD). The D1 and the left circumflex coronary artery (LCX) arise with a common trunk from the right sinus of Valsalva (R), which passes retroaortically between the aorta and the right atrium (RA) and the left atrium (LA) (*asteriks* in **Panel D**). This common trunk then splits into the D1 and LCX, which then pass to the anterolateral myocardium and the left atrioventricular sulcus, respectively. The RCA and the LAD arise from a common ostium also from the right sinus of Valsalva (**Panels C and D**). The RCA takes the typical course, whereas the LAD passes anterior to the pulmonary outflow tract to the anterior interventricular sulcus. Coronary CT angiography of this 64-year-old male patient with known severe coronary artery disease was done after conventional coronary angiography for further imaging of the courses of the anomalous vessels. The patient then received two stents into the LCX due to high grade stenosis. **Panels A** and **B** show three-dimensional volume renderings of the heart from two different viewing angles, which do not allow full identification of the coronary anatomy. The three-dimensional reconstruction of the coronary tree in **Panel C** also fails to clearly show the course of the coronary arteries. The most distinct anatomical depiction is given by the globe view in **Panel D**, which resolves the origins and courses of the anomalous coronary arteries

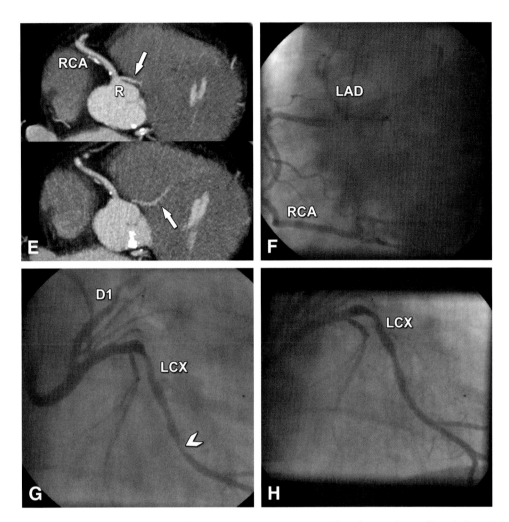

◘ **Fig. 17.6** (continued) **Panel E** shows para-axial maximum-intensity projections of another small septal branch that originates from the proximal RCA and takes an intramyocardial path into the anterior interventricular septum (*arrow*). **Panels F** and **G** show the corresponding conventional coronary angiography with the coronary stenosis in the LCX (*arrowhead*). **Panel H** demonstrate the LCX after successful stenting of the stenosis. *N* noncoronary sinus

17.3.2   Malignant Coronary Anomalies

Malignant coronary anomalies with an interarterial course have the highest potential for cardiac events. In those cases the anomalous coronary artery arises from the opposite sinus of Valsalva and takes an interarterial course between the aorta and the pulmonary artery (**Figs. 17.7–17.10**). These anomalies are made responsible for sudden cardiac death, especially in young persons, during or shortly after physical exercise. This is probably due to increased blood flow in the aorta and the pulmonary artery during physical activity, resulting in a compression of the aberrant vessel, thereby inducing myocardial ischemia. Additionally, the origin of the anomalous artery may be narrowed and form an acute angle with the aorta,

making it more likely that the blood flow is compromized. An intramural proximal intussusception of the aberrant artery at the wall of the aortic root has been reported in intravascular ultrasound studies and might also be an important pathophysiological mechanism.

Under certain conditions, benign courses of the anomalous coronary arteries that are usually not associated with myocardial ischemia can reduce myocardial blood flow. If for instance the left anterior descending coronary artery (LAD) or right coronary artery (RCA) passes anterior to a dilated right ventricular outflow tract, as in pulmonary hypertension, the anomalous vessel can be stretched and the lumen narrowed. Other coronary anomalies can predispose to clotting, spasm or atherosclerotic build-up.

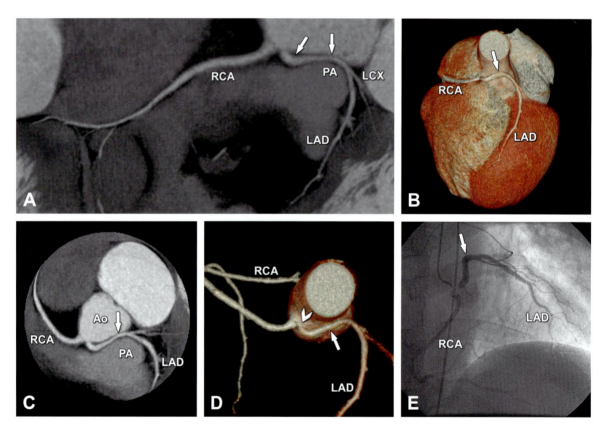

17

◘ **Fig. 17.7** Interarterial (malignant) course of the left coronary artery (*arrow*) with origin from the right sinus of Valsalva next to the ostium of the right coronary artery (RCA). After the interarterial course, the anomalous vessel splits into the left anterior descending coronary artery (LAD) and left circumflex coronary artery (LCX). **Panel A** shows the two-dimensional map view and **Panel B** the corresponding three-dimensional volume-rendered image. **Panel C** presents an additional globe view showing the course similar to the map view while **Panels D** shows the ostium of the left coronary artery (*arrowhead*) next to the one of the RCA. **Panel E** is the conventional coronary angiography which was done in this 36-year-old patient with hypertension because of a positive stress test at high exertion levels with ST-segment depression in the anteroseptal wall. Conventional angiography showed a coronary anomaly with all three coronary arteries arising from the right sinus of Valsalva; however, the course of the left coronary artery was unclear. Therefore CT was performed. Due to the positive stress test the patient received an off-pump single bypass operation connecting the left internal mammary artery (LIMA) to the LAD. *Ao* aorta; *PA* pulmonary artery

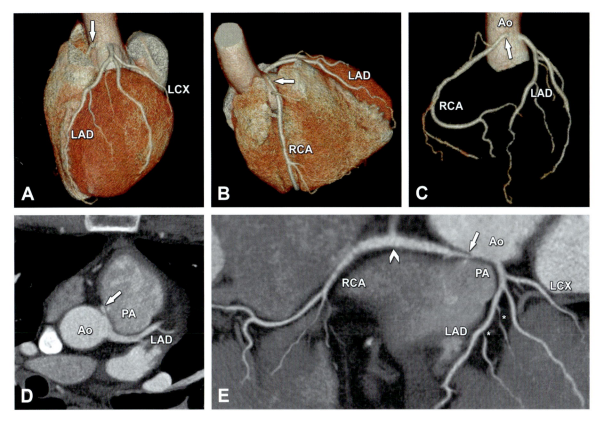

Fig. 17.8 Malignant interarterial course of the right coronary artery (RCA), which originates separately from the ostium of the left coronary artery from the left sinus of Valsalva (*arrow* in **Panels A–E**). The 31-year-old male patient came for further clarification after conventional coronary angiography, which was performed for atypical chest pain. Stress testing revealed no signs of myocardial ischemia and conservative treatment was recommended. The three-dimensional volume-rendered reconstructions of the heart (**Panels A** and **B**) and the coronary tree (**Panel C**) show the small ostium of the RCA (*arrow*), which forms an acute angle with the aorta (Ao). The maximum-intensity projection in **Panel D** shows that already the ostium of the RCA is located between the aorta and the pulmonary artery (PA). An overview is given in the two-dimensional map view (**Panel E**). The narrowings of the diagonal branches (*asterisks*) of the left anterior descending coronary artery (LAD) as well as the bulging out of the RCA (*arrowhead*) are artifacts of the map reconstruction (compare with **Panel A**). *LCX* left circumflex coronary artery

In a patient with a potentially malignant course of a coronary artery, further treatment is based on the clinical symptoms and the result of stress testing. In symptomatic patients with positive stress testing bypass surgery is usually recommended (**Fig. 17.7**). However, many patients with a potentially malignant course are asymptomatic and have a negative stress test. In these patients conservative treatment is possible. In equivocal cases, intravascular ultrasound is usually recommended for further analysis.

A very rare but severe congenital coronary anomaly is the anomalous left coronary artery off the pulmonary artery (ALCAPA), also called Bland-White-Garland syndrome (**Fig. 17.11**). It occurs in approximately 0.25–0.5% of all congenital heart disease patients (Chap. 18). Most patients show first symptoms of myocardial ischemia or infarction in infancy or early childhood because the entire perfusion territory of the left coronary artery is supplied with venous blood. In untreated cases, mortality within the first year is approximately 90%. Surgical reconstruction is the appropriate treatment.

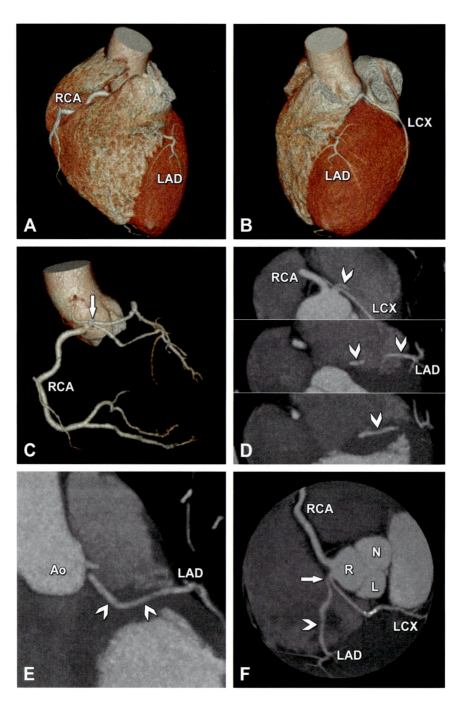

■ **Fig. 17.9** Origin of the left anterior descending coronary artery (LAD) and the left circumflex coronary artery (LCX) from the right sinus of Valsalva (*arrow*) next to the origin of the right coronary artery (RCA) with a malignant course (**Panels A–C**). The LCX passes between the aorta (Ao) and the pulmonary artery (interarterial), whereas the proximal LAD shows myocardial bridging on its way through the proximal interventricular septum (*arrowheads*) without recognizable compression of the lumen during systole. **Panels A** and **B** show a three-dimensional volume rendering, where the anomalous coronary course cannot be recognized. The volume-rendered coronary tree in **Panel C** gives a good view of the origin of the left coronary artery. The maximum-intensity projections in **Panel D** (axial orientation) and **Panel E** (parasagittal orientation) best show the intraseptal course of the LAD (*arrowheads*). The globe view in **Panel F** gives the best overview of the anatomical situation

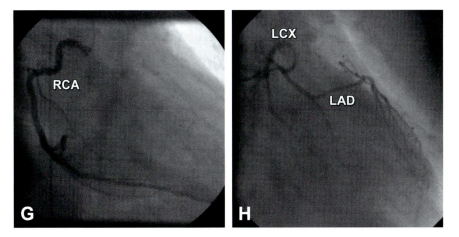

▫ **Fig. 17.9** (continued) **Panels G** and **H** show the corresponding conventional coronary angiography in right anterior oblique projections. This 53-year old male patient was sent to CT for further imaging of the coronary anomaly after coronary angiography. Conservative medical treatment was recommended because stress testing revealed no signs of myocardial ischemia and presence of a dominant nonobstructed RCA. *R* right sinus of Valsalva; *L* left sinus of Valsalva; *N* noncoronary sinus

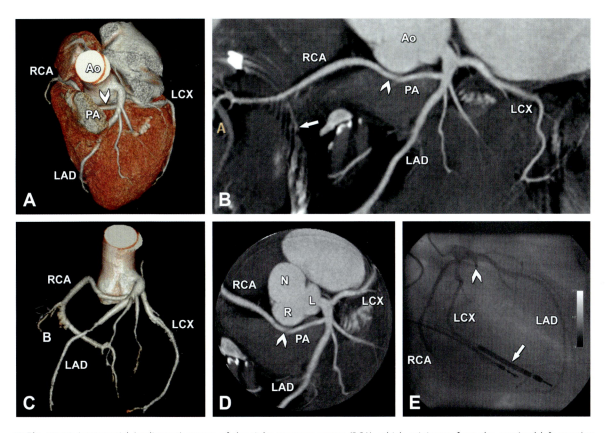

▫ **Fig. 17.10** Interarterial (malignant) course of the right coronary artery (RCA), which originates from the proximal left anterior descending (LAD) and passes between the aorta (Ao) and the pulmonary artery (PA, *arrowhead* in **Panels A** and **B**). The 45-year-old male patient with known hypertrophic obstructive cardiomyopathy (HOCM) came for a second imaging for better depiction of the known coronary anomaly. **Panel A** shows a top view on the three-dimensional volume rendering with the corresponding volume-rendered coronary tree in **Panel C**. The two-dimensional map view (**Panel B**) gives the best overview of the coronary anomaly while the globe view in **Panel D** best shows the aortic valve with its sinuses (*R* right sinus of Valsalva; *L* left sinus of Valsalva; *N* noncoronary sinus). **Panel E** shows the conventional coronary angiography of the patient, confirming the narrowing of the anomalous interarterial vessel (*arrowhead*). The **arrow** in **Panel B** indicates an artifact of the electrode of the implantable cardioverter-defibrillator (ICD) also shown in **Panel E** (*arrow*). The patient was listed for heart transplantation due to HOCM

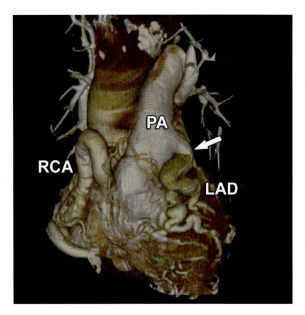

● **Fig. 17.11** Volume-rendered image of a Bland-White-Garland syndrome in a right anterior oblique view. The right coronary artery (RCA) is dilated. The left anterior descending (LAD) originates from the pulmonary artery (*arrow*) and is also markedly dilated and tortuous. *PA* pulmonary artery. With permission from Komatsu and Sato et al. Heart Vessels 2008

17.3.3 Further Anomalies

Anomalies of the intrinsic coronary anatomy summarize several anomalies (**Table 17.1**) which do not primarily affect the origin or general course of the coronary arteries, such as congenital stenosis or atresia, aplasia or hypoplasia, or coronary ectasia or aneurysm formation. Aneurysms, however, most commonly develop secondary to atherosclerosis and occur in about 5% of patients with coronary artery disease (**Fig. 17.12**). Angelini did not explicitly mention aneurysms of the coronary ostium or sinus of Valsalva (**Fig. 17.13**) in the intrinsic coronary anatomy group of anomalies but these anomalies best fit into this category. Anomalies of coronary termination (**Table 17.1**) include all kinds of fistulas between coronary arteries and other cardiac vessels or cavities (**Figs. 17.14 and 17.15**).

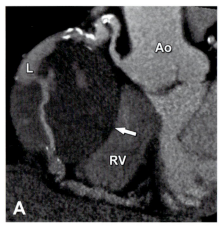
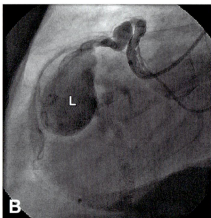

● **Fig. 17.12** Coronary aneurysm of the right coronary artery (*arrow*) in a 63-year-old male patient who was referred for a right ventricular biopsy after a tentative diagnosis of a malignant tumor of the right ventricular and atrial wall was made. The patient had a history of posterior myocardial infarction. Therefore, cardiac CT (**Panel A**) was performed, which revealed a huge aneurysm of the right coronary artery (*arrow*) measuring 5.6×6.6×5.8 cm, which was filled with thrombotic material and had a residual lumen (L). No significant stenosis was found (the gap in the distal right coronary artery is an artifact from the cath view reconstruction). The aneurysm obstructed the right ventricle (RV) from outside. Conventional coronary angiography confirmed the huge aneurysm (*arrow* in **Panel B**) and the patient was sent to surgery

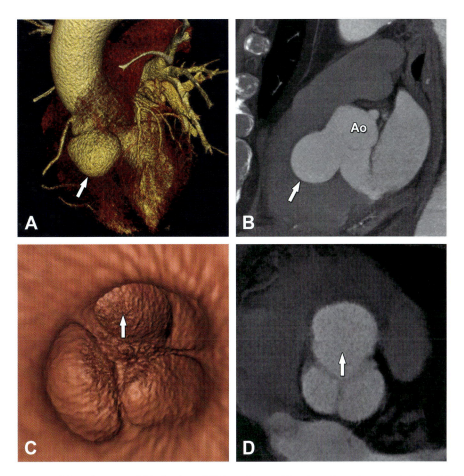

◩ **Fig. 17.13** Aneurysm of the right sinus of Valsalva (**Panel A**) in a 79-year-old male patient who was admitted with atypical angina pectoris. This 3.2 cm aneurysm (*arrow*) protrudes into the right ventricle (**Panels A** and **B**). An endoluminal view (**Panel C**) and a minimum intensity projection (**Panel D**) are shown for comparison; CT did not detect any significant coronary artery stenosis. No fistula or pericardial effusion was seen on CT. Because of the patient's age and normal global function on CT and transthoracic echocardiography, surgery was not considered further. *Ao* aorta

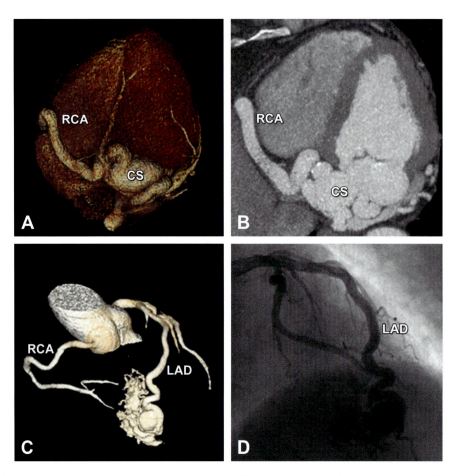

□ **Fig. 17.14** Examples of abnormal termination of coronary arteries. Fistula between the right coronary artery (RCA) and the coronary sinus (CS) depicted by three-dimensional reconstruction (**Panel A**) and multiplanar reformation (**Panel B**). Fistula in a different patient between the left anterior descending coronary artery (LAD) and the right ventricle displayed on three-dimensional reconstructions (**Panel C**) and the corresponding conventional angiogram (**Panel D**). With permission from Cademartiri et al. European Radiology 2007

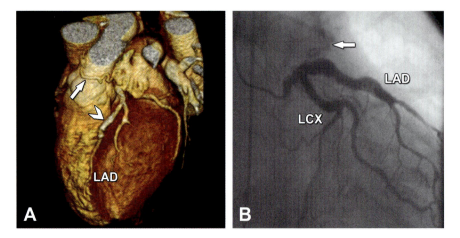

□ **Fig. 17.15** Coronary-pulmonary shunt in a 65-year-old patient who was referred to evaluate the patency of a stent in the proximal left anterior descending coronary artery (LAD) (*arrowhead* in **Panel A**). Additionally, a small shunt vessel between the LAD and pulmonary artery (*arrow*) is seen (**Panel A**), which was verified by conventional coronary angiography (**Panel B**). **Panel A** is a three-dimensional volume rendering. *LCX* left circumflex coronary artery. Images courtesy of Thorsten Bley, Hamburg

17.4   Cardiac CT

The major advantage of coronary CT in the diagnostic workup of a suspected coronary anomaly is the better anatomic depiction of the origin and course of the coronary arteries. CT is often performed after conventional coronary angiography, either because the latter could not detect a coronary artery or because the course of an anomalous coronary artery did not become absolutely clear.

A CT examination performed for delineation and evaluation of coronary anomalies is similar to standard coronary CT angiography. Emphasis has to be put on secondary reformations, which are important to capture the path of the anomalous vessels, e.g., with double-oblique maximum-intensity projections, curved multiplanar reformations, globe views, map views, cath views, and angiographic emulations. In patients with suspected coronary artery anomalies, coronary CT angiography is considered an appropriate indication (Chap. 6). Nevertheless, magnetic resonance imaging should be preferred in younger patients if no contraindications exist.

Recommended Reading

1 Angelini P (2007) Coronary artery anomalies: an entity in search of an identity. Circulation 115:1296–1305

2 Angelini P, Velasco JA, Flamm S (2002) Coronary anomalies: incidence, pathophysiology, and clinical relevance. Circulation 105:2449–2454

3 Bernanke DH, Velkey JM (2002) Development of the coronary blood supply: changing concepts and current ideas. Anat Rec 269:198–208

4 Borjesson M, Pelliccia A (2009) Incidence and aetiology of sudden cardiac death in young athletes: an international perspective. Br J Sports Med 43:644–648

5 Cademartiri F, La Grutta L, Malagò R et al (2008) Prevalence of anatomical variants and coronary anomalies in 543 consecutive patients studied with 64-slice CT coronary angiography. Eur Radiol 18:781–791

6 Cheitlin MD, MacGregor J (2009) Congenital anomalies of coronary arteries: role in the pathogenesis of sudden cardiac death. Herz 34:268–279

7 Davies JE, Burkhart HM, Dearani JA et al (2009) Surgical management of anomalous aortic origin of a coronary artery. Ann Thorac Surg 88:844–847

8 Dodd JD, Ferencik M, Liberthson RR et al (2007) Congenital anomalies of coronary artery origin in adults: 64-MDCT appearance. AJR Am J Roentgenol 188:W138–W146

9 Kang JW, Seo JB, Chae EJ et al (2008) Coronary artery anomalies: classification and electrocardiogram-gated multidetector computed tomographic findings. Semin Ultrasound CT MR 29:182–194

10 Kim SY, Seo JB, Do KH et al (2006) Coronary artery anomalies: classification and ECG-gated multi-detector row CT findings with angiographic correlation. Radiographics 26:317–333, discussion 333-4

11 Kini S, Bis K, Weaver L (2007) Normal and variant coronary arterial and venous anatomy on high-resolution CT angiography. AJR Am J Roentgenol 188:1665–1674

12 von Kodolitsch Y, Ito WD, Franzen O, Lund GK, Koschyk DH, Meinertz T (2004) Coronary artery anomalies. Part I: Recent insights from molecular embryology. Z Kardiol 93:929–937

13 Loukas M, Groat C, Khangura R, Owens DG, Anderson RH (2009) The normal and abnormal anatomy of the coronary arteries. Clin Anat 22:114–128

14 Maron BJ, Doerer JJ, Haas TS, Tierney DM, Mueller FO (2009) Sudden deaths in young competitive athletes: analysis of 1866 deaths in the United States, 1980-2006. Circulation 119:1085–1092

15. Schmitt R, Froehner S, Brunn J et al (2005) Congenital anomalies of the coronary arteries: imaging with contrast-enhanced, multidetector computed tomography. Eur Radiol 15:1110–1121

16 Swaye PS, Fisher LD, Litwin P et al (1983) Aneurysmal coronary artery disease. Circulation 67:134–138

17 Yamanak O, Hobbs RE (1990) Coronary artery anomalies in 126,595 patients undergoing coronary arteriography. Cathet Cardiovasc Diagn 21:28–40

Congenital and Acquired Heart Disease

S. Ley and R. Arnold

Abstract

This chapter outlines imaging strategies for congenital heart disease and gives an insight into therapeutic approaches and the follow-up of patients.

18.1   Introduction

Congenital heart disease (CHD) is the collective term for congenital malformations affecting the heart, pulmonary arteries, aorta, and coronary arteries. Most cases of CHD are thought to be multifactorial in origin, resulting from an interaction of genetic predisposition and environmental stimulus. In general, CHD occurs in 0.5–0.8% live births, meaning that about 1.5 million children are born with a cardiac malformation worldwide each year. The spectrum of anatomic malformations ranges from relatively simple to very complex entities. About two to three out of 1,000 newborns will become symptomatic with heart disease in the first year of life. Today most cases of CHD are diagnosed in the first month of life. Of note, the most frequent disorders such as ventricular and atrial septal defects are no indications for CT assessment. In Ebstein anomalies the focus of diagnostic evaluation is on cardiac function, which is why echocardiography and magnetic resonance imaging (MRI) are the preferred diagnostic modalities.

Congenital anomalies of the coronary arteries are rare and usually associated with additional cardiac abnormalities. Most of them are asymptomatic and do not have clinical significance. In contrast, coronary malformations are severe forms of CHD that lead to congestive heart failure. They are associated with sudden cardiac death in young athletes, even when no other cardiac anomalies are present.

Many children with CHD require surgical or catheter interventions, either corrective or palliative. With technical improvement, the survival rate has increased dramatically, leading to a growing number of patients requiring serial postoperative follow-up. Pre- and postinterventional imaging should be done as gently as possible, avoiding invasive techniques if possible. Furthermore, high-quality imaging (with three-dimensional visualization of the anatomy) is an essential part of treatment planning.

M. Dewey, *Cardiac CT*,
DOI: 10.1007/978-3-642-14022-8_21, © Springer-Verlag Berlin Heidelberg 2011

CT of the great thoracic vessels and coronary arteries in children is limited to complex cases. Single pathologies such as atrial or ventricular septal defects are best evaluated by echocardiography and do not require visualization by CT. They can be seen as incidental findings on CT in adulthood (**Fig. 18.1**). For patients scheduled for follow-up examinations either echocardiography or MRI should be considered the methods of choice to keep the radiation burden in these patients as low as possible. With the increased live expectancy of patients after CHD correction, radiation exposure is an increasingly important issue. There are only a few conditions that require CT follow-up. This is mainly the case if the morphology of the coronary arteries has to be imaged (like in Kawasaki disease). Visualization of the pulmonary arterial anastomoses to pulmonary arterial grafts in young children is also challenging for MRI. In general, a detailed description of the surgical procedures performed and the precise clinical question are mandatory to know before the examination. This chapter focuses on the most frequent CHD and their typical imaging findings.

18.2 Technical Considerations

When cardiac CT is considered in children, many aspects are different from imaging adults.

18.2.1 Size of Vascular Structures

The small size of vascular structures in children is a challenge for noninvasive imaging. As the children get older, the diameters of great arteries are constantly increasing (**Table 18.1**). For instance, the increase is 0.43 mm per kg body weight gain for the ascending aorta.

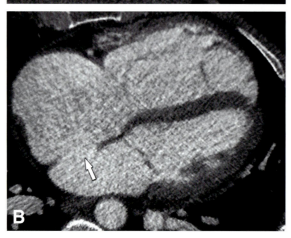

■ **Fig. 18.1** Two examples of atrial septal defect. **Panel A** shows a double-oblique maximum-intensity projection along the left atrium (LA) and right atrium (RA) in a 47-year-old male patient who was referred for rule-out of coronary artery disease (reformations along the nonobstructed coronary arteries not shown). There is a left-to-right shunt seen in this patient with a small patent foramen ovale (*arrow* in **Panel A**). A larger atrial defect (*arrow*) in a 44-year-old male patient is shown in a four-chamber view (**Panel B**). A patient with a ventricular septal defect is shown in **Fig. 18.7**

■ **Table 18.1** Age-related diameters and growth rate of great arteries in children

Vessel	Day 1 (mean weight: 2.2 kg)	3 years (mean weight: 20 kg)	Weight-adapted growth per kg weight gain
Ascending aorta	8.4 mm	14 mm	0.43 mm
Aortic arch	6.8 mm	14.4 mm	NA
Aortic isthmus	4.7 mm	8.3 mm	NA
Main pulmonary artery	7.5 mm	14 mm	0.5 mm
Right pulmonary artery	4.3 mm	8.6 mm	0.33 mm
Left pulmonary artery	4.2 mm	8.8 mm	0.35 mm

Data were obtained in 130 normal newborns and infants by Trowitzsch et al.; diameters were measured by echocardiography. Linear growth of the great arteries within the first 3 years of life was found. NA – not available

18.2.2   Heart Rate and Premedication

Children's hearts beat much faster than those of adults, e.g., babies have heart rates of up to 160 beats per min (**Table 18.2**). A low heart rate is advantageous for image quality. However, due to the fast rotation times and/or multisegment reconstruction available today, even pediatric hearts can be imaged without significant motion artifacts. In our experience, the ascending aorta and pulmonary arteries can be nicely visualized without reduction of heart rate, even in newborns. With sedation, the heart rate is usually reduced to around 130 beats per min. More important for image quality is a regular cardiac rhythm. In case of severe arrhythmia image quality will be clearly hampered by pulsation artifacts and CT imaging should be avoided.

Image quality of the coronary arteries is more dependent on the heart rate. The segments most often affected are the mid-segment of the right coronary artery, distal segments of the left anterior descending, and the left circumflex coronary artery. These motion artifacts do not disturb evaluation of larger cardiac structures but hamper evaluation of coronary artery plaques, which, however, play no role in children.

Younger children requiring cardiovascular and especially coronary artery imaging are often critically ill. The use of beta-blockers to lower the heart rate should thus be avoided because of reduced coronary blood flow and blood pressure. With the development of volume scanners such as 320-row CT, the whole heart can be assessed within one rotation. However, even 16-row CT with multisegment reconstruction allows cardiac examinations of newborns (**Fig. 18.2**). Also, premedication with nitroglycerin is not necessary since an in-depth analysis of coronary arteries and their wall is not essential in the work-up of CHD.

Table 18.2 Age-related heart rate in children

Age (years)	Heart rate (beats per min)
<1	110–160
1–2	100–150
2–5	95–140
5–12	80–120
>12	60–100

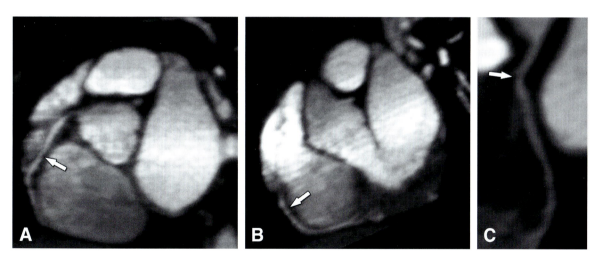

Fig. 18.2 Exclusion of coronary artery anomalies using CT (60% phase) in a 10-week-old girl with laryngomalacia who presented with a heart rate of 133 beats per min (no beta-blockers were given). 5 ml of an iodinated contrast agent (250 mg iodine/ml) were injected via a peripheral venous line at an injection speed of 0.5 ml/s, and imaging was performed using retrospective ECG gating on a 16-row CT scanner using adaptive multisegment reconstruction. All vascular territories are visualized and the anatomy of the coronary arteries can be examined. Image quality is slightly reduced due to blurry edges of the vessels (*arrow*). However, detailed analysis of the vessel wall (as in plaque imaging) is not required in children. The proximal right coronary artery is shown in **Panel A** and the distal segment in **Panel B** (oblique maximum-intensity projections). **Panel C** shows the left main and left descending artery on a curved multiplanar reformation

18.2.3 Respiratory Artifacts

The scan time of 64-row CT scanners to cover the heart in children is less than 3 s. Noncooperative younger children have a relatively fast respiratory rate and irregular rhythm. However, sedation will slow the respiratory rate, and the rhythm becomes more regular. The fast scan times in conjunction with such regular breathing patterns usually allow artifact-free CT imaging without intubation.

18.2.4 Speed of Contrast Agent Injection

Usually children are only equipped with a peripheral, tiny intravenous cannula (26 or 24G). This is sufficient for visualization of the large thoracic vessels, for optimal imaging of the coronary arteries a larger intravenous cannula in an antecubital position or even a central line is beneficial (**Table 18.3**). If the venous line is placed in a head vein, sedation has to be rather deep, as patients are sensitive at this location and usually move during injection of iodinated contrast agent.

Contrast agent injection can be done using a power injector without negative effects. An injection rate of 0.5 ml/s was found to be reliably possible through a central line in newborns. Besides technical considerations, the patients' cardiac condition has to be taken into account. In severe cardiac malformation the combination of high flow rate and high volume can affect a patient's circulation. Therefore, the contrast agent injection speed and volume should be discussed with the pediatrician/pediatric cardiologist before the examination.

18.2.5 Iodine Concentration of Contrast Agent

Another issue to be considered is the iodine concentration of the contrast agent used. Infants and young children should be given a low-osmolar contrast agent (usually combined with a low iodine concentration of 200–250 mg iodine/ml). Children above the age of 3 without any cardiac malformations tolerate an injection rate of 2 ml/s (350 mg iodine/ml). The volume for optimal aortic enhancement should not exceed 1.5 ml/kg body weight.

18.2.6 Scanning Protocol

One of the most important points to keep in mind is that the automatic dose modulation of the CT scanner cannot be reliably used in children. Manual setting of parameters is recommended instead. During the past years the number of CT scanners and slices has increased dramatically, and all vendors have different strategies for dose reduction. Therefore, no global recommendation for kV and mAs settings can be given. Furthermore, for dose comparison, the dose length product (DLP) is recommended. In our experience, a DLP as low as 8 mGy*cm (80kV) is sufficient for imaging a baby with a weight of 3–4 kg. Only a minor increase in DLP is necessary with increasing weight, as the thoracic diameter stays rather constant during the first years of life.

18.3 Congenital Heart Disease

The most common congenital anomalies are atrial (7%) and ventricular septal (31%) wall defects. However, the role of CT in patients who are referred for preoperative evaluation of ventricular or atrial septal wall defects is limited with echocardiography and MRI being the main clinical players in that regard. Still, one might encounter those defects in patients referred, e.g., for rule-out of coronary artery disease, and **Fig. 18.1** shows two examples.

◘ **Table 18.3** Recommended contrast agent injection protocols in children

Age (years)	Preparation (64-row CT)
<1	24G venous line as proximal as possible (preferred: central line), contrast agent injection: 0.5 ml/s, 250 mg iodine/ml, volume 5 ml, saline chaser: 10 ml at 0.5 ml/s
1–2	24G venous line as proximal as possible (preferred: central line), contrast agent injection: 1 ml/s, 250 mg iodine/ml, volume 5 ml, saline chaser: 10 ml at 1 ml/s
≥2–5	22G venous line (antecubital vein), contrast agent injection: 2 ml/s, 300 mg iodine/ml, volume 15 ml, saline chaser: 20 ml at 2 ml/s
>5	20G venous line (antecubital vein), contrast agent injection: 3 ml/s, 350 mg iodine/ml, volume 20 ml, saline chaser: 25 ml at 2 ml/s

List 18.1. Aortic anomalies and defects

1. Persistent ductus arteriosus (PDA, **Fig. 18.3**)
2. Anomalies of the ascending aorta and of the aortic arch
   (a) Hypoplastic arch (**Fig. 18.3**)
   (b) Aortic rings
      i. Double aortic arch
      ii. Right-sided aortic arch with aberrant left subclavian artery and left-sided ductus arteriosus
      iii. Left-sided aortic arch with Lusoria artery
   (c) Interrupted aortic arch
   (d) Truncus arteriosus
3. Aortic stenosis and coarctation
   (a) Coarctation (**Fig. 18.5**)
   (b) Other aortic stenosis, e.g., subvalvular
4. Rare anomalies, e.g., aneurysm of the ductus arteriosus
5. Complications after interventions and/or surgery (**Fig. 18.4**)
6. Marfan syndrome (development of aortic root dilatation)
7. Ulrich–Turner syndrome (associated with aortic coarctation)

18.3.1 Aortic Arch

Congenital anomalies of the aorta are one of the most frequent cardiovascular malformations. They include a wide spectrum of diseases (**List 18.1**), e.g., patent ductus arteriosus (**Fig. 18.3**) (5–10% of all CHD) or aortic coarctation (8–10%). The initial diagnosis is usually established by echocardiography. Beside the morphological configuration of the aorta, the pressure gradient is determined for surgery. Therefore, catheterization is necessary. With these techniques all critical stenoses are detected. Noncritical stenosis is often detected in grown-ups, usually due to arterial hypertension and blood pressure differences between arms and legs. Clinical indications for follow-up examinations are re-coarctation (<3%, higher when operated on in infancy) or postoperative aneurysms (24% after patch angioplasty) or dissection (5–50% after patch angioplasty, **Fig. 18.4**). Because of the lack of radiation exposure and the option to assess function (e.g., flow quantification), MRI is the preferred test in suspected coarctation (**Fig 18.5**). With increasing age, it becomes more and more difficult to obtain an adequate acoustic window. CT is indicated for follow-up of patients who underwent stent implantation for aortic coarctation, as MRI is limited in visualizing the stent lumen. In complex aortic

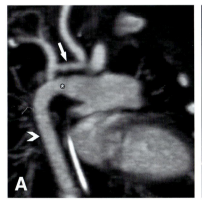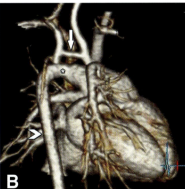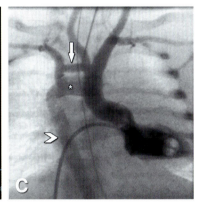

■ **Fig. 18.3** Hypoplastic aortic arch (*arrow*) and large persistent ductus arteriosus Botalli (*asterisk*) in a 2-day-old child prenatally diagnosed with a cardiac malformation. On a double oblique maximum-intensity projection (**Panel A**) the large persistent ductus arteriosus and the hypoplastic aortic arch (*arrow*) is shown. The persistent ductus arteriosus connects the main pulmonary artery and the descending aorta (*arrowhead*), which is normal. For operative planning the CT images were additionally demonstrated to the surgeon as three-dimensional volume renderings (**Panel B**). **Panel C** presents the corresponding image from left ventricular catheterization

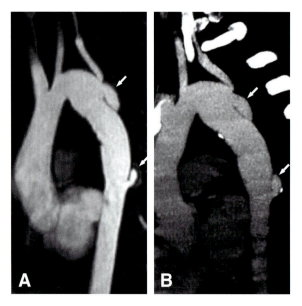

☐ **Fig. 18.4** Dissection as a complication after aortic arch operation in a 24-year-old female patient with congenital hypoplasia of the distal aortic arch and patch angioplasty at the age of 2 years. Eight years later a restenosis was diagnosed and a vascular prosthesis (16-mm Hemashield) was implanted. Regular follow-up was performed by MRI. **Panel A** is an MR angiography after intravenous contrast agent administration (10-mm double-oblique maximum-intensity projection) that shows new dissections at the proximal and distal anastomosis of the prosthesis (*arrows*). For further surgical planning a nongated CT was performed (**Panel B**, 5-mm maximum-intensity projection), which confirmed the MRI findings

arch abnormalities (i.e., double aortic arch), surgeons prefer three-dimensional visualization of the anatomic relationship between the trachea and the vascular structures. This information can be nicely provided by CT, even in critically ill children.

18.3.2   Persistent Ductus Arteriosus (PDA)

During fetal life the ductus arteriosus connects the main pulmonary artery near its bifurcation to the aorta just beyond the origin of the left subclavian artery. The ductus arteriosus usually closes functionally soon after birth through muscular contractions. A persistent ductus arteriosus is encountered in approximately 7% of all congenital heart defects. Echocardiography is the modality of choice for assessment of the ductus arteriosus in infants. CT is only performed if a complex malformation is suspected (**Fig. 18.3**).

18.3.3   Transposition of the Great Arteries

Dextrotransposition of the great arteries is a cyanotic CHD found in approximately 3–5% of all newborns with CHD. Arterial switch operation restores the normal anatomic arrangement of the circulation and, as such, promises a lifelong perfect postoperative anatomy and physiology. From its first description by Jatene in 1976, it has steadily

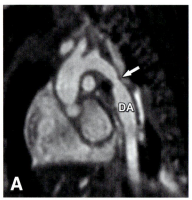
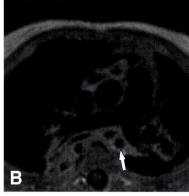
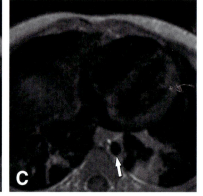

☐ **Fig. 18.5** Coarctation of the aorta in a 5-month-old male baby. **Panel A** is an ECG- and respiratory-gated steady-state free precession three-dimensional sequence (MR angiography) without contrast enhancement and demonstrates a focal narrowing (*arrow*) of the descending aorta (DA). **Panel B** is a spin-echo MR sequence with dark-blood pulse preparation that shows the narrowing of the aorta in transverse orientation (*arrow*), while **Panel C** shows the normal lumen of the descending aorta (*arrow*) on the same sequence at the level of the diaphragm. Note that the consolidation in the left lower lung seen on **Panel C** is due to a prior pneumonia in this patient

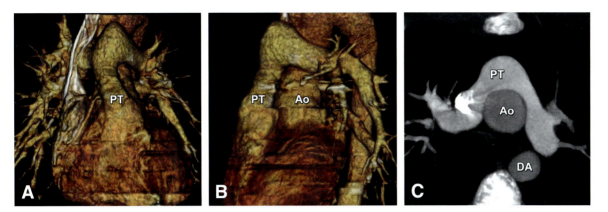

Fig. 18.6 Status post arterial switch operation for dextro-transposition of the great arteries in a 12-year-old boy. **Panels A** and **B** show three-dimensional volume renderings after surgery (anterior and lateral view, PT = pulmonary trunk, Ao = ascending aorta). No stenoses or aneurysms were found. An axial maximum-intensity projection (**Panel C**) demonstrates the main pulmonary artery anterior to the ascending aorta (Ao), whereas there is a normal position of the descending aorta (DA)

become the procedure of choice when the anatomy is appropriate and is usually performed in the first month of life. The outcome of arterial switch operations is usually uneventful and a number of studies show excellent results concerning general health status (**Fig. 18.6**). Despite excellent early outcome, however, arterial switch operation still remains a complex surgical procedure with the potential for significant short-, mid- and long-term complications such as coronary and pulmonary stenoses in the early- and mid-term and aortic root dilation with aortic regurgitation in the long-term. The incidence of pulmonary arterial stenosis is 3–30%. It is usually a branch stenosis, which is characterized by an oval shape. The development of aortic root dilation leading to progressive aortic regurgitation is still not fully understood. Seventy percent of the children after arterial switch operation show dilation 10 years after corrective surgery.

Transposition of the great arteries is associated with a huge variety of coronary abnormalities, most of them without clinical impact. Coronary anomalies affect the surgical procedure because transfer of the coronary vessels may be necessary. Coronary anatomy is sufficiently visualized preoperatively using echocardiography. The incidence of coronary stenosis after switch leading to impaired ventricular function ranges from 2% to 20%.

In a large study (130 children, age 5.6 ± 1.1 years) after arterial switch operation, 64-row CT correctly identified all children (9.2%) with coronary artery stenosis compared to conventional coronary angiography. One noteworthy issue, however, was the significantly higher radiation dose of CT (4.5 ± 0.5 mSv) compared to conventional angiography (3.1 ± 1.6 mSv). On the other hand, in six patients (4.6%), relevant complications occurred after conventional angiography (bleeding, femoral hematoma at the arterial access site, femoral artery aneurysm, and transient ischemic stroke). Cardiac function and aortic regurgitation is best determined by MRI, while gross anatomy and the orifice of the coronary arteries hare better delineated by CT. A prospectively ECG-gated CT angiography is recommended whenever feasible to reduce effective dose (Chap. 8).

18.3.4   Tetralogy of Fallot

Tetralogy of Fallot (5–7% of all CHD) typically includes four malformations: ventricular septal defect (**Fig. 18.7A**), pulmonary stenosis (**Fig. 18.7B**), right ventricular hypertrophy, and aortic striding. In patients with tetralogy of Fallot, pulmonary stenosis leads to diminished blood flow to the pulmonary arteries causing severe cyanosis. In extreme forms, associated with pulmonary atresia and pulmonary artery hypoplasia, pulmonary blood flow is dependent on a patent ductus arteriosus or collateral vessels arising from the aortic arch (**Fig. 18.7C**). Lung perfusion is partly established by these systemic vessels. In this particular situation surgeons are especially interested if these vessels are suitable for connection to the pulmonary arteries or if they provide an unbalanced, high pressure blood flow situation, leading to pulmonary hypertension.

The architecture of the pulmonary vessels is most important to identify patients in whom primary correction is possible. In pulmonary artery hypoplasia sufficient pulmonary blood flow needs to be established early to ensure growth of the pulmonary arteries. Therefore, a stable aortopulmonary connection needs to be established. Later, further corrective or palliative operations are usually possible. The first aortopulmonary shunt described was the so called Blalock–Taussig shunt (1944). Here, the right or left subclavian artery and the ipsilateral pulmonary artery are connected in cyanotic patients with tetralogy of Fallot. This operation is no performed because only one pulmonary artery will be sufficiently perfused. Central aortopulmonary shunts (using Goretex[R]) or a direct connection of the hypoplastic pulmonary trunk to the aorta are preferred as they lead to a balanced growth of both pulmonary arteries (**Fig. 18.8**).

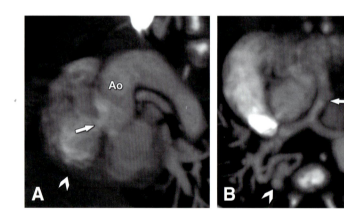
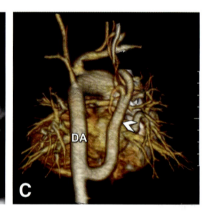

◘ **Fig. 18.7** Tetralogy of Fallot in a 1-month-old male baby. ECG-gated CT (16 rows) was performed using 30 ml of contrast agent with 250 mg I/ml followed by 10 ml saline at an injection rate of 1 ml/s through a venous line at the head. A larger amount of contrast agent was used to opacify the pulmonary arteries as well as the descending aorta and potential collaterals. **Panel A** (double oblique reformation) shows the ventricular septal defect (*arrow*), the overstriding ascending aorta (Ao), and the right ventricular hypertrophy (*arrowhead*). **Panel B** (transverse maximum-intensity projection) shows the hypoplastic main (*arrow*), right and left pulmonary arteries, and a large major aortopulmonary collateral artery (MAPCA) draining into the pulmonary arteries (*arrowhead*). The volume rendering (**Panel C**) shows the descending aorta (DA) and the large MAPCA (*arrowhead*), which is directed upwards. In this case the MAPCAs were too large for embolization and had to be clipped surgically

18

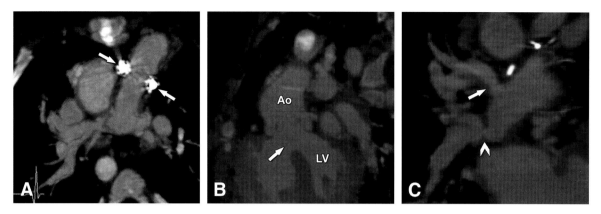

⬚ **Fig. 18.8** Status post implantation of a pulmonary valved conduit (*arrows*) in a 2-year-old boy with tetralogy of Fallot (**Panel A**). **Panel B** shows the position of the ascending aorta (Ao) overstriding the large ventricular septal defect (*arrow*) between the right and left ventricle (LV). The examination was indicated to evaluate the anastomosis of the conduit to the native pulmonary arteries (*arrow* and *arrowhead* in **Panel C**). A focal stenosis of the lower lobe pulmonary artery (*arrowhead* in **Panel C**) can be seen. Interestingly, using MRI the spatial resolution was insufficient for precise visualization of the anastomoses and interpretation was additionally impaired by artifacts from the mediastinal clips

After corrective surgery, pulmonary insufficiency has been identified as a factor that particularly limits right ventricular function and, accordingly, the quality of life and life expectancy. The time of reintervention should be determined without serial catheterization (i.e., by echocardiography or MRI).

The incidence of additional coronary arterial anomalies in patients with tetralogy of Fallot is between 8% and 36%. The following anomalies in the course and/or distribution of the coronary arteries have been described: single coronary ostium, left anterior descending artery arising from the right coronary artery, circumflex artery arising from the right coronary artery, small fistulas between coronary arteries and the pulmonary artery, fistulas between coronary and bronchial arteries or right atrium. CT in children with tetralogy of Fallot was found to have a high diagnostic accuracy of 95.5% for all disease-related issues (compared to surgical findings) in a pilot study.

Preoperative assessment of vascular structures (pulmonary arteries, aorta, and collaterals) is possible with MRI and CT. Echocardiography alone can also provide adequate information if pulmonary and coronary anatomy can be visualized sufficiently. Still some centres perform conventional angiography despite the potential risk of a cyanotic spell caused by catheter manipulation (during a cyanotic spell, the child develops very rapid deep breathing and sweating, and the child may become limp and lose consciousness) emphasizing the necessity of high-quality coronary imaging in very small infants.

18.3.5 Sequestration

Pulmonary sequestration is a malformation defined as a segment of lung parenchyma that is separated from the tracheobronchial tree and is supplied with blood from a systemic artery. Sequestration has an estimated incidence between 0.15% and 1.7% in the general population. The blood supply usually comes from the descending thoracic aorta, but in about 20% of cases it comes from the upper abdominal aorta, celiac artery, or splenic artery. All pulmonary sequestrations should be treated surgically or interventionally because the high blood flow through the lesion can cause heart failure. Surgical procedures include ligation of the afferent vessels and/or resection of the pulmonary malformation.

In pulmonary sequestration CT is superior to most other techniques, providing excellent information on both the arterial and venous vessels supplying and draining the malformation and the structure of the lung parenchyma inside the malformation (**Fig. 18.9**). The spatial resolution of MR angiography may be too low to achieve adequate visualization of all vascular structures. Also, visualization of the lung parenchyma is difficult using MRI.

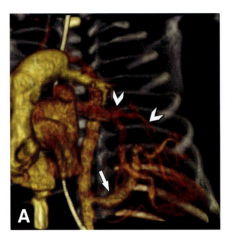
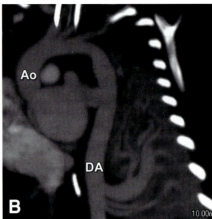

Fig. 18.9 Lung sequestration in a 15-day-old female baby with a prenatally diagnosed anomaly of the left lung. ECG-gated CT was performed using 7 ml contrast agent with 250 mg I/ml at an injection rate of 0.3 ml/sec. **Panel A** shows a volume rendering of the arterial supply (3 vessels) of the sequestration from the descending aorta (*arrows*). The venous drainage is to the left atrium (*arrowheads*). **Panel B** is a double-oblique maximum-intensity projection along the ascending aorta (Ao) and descending aorta (DA) showing the three arteries supplying the sequestration from the DA. Due to the large size of the arterial supply the patient went to surgery for clipping of the arteries

18.3.6 Origin of the Left Pulmonary Artery from the Right Pulmonary Artery (Pulmonary Sling)

The left pulmonary artery arises aberrantly from the right pulmonary artery and runs between the trachea and esophagus to the left side, which either leads to an acute and severe airway compression (infants) or signs of chronic obstructive lung disease (children and young adults). Echocardiography is feasible in infants but further visualization of the airways is mandatory. Therefore, CT is the recommended technique for visualization of the pulmonary arteries and the tracheobronchial tree (**Fig. 18.10**). Surgical correction is always performed with attachment of the left pulmonary artery to the pulmonary trunk anterior to the aorta.

18.4 Coronary Artery Anomalies

Coronary anomalies are classified according to their origin, course, and termination. For further details on coronary anomalies pertaining to adults see Chap. 17. An abnormal coronary origin from the opposite sinus of Valsalva is the second most common cause of sudden death on the athletic field in the US, while the most frequent cause is hypertrophic cardiomyopathy. Although

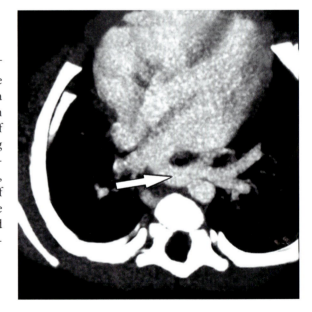

Fig. 18.10 Sling left pulmonary artery in a 5-month-old boy with a history of lower airway obstruction. Maximum-intensity projection in the axial plane demonstrates a sling left pulmonary artery (*arrow*) that arises from the right pulmonary artery and courses posterior to the left main bronchus to supply the left lung. The child underwent reimplantation of the sling left pulmonary artery to the main pulmonary artery anterior to the trachea, relieving compression on the left main bronchus. With permission from A.-M. du Plessis et al. Pediatr Radiol 2008

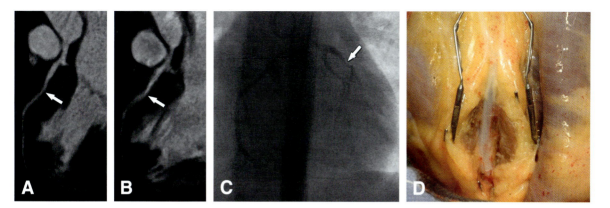

Fig. 18.11 11-year-old girl with myocardial bridging of the left anterior descending coronary artery (LAD) due to hypertrophic cardio-myopathy. She was admitted to the hospital after a heart attack and resuscitation and was thus referred for CT, which was performed on a dual-source CT scanner at a heart rate of 103 beats per min. The patient showed only limited breath-hold capabilities, leading to arti-facts on the reconstructed images. ECG-gated CT angiography using 50 ml of an iodinated contrast agent (370 mg iodine/ml) shows the intramural segment (*arrows*) of the left anterior descending coronary artery displayed as curved multiplanar reformations during systole (**Panel A**) and diastole (**Panel B**). Note the narrow lumen (*arrow*) of the intramural segment during systole and diastole (**Panels A** and **B**). This finding was confirmed on conventional angiography (*arrow* in **Panel C**). **Panel D** shows the intraoperative situs after dissection of the myocardium. The further clinical course was uneventful. **Panel D** is courtesy of Dr. C. Sebening, Heidelberg

the right coronary artery arising from the left coronary sinus is four times as common as the left coronary artery arising from the anterior sinus, it is the latter that is by far the more common cause of sudden death during or shortly after vigorous physical activity. In a continuous series of 6.3 million 18-year-old recruits who underwent intense military training for 8 weeks, a group at the American Armed Forces Institute of Pathology identi-fied 277 deaths unrelated to trauma. A review of the clinical and necropsy charts showed that, of 64 cardiac deaths, 21 (33%) were related to anomalous origination of a coronary artery from the opposite sinus.

Myocardial bridging most often affects the left ante-rior descending coronary artery. Mild bridging (less than 20% diameter stenosis) is often undetectable, as the blood usually flows through the coronaries while the heart is relaxing in diastole. A constriction of up to 50% is probably benign. A narrowing of 70% or more (during diastole) usually causes angina pectoris. Visualization of the coronary arteries during diastole and systole is mandatory to analyze the percentage diameter stenosis and measure the length of the tun-neled part for planning the surgical strategy in patients with ischemia (**Fig. 18.11**).

18.4.1 Myocardial Bridging

Normally, coronary arteries have an epicardial course. A myocardial bridge is a congenital condition in which a segment of coronary artery runs intramurally, through the myocardium, beneath a muscular bridge. The coro-nary artery segment covered by the myocardial bridge is called a tunneled artery. As the heart contracts to pump blood, the muscle exerts pressure across the bridge and may constrict the artery. This can lead to premature ven-tricular contractions and angina pectoris. There are only case reports on the use of CT for diagnosing a myocardial bridge in children, and bridging is most commonly seen in children with hypertrophic cardiomyopathy.

18.4.2 Anomalous Origin of the Left Coronary Artery from the Pulmonary Artery (ALCAPA or Bland-White-Garland Syndrome)

The anomalous origin of the left coronary artery from the pulmonary artery (ALCAPA) is a rare congenital malformation reported to occur in 0.25–0.5% of all CHD. Most of the times, the anomaly is the only cardiac mal-formation; in those less common cases where it is associ-ated with with other structural abnormalities, these may conceal the clinical findings and make the diagnosis even more difficult. Chronic myocardial ischemia leads to early progressive left heart failure and cardiac death.

Children can survive if sufficient collaterals between the right coronary artery with a normal origin and the left coronary artery exist (formerly called adult type). This is only the case in 15–20% of patients. The other 80–85% do not have sufficient collaterals and develop progressive heart failure with subsequent death at the age of 3–6 months. Usually, symptoms occur late and the clinical examination is inconspicuous. If there is a clinical suspicion, at this point CT can reliably detect the anomalous origin of the left coronary artery. It must be kept in mind that scanning should be started when the contrast agent is in the ascending aorta (as usual) as the left coronary artery is filled retrogradely by the right coronary artery (**Fig. 18.12**).

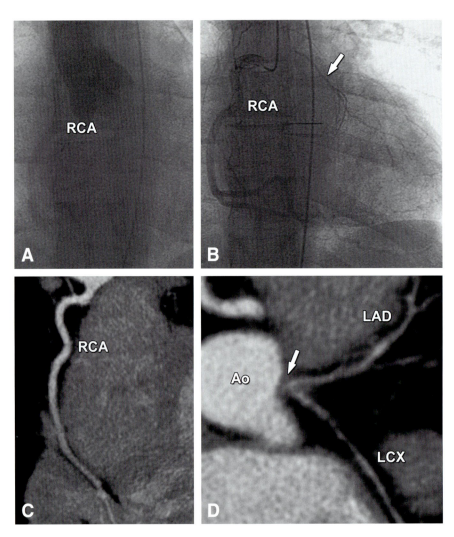

Fig. 18.12 Surgically corrected Bland-White-Garland syndrome in a 16-year-old girl. The left main coronary artery originated from the pulmonary artery and was surgically transferred to the aortic root during infancy to restore normal anatomy. Additionally, a mechanical mitral valve was placed. Conventional angiography (aortography) at follow-up demonstrated the right coronary artery (RCA, **Panel A**) but not the ostium of the left coronary artery. A late phase of the dedicated angiography of the RCA demonstrated retrograde filling of the left coronary arterial system (*arrow* in **Panel B**) as an indirect sign of left main occlusion. The patient had no clinical symptoms or ECG changes. 16-row CT using adaptive multisegment reconstruction ruled out stenosis of the dominant RCA (**Panel C**, curved multiplanar reformation) but also confirmed the occlusion of the reinserted left main coronary artery (*arrow* in **Panel D**, curved multiplanar reformation; Ao = ascending aorta). Both the left anterior descending (LAD) and the left circumflex coronary artery (LCX) were contrasted on CT due retrograde filling via collaterals from the RCA

18.4.3   Kawasaki Disease

Kawasaki disease is an acute, self-limiting vasculitis of unknown etiology that occurs predominantly in infants and young children. It was first described in 1967 by Dr. Tomisaku Kawasaki in the Japanese literature (Arerugi). The specific cause of the disease is still unknown; current theories center primarily on immunological causes. Classically, five days of fever plus four of five diagnostic criteria must be met to establish the diagnosis. Japan has by far the highest incidence of Kawasaki disease (175 per 100,000 patients under 5), though its incidence in the US is increasing (approximately 2,000–4,000 cases are identified in the US each year). Kawasaki disease is predominantly a disease of young children, with 80% of patients being younger than five. The disease affects more boys than girls. Kawasaki was extremely uncommon in Caucasians until the last few decades.

Cardiac complications are the most important aspect of the disease. Kawasaki disease can cause vasculitis in the coronary arteries and subsequent coronary artery aneurysms. These aneurysms can lead to myocardial infarction even in young children. Overall, about 5–20% of children with Kawasaki disease develop coronary artery aneurysms with much higher prevalence among patients who are not treated early in the course of illness. Virtually all deaths in patients with Kawasaki disease result from its cardiac sequelae. Mortality is highest 15–45 days after the onset of fever; during this time coronary vasculitis occurs concomitantly with a marked elevation of the platelet count and a hypercoagulable state. However, sudden death from myocardial infarction may also occur many years later in individuals presenting with stenosis after having developed coronary artery aneurysms as children. Many cases of fatal and nonfatal myocardial infarction in young adults have been attributed to "missed" Kawasaki disease in childhood.

Evaluation of the coronary arteries should include quantitative assessment of the internal vessel diameters. Aneurysms are at least 1.5 times larger than the surrounding reference vessel diameter and are classified as saccular if axial and lateral diameters are nearly equal or as fusiform if symmetric dilatation with gradual proximal and distal tapering is seen. When a coronary artery is larger than normal without a segmental aneurysm, it is considered ectatic. Care must be taken in making the diagnosis of ectasia because of considerable normal variation in coronary artery distribution and dominance. The Japanese Ministry of Health criteria classify coronary arteries as abnormal (ectatic) if the internal lumen diameter is >3 mm in children <5 years of age or >4 mm in children ≥5 years of age, if the internal diameter of a segment measures ≥1.5 times that of an adjacent segment, or if the coronary lumen is clearly irregular.

Evaluation of the proximal parts of the left and right coronary artery can be done by echocardiography. However, for evaluation of the more distal segments either conventional coronary angiography or CT is required. Small studies in follow-up patients (mostly teenagers) have confirmed an almost 100% diagnostic accuracy of CT for detection of aneurysms with conventional coronary angiography as the reference standard (**Fig. 18.13**). Thus, recent CT scanners can be recommend for noninvasive follow-up after childhood Kawasaki disease, while severe calcifications may still challenge the interpretation of the degree of coronary stenoses (**Fig. 18.14**).

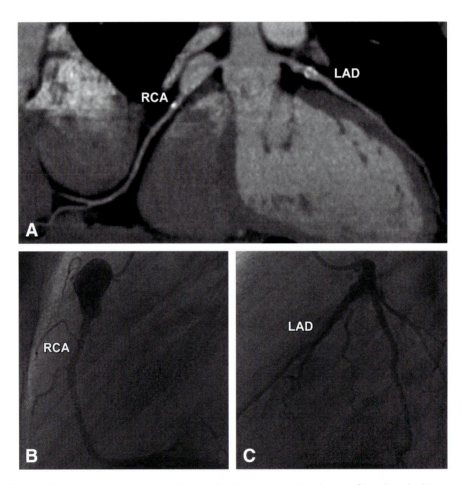

Fig. 18.13 25-year-old male patient with Kawasaki disease. The disease occurred at the age of 2 and resulted in a giant aneurysm of the proximal right coronary artery (RCA) and a fusiform aneurysm in the left anterior descending coronary artery (LAD) seen at CT follow-up (curved multiplanar reformation, **Panel A**). Conventional coronary angiography confirmed these findings in the RCA (**Panel B**) and LAD (**Panel C**). The RCA aneurysm was 25 mm long and had a diameter of 12.5 mm on CT. Used with permission from Arnold et al. Pediatr Radiol 2007

18

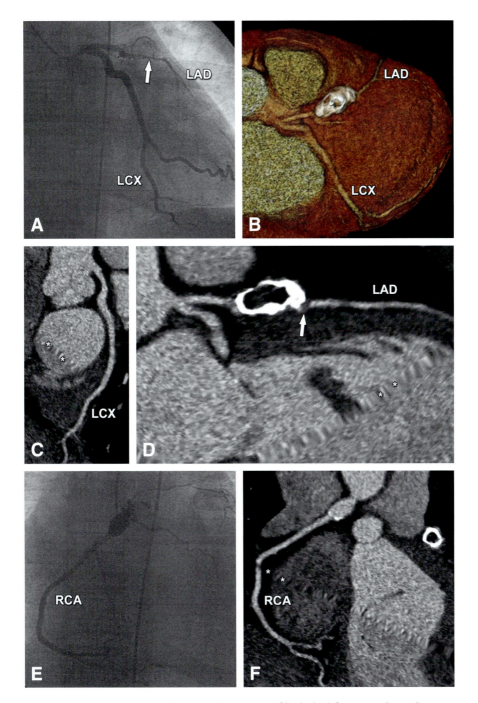

□ **Fig. 18.14** 21-year-old patient with Kawasaki disease and aneurysms of both the left anterior descending coronary artery (LAD, **Panels A–D**) and the right coronary artery (RCA, **Panels E** and **F**). The LAD aneurysm was severely calcified (**Panel B**, curved multiplanar reformation) and stenosis was demonstrated distal to the aneurysm (*arrow* in **Panels A** and **D**). However, the percent diameter stenosis was difficult to evaluate using CT due to the aneurysmal calcification (**Panel D**). There was no stenosis and aneurysm in the left circumflex coronary artery (LCX) both on conventional coronary angiography (**Panel A**) and prospectively ECG-gated dual-source CT (**Panel C**). There was no significant stenosis in the RCA as seen on conventional coronary angiography (**Panel E**). The CT examination was superior in visualizing the calcifications in the aneurysm and also did not show any stenosis (**Panel F**). However, there was an artifact on CT as seen in **Panels C, D**, and **F** (*asterisks*), which was due to arrhythmia

Recommended Reading

1 Arnold R, Ley S, Ley-Zaporozhan J et al (2007) Visualization of coronary arteries in patients after childhood Kawasaki syndrome: value of multidetector CT and MR imaging in comparison to conventional coronary catheterization. Pediatr Radiol 37:998–1006

2 Bae KT, Shah AJ, Shang SS et al (2008) Aortic and hepatic contrast enhancement with abdominal 64-MDCT in pediatric patients: effect of body weight and iodine dose. AJR Am J Roentgenol 191:1589–1594

3 Bland EF, White PD, Garland J (1933) Congenital anomalies of the coronary arteries: report of an unusual case associated with cardiac hypertrophy. Am Heart J 8:787–801

4 Burns JC, Glode MP (2004) Kawasaki syndrome. Lancet 364:533–544

5 du Plessis AM, Andronikou S, Goussaard P (2008) Bridging bronchus and sling left pulmonary artery: a rare entity demonstrated by coronal CT with 3-D rendering display and minimal-intensity projections. Pediatr Radiol 38:1024–1026

6 Ferguson EC, Krishnamurthy R, Oldham SA (2007) Classic imaging signs of congenital cardiovascular abnormalities. Radiographics 27:1323–1334

7 Frush DP, Siegel MJ, Bisset GS 3rd (1997) From the RSNA refresher courses. Challenges of pediatric spiral CT. Radiographics 17:939–959

8 Haramati LB, Glickstein JS, Issenberg HJ, Haramati N, Crooke GA (2002) MR imaging and CT of vascular anomalies and connections in patients with congenital heart disease: significance in surgical planning. Radiographics 22:337–347, discussion 48-9

9 Hoffmann A, Engelfriet P, Mulder B (2007) Radiation exposure during follow-up of adults with congenital heart disease. Int J Cardiol 118:151–153

10 Jatene AD, Fontes VF, Paulista PP et al (1976) Anatomic correction of transposition of the great vessels. J Thorac Cardiovasc Surg 72:364–370

11 Ley S, Zaporozhan J, Arnold R et al (2007) Preoperative assessment and follow-up of congenital abnormalities of the pulmonary arteries using CT and MRI. Eur Radiol 17:151–162

12 Ou P, Celermajer DS, Marini D et al (2008) Safety and accuracy of 64-slice computed tomography coronary angiography in children after the arterial switch operation for transposition of the great arteries. JACC Cardiovasc Imaging 1:331–339

13 Rigsby CK, Gasber E, Seshadri R, Sullivan C, Wyers M, Ben-Ami T (2007) Safety and efficacy of pressure-limited power injection of iodinated contrast medium through central lines in children. AJR Am J Roentgenol 188:726–732

14 Trowitzsch E, Berger T, Stute M (1991) The diameter of the large arteries in the first 3 years of life. An echocardiography study. Monatsschr Kinderheilkd 139:355–359

15 Warnes CA (2006) Transposition of the great arteries. Circulation 114:2699–2709

Typical Clinical Examples

M. Dewey

Abstract

This chapter summarizes the most common clinical examples of cardiac CT.

19.1   Normal Coronary Arteries

The normal anatomy of different coronary artery distribution types as seen with multislice CT is presented in **Figs. 19.1–19.3**.

19.2   Coronary Artery Plaques

Coronary artery plaques of potentially different clinical importance are shown in **Figs. 19.4 –19.7**.

19.3   Coronary Artery Stenoses

Significant coronary artery stenoses and occlusions and their variable appearance on cardiac CT, when compared with conventional invasive angiography, are shown in **Figs. 19.8–19.17**. See Chap. 20 for a summary of the diagnostic performance of coronary CT angiography in this application.

19.4   Coronary Artery Bypass Grafts

Arterial and venous coronary artery bypass grafts differ in diameter and are therefore more or less amenable to evaluation by CT. Examples are shown in **Figs. 19.18–19.26**. See Chap. 20 for a summary of the diagnostic performance of coronary CT angiography in this application.

19.5   Coronary Artery Stents

Evaluation of coronary artery stents is limited using today's technology, and if recommended at all, CT should only be used in patients with a single large-diameter (at least 3.5 mm) coronary stent. Typical results and issues involved in coronary CT stent imaging are shown in **Figs. 19.27–19.36**. See Chap. 20 for a summary of the diagnostic performance of coronary CT angiography in this application.

19.6   Noncardiac Findings

Noncardiac findings on cardiac CT are not uncommon and must be analyzed as meticulously as possible to ensure that important findings that might be responsible for a patient's symptoms are not missed and that unnecessary follow-up examinations are avoided. Common examples of noncardiac findings are provided in **Figs. 19.37–19.51**.

19.7   Extracoronary Cardiac Findings

Extracoronary cardiac findings are also quite common on cardiac CT and are important, in that they are often associated with the coronary findings and can be responsible for a patient's symptoms. Examples of typical extracoronary cardiac findings are provided in **Figs. 19.52–19.60**.

M. Dewey, *Cardiac CT*,
DOI: 10.1007/978-3-642-14022-8_22, © Springer-Verlag Berlin Heidelberg 2011

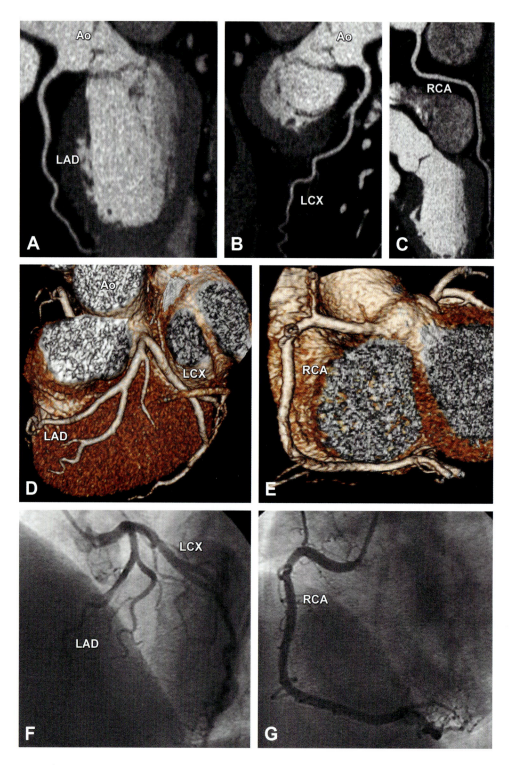

☐ **Fig. 19.1** Normal coronary arteries in a 56-year-old female patient presenting with nonanginal chest pain (see Chap. 6 for a description of angina types) and 0.2 mV (2 mm) ST segment depression in II, III, and aVF during stress testing (bicycle). **Panels A–C** show the curved multiplanar reformations along the left anterior descending (LAD), left circumflex (LCX), and right coronary (RCA) artery, respectively. Three-dimensional reconstructions of the left (**Panel D**) and right (**Panel E**) coronary artery are also unremarkable and demonstrate a codominant coronary distribution in this patient, which is found in 7–20% of all individuals. This distribution type is also seen on the corresponding conventional coronary angiograms of the left (**Panel F**) and right coronary artery (**Panel G**). Ruling out coronary artery disease in patients with low-to-intermediate pretest likelihood is the main application of coronary CT angiography. *Ao* aorta

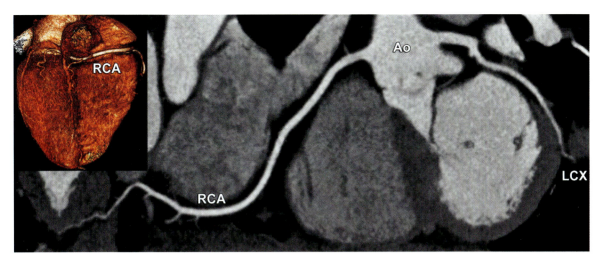

Fig. 19.2 Right coronary artery dominance, which is found in 60–85% of all individuals, as seen with CT using a curved multiplanar reformation along the right coronary (RCA) and left circumflex (LCX) coronary artery (inset shows the base of the heart with RCA dominance). *Ao* aorta

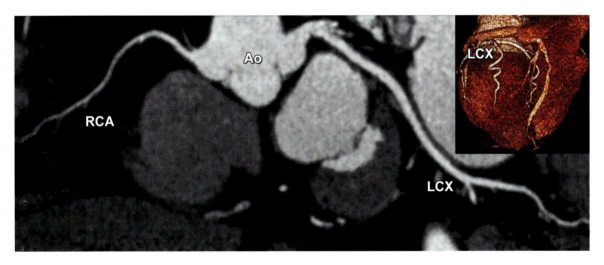

Fig. 19.3 Left coronary artery dominance, which is found in 7–20% of all individuals, as seen with CT using a curved multiplanar reformation along the right coronary (RCA) and left circumflex (LCX) coronary artery (inset shows the base of the heart with dominance of the LCX). *Ao* aorta

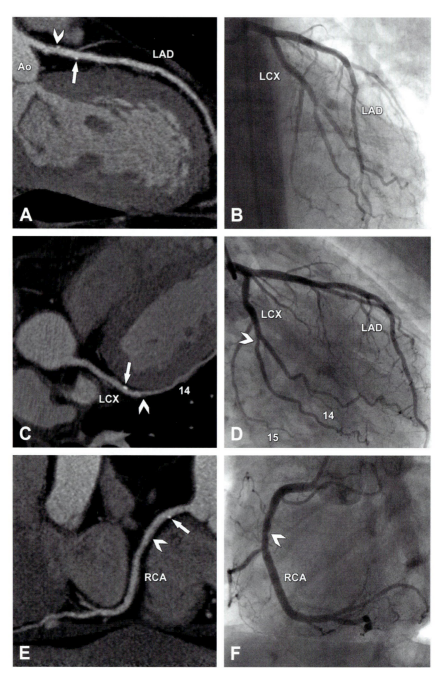

19

◘ **Fig. 19.4** No significant coronary artery stenoses, but small calcified plaques ("calcium spots") and noncalcified plaques in all coronaries in a 65-year-old male patient. The curved multiplanar reformation along the left anterior descending (LAD) coronary artery (**Panel A**) shows a calcium spot (*arrow*) and a mixed plaque (consisting of calcified and noncalcified components, *arrowhead*), which do not cause any indentation of the coronary lumen, as demonstrated by conventional coronary angiography (**Panel B**). There is another calcium spot (*arrow*) in the middle segment of the left circumflex coronary artery (LCX, **Panel C**) that does not cause any visible luminal narrowing on conventional angiography (**Panel D**), whereas a purely noncalcified plaque in the second obtuse marginal branch (*arrowhead*, segment 14) causes slight indentation of the coronary lumen (*arrowhead* in **Panel D**). The curved multiplanar reformation along the right coronary artery (RCA) shows the same findings (**Panel E**) with a calcium spot (*arrow*) not causing luminal narrowing, whereas the more distal noncalcified plaque in segment 2 (*arrowhead* in **Panel E**) is the cause of slight indentation (*arrowhead* in **Panel F**). *Ao* aorta; 15 = segment 15 (distal LCX)

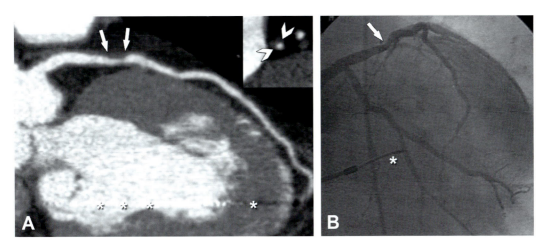

☐ **Fig. 19.5** Large noncalcified plaque in the proximal left anterior descending coronary artery (*arrows* in **Panel A**) of a 72-year-old male patient with typical angina pectoris (see Chap. 6 for a description of angina types). The plaque causes positive remodeling of the outer vessel wall (see inset in **Panel A**; *arrowheads* demarcate the boundaries of this plaque). The so-called remodeling index is defined as the ratio of the vessel area at the plaque site (including plaque and lumen area) to the mean of the vessel area at the reference site proximal and distal to the plaque. Positive remodeling, as in this case, is present if the index is >1.05 and indicates an increased risk for unstable presentation of patients. However, the value of potential clinical consequences (e.g., initiation or increase in statin therapy) in patients with noncalcified plaques without significant luminal narrowing but positive remodeling has not been established. This plaque (*arrow*) caused a 35% diameter stenosis, as measured with quantitative analysis of coronary angiography (**Panel B**). Note the artifacts in CT (*asterisks* in **Panel A**) arising from the cardiac pacemaker lead (*asterisk* in **Panel B**)

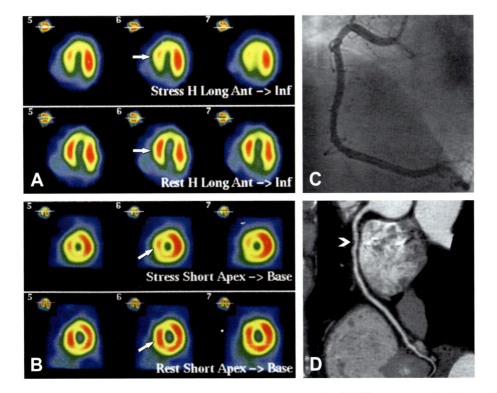

☐ **Fig. 19.6** Example of a false-positive single-photon emission computed tomography (SPECT) examination with ⁹⁹ᵐTc in a 68-year-old male patient with reduced septal and inferior stress perfusion (*arrows* in **Panels A** and **B**). These findings were suggestive of a significant stenosis in the right coronary artery. The right coronary artery, however, was normal and without signs of significant stenosis on conventional coronary angiography (**Panel C**) or coronary CT angiography (curved multiplanar reformation, **Panel D**). However, there was a noncalcified coronary plaque in the midsegment of the right coronary artery on CT (*arrowhead* in **Panel D**) that was not visible on conventional angiography and might have been responsible for the SPECT findings

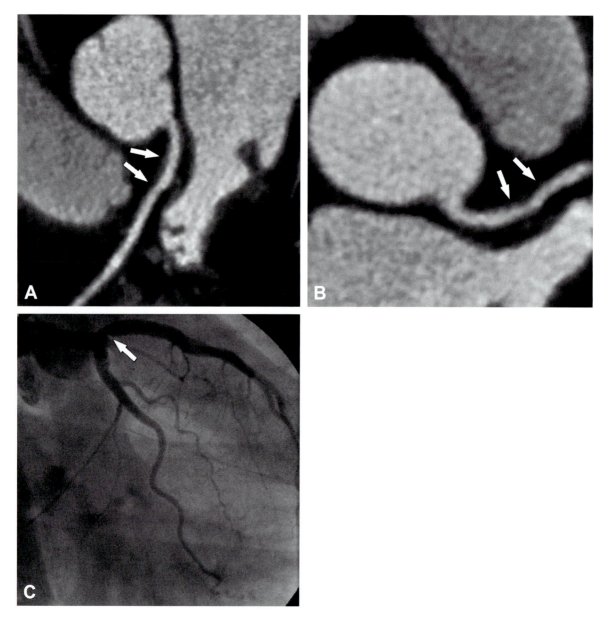

◘ **Fig. 19.7** Large noncalcified plaque (*arrows* in **Panels A** and **B**) in the proximal left anterior descending coronary artery in a 58-year-old female patient with typical angina pectoris. The CT results are illustrated using a curved multiplanar reformation (**Panel A**) and maximum-intensity projection (**Panel B**). This plaque also results in positive remodeling (remodeling index of >1.05), but the indentation of the coronary artery lumen (from below, *arrow* in **Panel C**) is not significant (30% diameter stenosis onquantitative analysis)

19

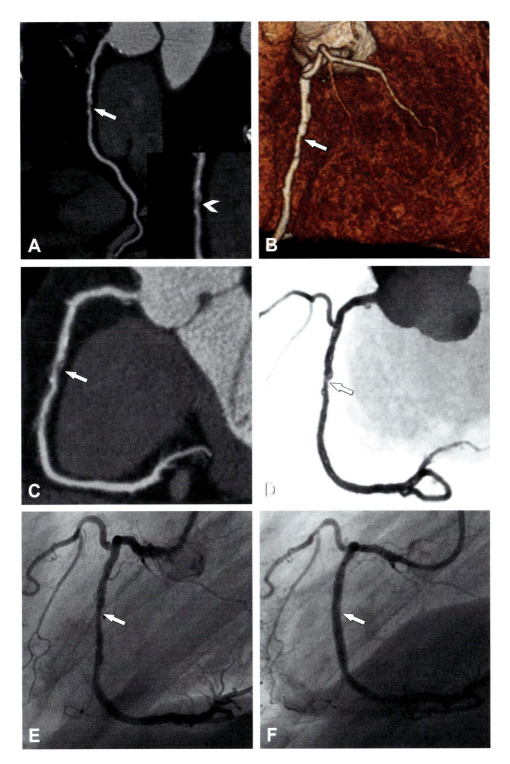

■ **Fig. 19.8** Significant stenosis in the mid-segment of the right coronary artery (*arrows*) on different CT reconstructions (**Panels A–D**) in a 62-year-old male patient with typical angina pectoris but unremarkable exercise ECG. Reconstructions of CT include curved multiplanar reformation (**Panel A**, inset shows the stenosis (*arrowhead*) in a magnified view), volume-rendered three-dimensional reconstruction (**Panel B**), thin-slab maximum-intensity projection curved along the vessel path (so-called CATH view, **Panel C**), and angiographic emulation (**Panel D**). There was good correlation with the findings on subsequently performed conventional coronary angiography (*arrow* in **Panel E**). During the same invasive angiographic examination, this lesion was treated percutaneously with stent placement, with no residual stenosis (*arrow* in **Panel F**)

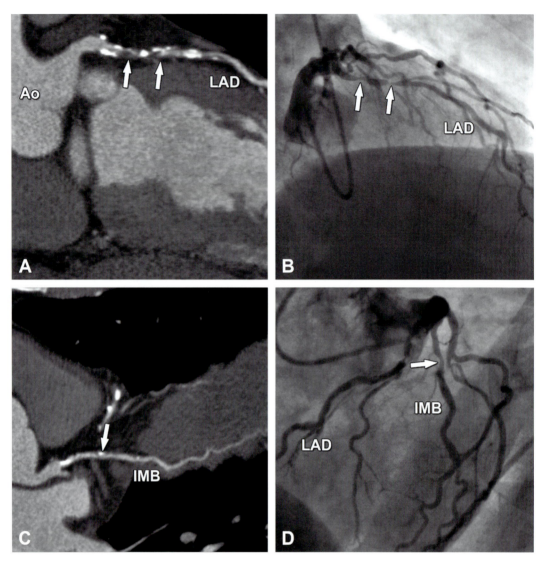

◘ **Fig. 19.9** Significant stenoses (*arrows*) in the four main coronary vessels in a 63-year-old male patient with typical angina pectoris and 0.2 mV (2 mm) ST segment depression on exercise ECG in II, III, and aVF indicating posterior ischemia. Coronary CT results are shown as curved multiplanar reformations along the vessels (left column) and are directly compared with conventional coronary angiography (right column, stenosis degrees obtained with quantitative analysis). There are two 80% diameter stenoses (*arrows*) in the proximal and mid-segment of the left anterior descending coronary artery (LAD, **Panels A** and **B**). These result mainly from noncalcified plaques in these two segments (**Panel A**). However, there are also severely calcified plaques that do not result in significant diameter reductions. An intermediate branch (IMB) is present in this patient and has a 65% diameter stenosis resulting from a calcified plaque (**Panels C** and **D**)

19

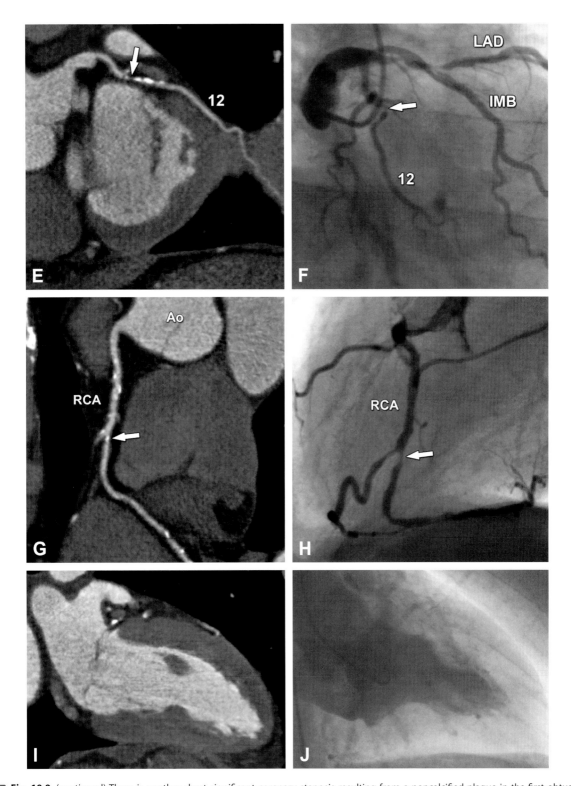

◻ **Fig. 19.9** (continued) There is another short significant coronary stenosis resulting from a noncalcified plaque in the first obtuse marginal branch (segment 12, **Panels E** and **F**), with a diameter stenosis on conventional coronary angiography of 75% that was clearly overestimated on CT (90–95%, **Panel E**). In contrast, the 80% diameter stenosis of the mid-right coronary artery (RCA, **Panel H**), as determined by quantitative coronary angiography, was underestimated by CT as only 65% (**Panel G**). Global left ventricular ejection fraction was 53% on CT (end-systolic two-chamber view, **Panel I**) and 50% on cineventriculography (end-systolic right anterior oblique view, **Panel J**). Thus, according to guidelines (Chap. 11) percutaneous stenting, rather than coronary bypass grafting, was initiated (beginning with the stenosis in the RCA responsible for the ischemic findings on exercise testing). *Ao* aorta

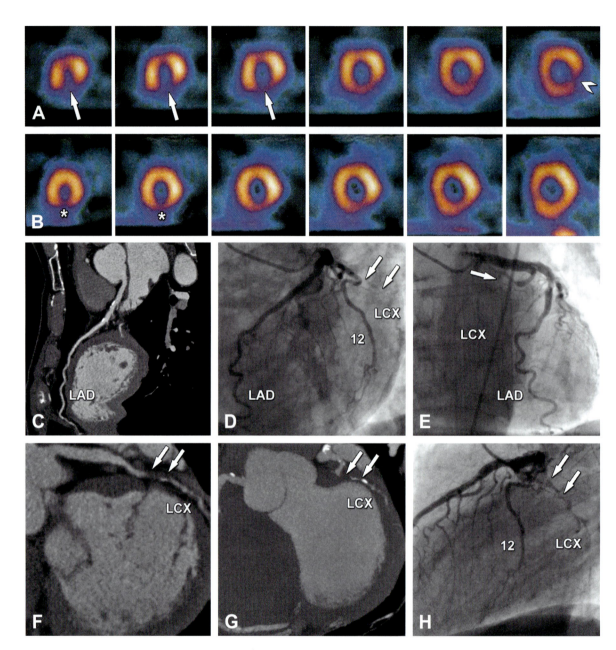

■ **Fig. 19.10** Two-vessel coronary artery disease correctly identified on single-photon emission computed tomography (SPECT) myocardial perfusion imaging (**Panels A** and **B**) and coronary CT angiography (**Panels C, F, G, I,** and **J**) in a 65-year-old male patient with a one-month history of atypical angina pectoris. SPECT shows ischemia in the apical and mid-inferior segments (*arrows* in **Panel A**, short-axis views) that correlates with less markedly reduced perfusion in the same segments at rest (*asterisks* in **Panel B**). In addition, SPECT shows ischemia in the basal inferolateral segment (*arrowhead* in **Panel A**). Coronary CT angiography shows no significant stenosis in the left anterior descending coronary artery, but only calcified plaques (LAD, **Panel C**). This finding is in agreement with conventional angiography (**Panels D** and **E**). However, there is a 10-mm-long occlusion of the mid-left circumflex coronary artery (LCX) caused by a mainly noncalcified plaque, as seen with CT (*arrows* in **Panels F** and **G**). **Panel F** is a curved multiplanar reformation along the vessel path, and **Panel G** is a maximum-intensity projection. Conventional coronary angiography confirms the presence of the occlusion but fails to exactly determine the length of the occlusion (*arrows* in **Panels D, E,** and **H**), while it nicely demonstrates the presence of right-to-left collaterals bridging the LCX occlusion (*asterisks* in **Panel K**)

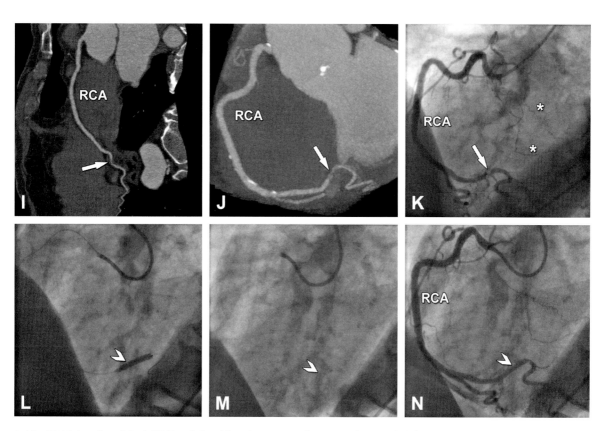

☐ **Fig. 19.10** (continued) Both CT (**Panels I** and **J**) and conventional angiography (**Panel K**) depict a rather short significant 80% diameter stenosis (*arrow*) at the crux cordis in the right coronary artery (RCA). Since the occlusion was considered to be a long-standing process, the recent onset of symptoms was most likely due to the reduction in collateral flow to the LCX because of the RCA stenosis. Thus, the RCA stenosis was stented (*arrowheads*) in the same angiographic session, with good technical success (**Panels L–N**)

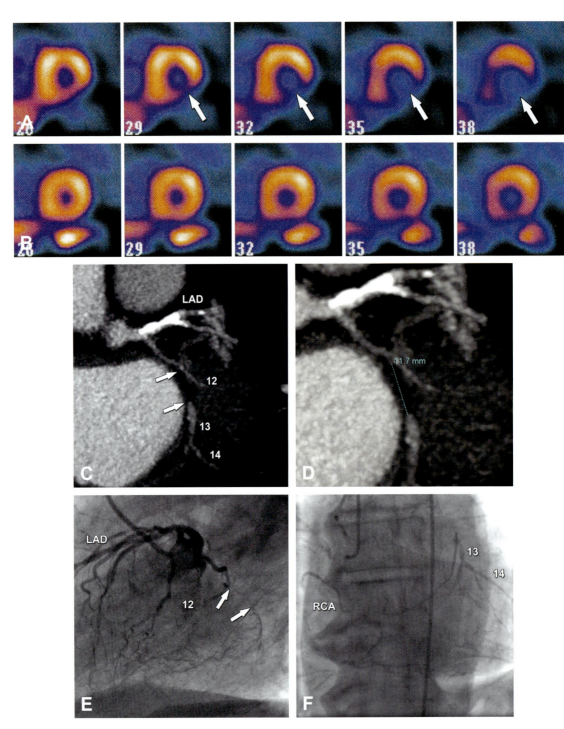

🔲 **Fig. 19.11** Occlusion of the left circumflex coronary artery (LCX) in a 72-year-old male patient with atypical angina pectoris. There is basal and mid-cavity inferolateral and posterior ischemia (*arrows*) on single-photon emission computed tomography (SPECT) myocardial perfusion imaging (**Panel A**, stress exam). There was no perfusion deficit during the examination of SPECT at rest (**Panel B**). Coronary CT angiography shows a 12 mm-long occlusion (*arrows* and measurement) of the mid-LCX (segment 13) as a result of a noncalcified plaque just distal to the branching of a small obtuse marginal artery (segment 12, **Panels C** and **D**, maximum-intensity projections). Conventional coronary angiography nicely shows the occlusion (*arrows* in **Panel E**) and demonstrates right-to-left collaterals, with filling of the middle and distal left circumflex coronary segments (**Panel F**). Despite the purely noncalcified occlusion, percutaneous revascularization failed, most likely because of the location at a branching obtuse marginal artery. Note that during this angiographic session, the left anterior descending coronary artery (LAD) was successfully revascularized. *RCA* right coronary artery

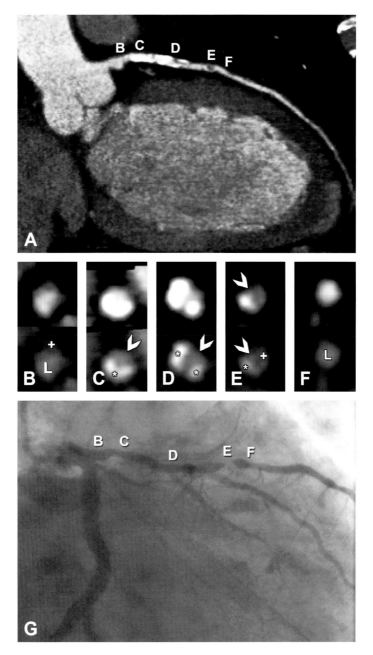

Fig. 19.12 Diffuse atherosclerotic changes in the left anterior descending coronary artery in a 63-year-old male patient with typical angina pectoris (curved multiplanar reformation of CT in **Panel A**). For correlation, cross-sections orthogonal to the curved multiplanar reformation along the vessel obtained by CT (**Panels B–F**) and conventional coronary angiography (**Panel G**) are provided. The letters from B to F indicate matching sites on CT (**Panel A**) and conventional angiography (**Panel G**). The corresponding cross-sections are provided in **Panels B–F** using standard coronary artery settings (*top row*) and bone-window-like settings (*bottom row*). Interestingly, despite the diffuse changes, there is only one significant luminal narrowing (90% diameter stenosis) of the coronary artery (*arrowhead* in **Panel E**), which is caused by a noncalcified plaque (*plus* in **Panel E**) and calcified plaque (*asterisk* in **Panel E**). Note that the residual lumen at the site of this plaque is better appreciated using the standard coronary artery window-level settings (*arrowhead* in the *upper row* in **Panel E**). In contrast, the stenosis diameter at the sites of highly calcified coronary artery plaques (*asterisks* in the *bottom row* in **Panels C** and **D**) is more easily evaluated using bone-window settings (*arrowheads* in the *bottom row* in **Panels C** and **D**). The proximal vessel segments (*B* in **Panel G**) and distal vessel segments (*F* in **Panel G**) appear very similar on conventional coronary angiography (**Panel G**). However, CT shows a relevant difference, with a large noncalcified plaque (*plus* in **Panel B**) proximally without luminal narrowing (*L* in **Panel B**), but no such atherosclerotic changes in the distal vessel segment (**Panel F**). This difference underscores the underestimation of the extent of atherosclerosis with conventional coronary angiography, which is well known from necropsy and intravascular ultrasound studies

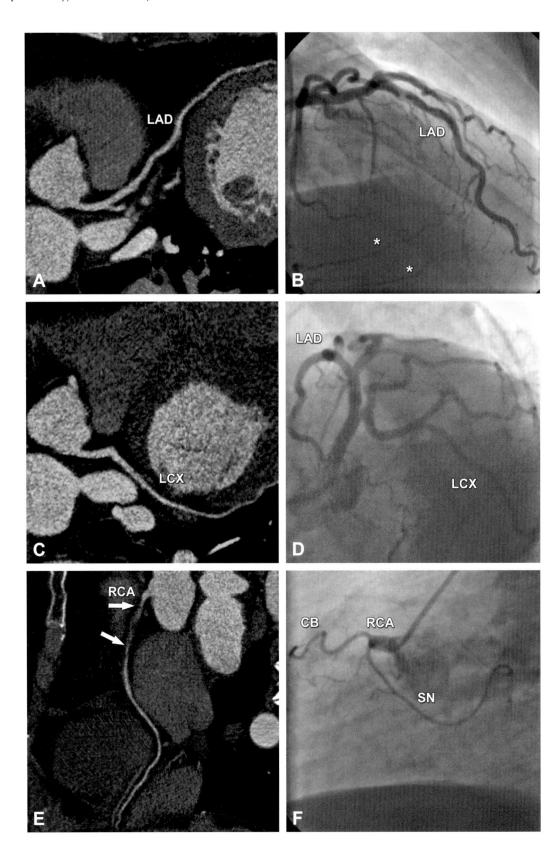

☐ **Fig. 19.13** Occlusion of the right coronary artery (RCA) in a 53-year-old male patient with rather atypical presentation (see Chap. 6 for a description of angina types) and 0.05 mV (0.5 mm) ST segment depression during stress testing in II, III, and aVF indicating posterior ischemia. There are no significant stenoses in the left anterior descending (LAD in **Panels A** and **B**) and left circumflex coronary artery (LCX in **Panels C** and **D**) as seen with coronary CT (curved multiplanar reformations in **Panels A** and **C**) and conventional coronary angiography (**Panels B** and **D**). The occlusion in the proximal and middle segments of the RCA extends over a length of 4 cm and is not calcified (*arrows* in **Panel E**). Because of the short distance from the ostium of the RCA to the beginning of the occlusion (0.5 cm, **Panel F**), percutaneous revascularization was unsuccessful. Note that CT is superior to invasive angiography in identifying the exact length of the occlusion (*arrows* in **Panel E**). Coronary bypass surgery was not considered as an option in this patient because there was good left-to-right collateralization of the occlusion (*asterisks* in **Panel B**), and the patient had only mild symptoms. However, medical therapy was optimized. *CB* conus branch; *SN* sinus node artery

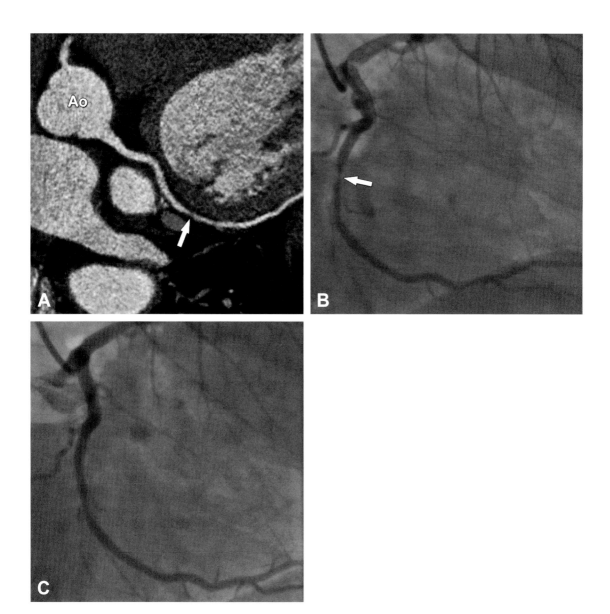

☐ **Fig. 19.14** Significant stenosis of the left circumflex coronary artery (*arrows*) in a 76-year-old male patient with typical angina pectoris, as seen with CT (**Panel A**) and conventional coronary angiography (**Panel B**). Measurement of the percent diameter stenosis resulted in values of 70% for CT and 75% for conventional angiography (with quantitative analysis). The stenosis was caused by a noncalcified plaque (*arrow* in **Panel A**). The outcome of percutaneous coronary intervention is shown in **Panel C**

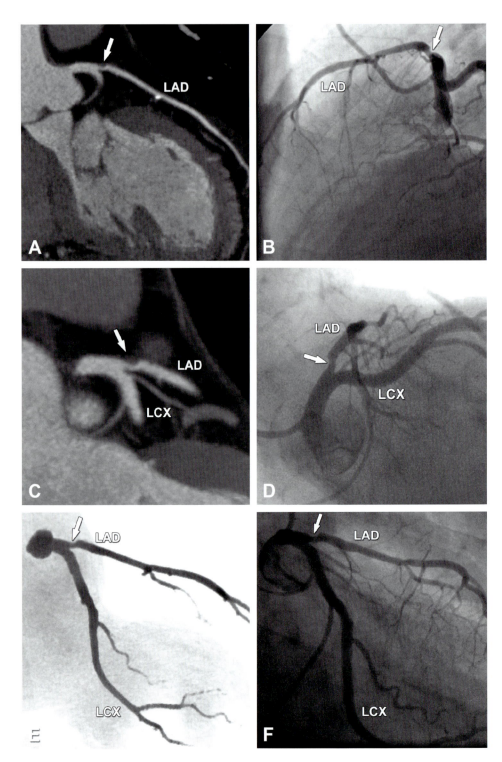

19

☐ **Fig. 19.15** Borderline stenosis (*arrows*) of the proximal left anterior descending coronary artery (LAD) in a 62-year-old male patient with typical angina pectoris, as seen with CT (*left column*) and conventional angiography (*right column*). Results of coronary CT angiography are shown as a curved multiplanar reformation (**Panel A**), thin-slab maximum-intensity projection (**Panel C**), and angiographic emulation (**Panel E**). There is good correlation with the corresponding invasive angiogram projections (**Panels B**, **D**, and **F**). Both CT and quantitative conventional coronary angiography estimated a percent diameter stenosis of 50%. Because there were no signs of ischemia on exercise ECG, no revascularization was attempted. With optimized medical management, the patient's angina pectoris resolved. Note that there is a small calcified plaque in the mid-LAD (**Panel A**). *LCX* left circumflex coronary artery

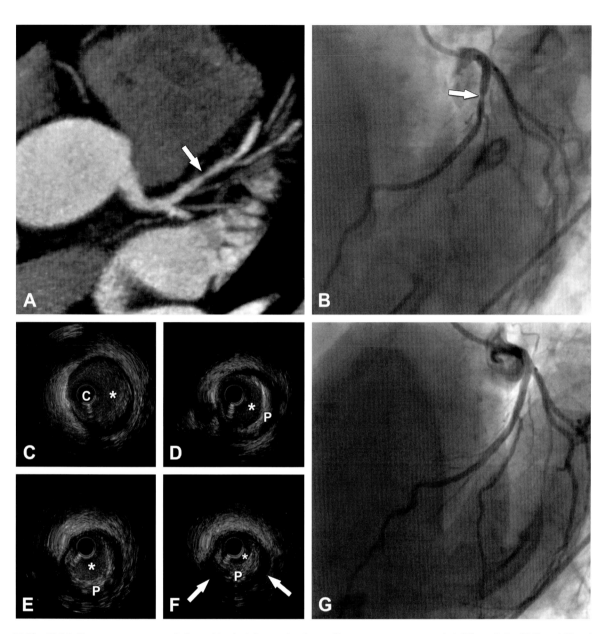

◻ **Fig. 19.16** Coronary artery stenosis (*arrow*) in the left anterior descending coronary artery, graded differently by CT (**Panel A**) and invasive angiography (**Panel B**) in a 62-year-old female patient with typical angina pectoris and ST segment depression of 0.15 mV (1.5 mm) in V4–6 during stress testing (bicycle) indicating anterior ischemia. CT shows a short 70% diameter stenosis caused by a noncalcified plaque in the proximal vessel segment with positive remodeling (**Panel A**, maximum-intensity projection), whereas quantitative analysis of conventional angiography shows only a 40% diameter reduction. Because of worsening angina pectoris and the coronary CT findings, repeat angiography, including intravascular ultrasound (**Panels C–F**), was performed 6 months later. Intravascular ultrasound (cross-sections), located from proximal LAD to the stenosis, confirmed the presence of the plaque (*P* in **Panels D–F**) that caused a short 70% diameter stenosis (*arrows* in **Panel F**) of the lumen (*asterisk* in **Panels C–F**). On the basis of these findings, percutaneous coronary intervention was performed (**Panel G**). *C* intravascular ultrasound catheter

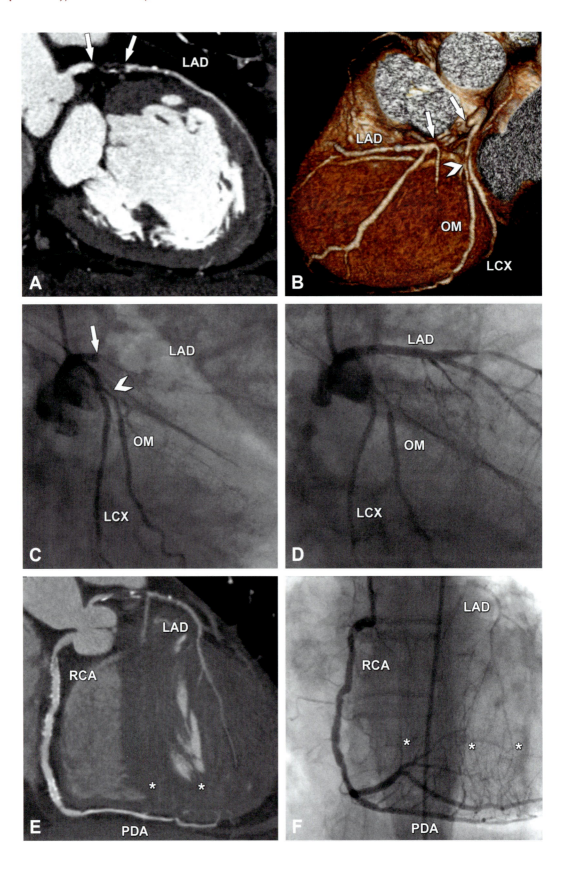

Fig. 19.17 Occlusion of the proximal left anterior descending coronary artery (LAD) in a 78-year-old female patient with a 2-week history of typical angina pectoris (*arrows* in **Panels A–C**). A curved multiplanar reformation of CT is shown in **Panel A**, while **Panel B** is a volume-rendered three-dimensional reconstruction. There is an excellent correlation with conventional coronary angiography, and the length (1.5 cm) of the occlusion, which was mainly caused by a noncalcified plaque, is better seen with CT (*arrows* in **Panel A**). Percutaneous coronary intervention was performed during the same angiographic session, and good revascularization was achieved (compare **Panel D** with **Panel C**). There was also a significant stenosis (*arrowhead* in **Panels B** and **C**) of the obtuse marginal artery (OM) of the left circumflex coronary artery (LCX). The LAD occlusion was collateralized via septal branches (*asterisks* in **Panels E** and **F**) arising from the posterior descending coronary artery (PDA). **Panel E** is a CATH view (curved thin-slab maximum-intensity projection) of coronary CT angiography along the right coronary artery (RCA). This CT reconstruction is superior in that it depicts both the RCA with the collaterals (*asterisks*) and the LAD (with the occlusion) in a single image

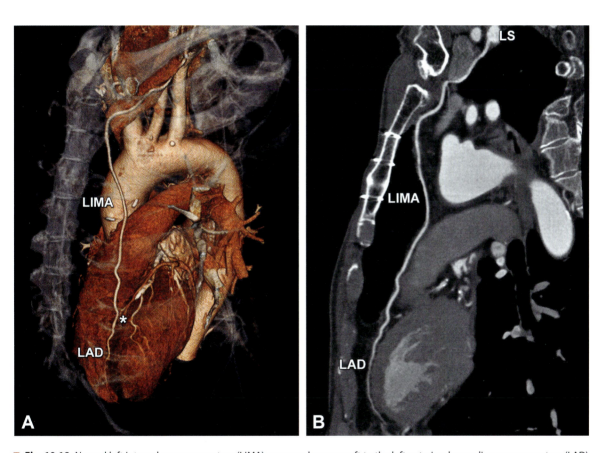

Fig. 19.18 Normal left internal mammary artery (LIMA) coronary bypass graft to the left anterior descending coronary artery (LAD). The CT data are shown in a three-dimensional volume-rendered reconstruction (left anterosuperior view, **Panel A**), with the distal anastomosis indicated by an *asterisk*. The curved multiplanar reformation along the arterial graft (including its origin from the left subclavian artery, LS) is shown in **Panel B**

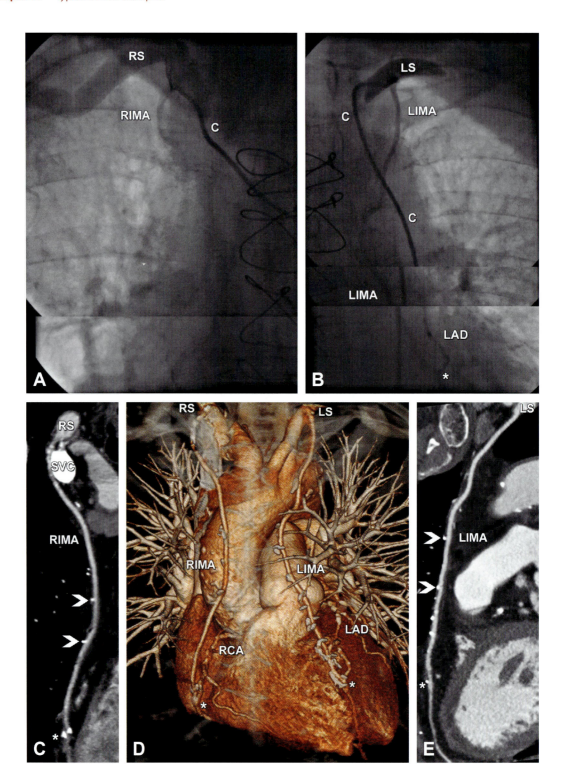

19

◘ **Fig. 19.19** Advantages of coronary CT angiography in depicting coronary bypasses. Example of patent coronary arterial bypass grafts in a 68-year-old male patient with typical angina pectoris who underwent bypass grafting 7 years earlier. Conventional coronary angiography failed to demonstrate patency of the graft because it was not possible to selectively insert the catheter into the right internal mammary artery (RIMA, **Panel A**). *C* indicates the position of the catheter. The left internal mammary artery (LIMA) coronary bypass to the left anterior descending coronary artery (LAD) including the distal anastomosis (*asterisk*) was normal on conventional angiography (**Panel B**). CT was initiated, and in contrast to the conventional angiograms, it was able to demonstrate a normal RIMA graft to the right coronary artery (RCA) on both a curved multiplanar reformation (**Panel C**) and a three-dimensional volume-rendered reconstruction (*anterior view*, **Panel D**). Coronary CT angiography also confirmed the patency of the LIMA to the LAD (**Panels D** and **E**). Note the metallic surgical clips along the arterial bypass grafts (*arrowheads* in **Panels C** and **E**) and the distal anastomoses (*asterisk* in **Panels C** and **E**). Very dense contrast material is still present in the superior vena cava (SVC) because the injection was performed via a right cubital vein. Deviating from the standard procedure of contrast injection into the right arm veins and using left-sided injection instead might have been preferable in this patient. This way, LIMA assessment might have been limited, but CT was primarily performed because conventional angiography was nondiagnostic with regard to the RIMA graft. *C* catheter; *LS* left subclavian artery; *RS* right subclavian artery

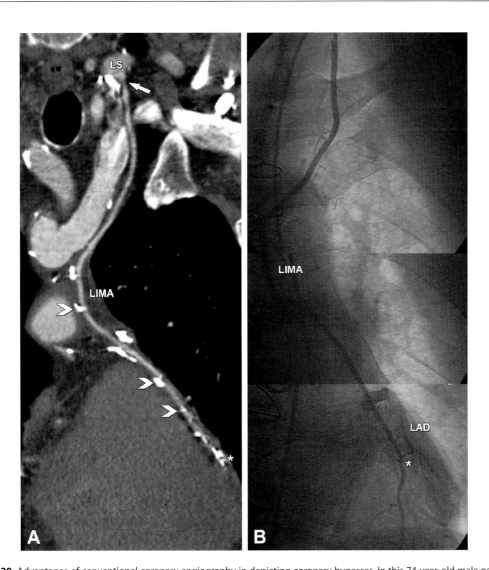

◘ **Fig. 19.20** Advantages of conventional coronary angiography in depicting coronary bypasses. In this 74-year-old male patient with atypical angina pectoris who underwent left internal mammary artery (LIMA) coronary bypass grafting to the left anterior descending coronary artery (LAD) 4 years ago, CT was unable to rule out significant stenoses because of artifacts arising from nearby dense contrast material in the veins (*arrow*) and surgical clips (*arrowheads* in **Panel A**, curved multiplanar reformation). Also, the distal anastomosis (*asterisk*) could not be reliably assessed with CT (**Panel A**). In contrast, subsequently performed conventional angiography shows a patent LIMA to LAD (**Panel B**). Newer surgical clips have a lower metal content and therefore tend to produce fewer artifacts on coronary CT

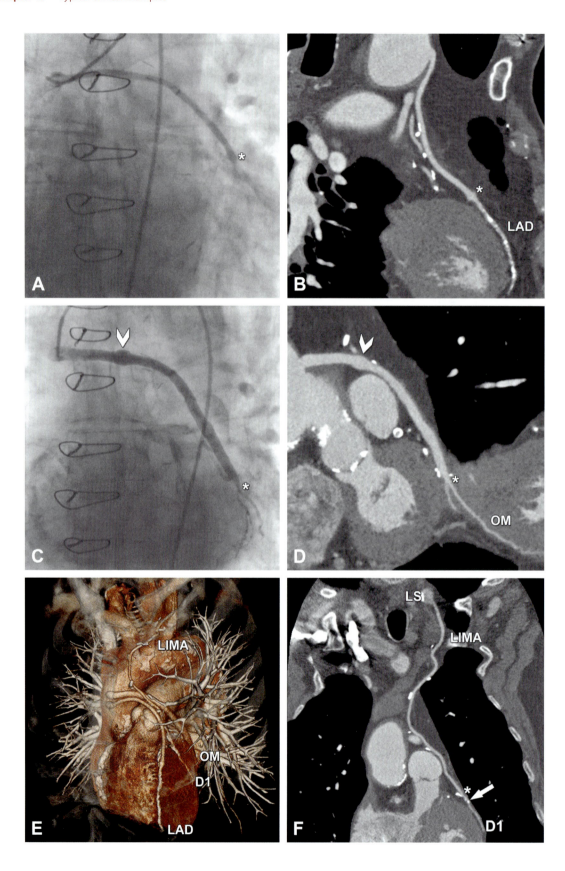

⬛ **Fig. 19.21** Normal coronary arterial and venous bypass grafts in a 79-year-old male patient. There is good correlation of conventional angiography (**Panels A** and **C**) and CT (**Panels B** and **D**) in the evaluation of the venous bypass grafts to the left anterior descending coronary artery (LAD, **Panels A** and **B**) and the obtuse marginal artery (OM, **Panels C** and **D**). There is focal dilatation of the venous graft to the OM due to a venous valve (*arrowhead* in **Panels C** and **D**), while the distal anastomoses (*asterisk*) are unremarkable (**Panels A–D**). However, conventional angiography was unsuccessful in aiding the selective insertion of a catheter into the left internal mammary artery (LIMA). Thus, CT was initiated and was able to visualize this graft to the first diagonal branch (D1). Three-dimensional and curved multiplanar reformations of the LIMA graft are shown in **Panels E** and **F**, respectively. The distal anastomosis of this graft was normal (*asterisk* in **Panel F**), but there was a significant stenosis of the D1 (*arrow* in **Panel F**), which was also seen on conventional coronary angiography. *LS* left subclavian artery

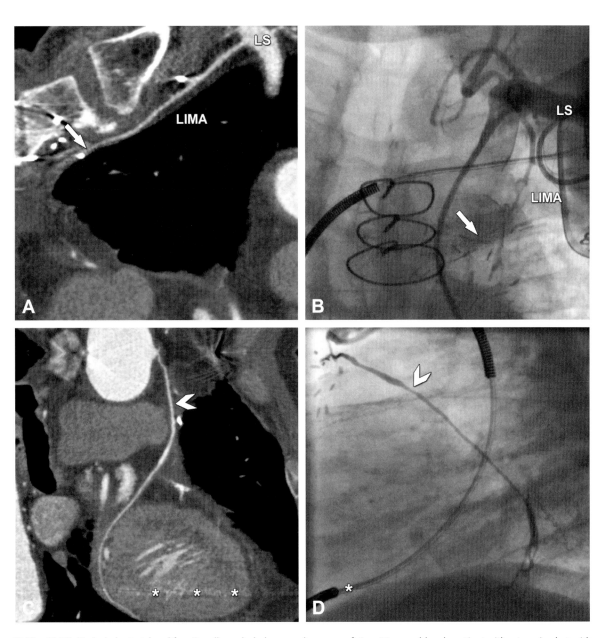

⬛ **Fig. 19.22** Occluded arterial and functionally occluded venous bypass graft in a 66-year-old male patient without angina but with severe dyspnea. Curved multiplanar reformation along the left internal mammary artery (LIMA) shows occlusion about 5–6 cm from the origin (*arrow* in **Panel A**). There is good agreement with the findings from conventional angiography (**Panel B**). The venous bypass graft to the obtuse marginal artery has a very small diameter of only 1 mm (*arrowhead*) and is functionally occluded, as seen on CT (**Panel C**, curved multiplanar reformation) and conventional angiography (**Panel D**). Note that the patient has an implanted cardiac defibrillator (*asterisk* in **Panel D**), which leads to minor artifacts on CT (*asterisks* in **Panel C**). *LS* left subclavian artery

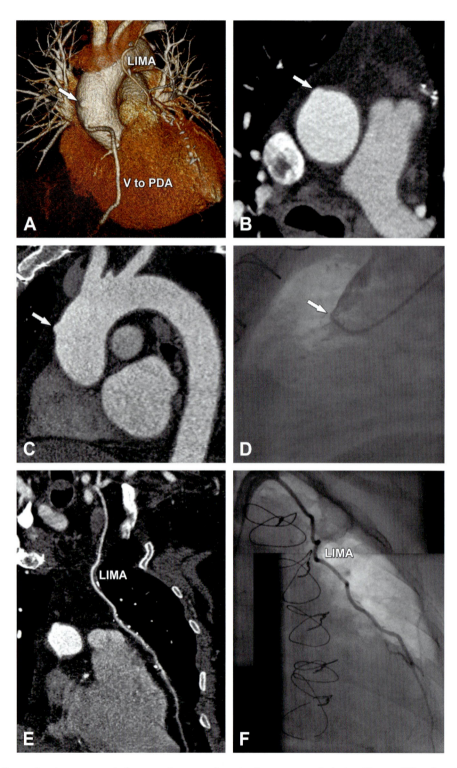

🔲 **Fig. 19.23** Comprehensive assessment of coronary bypass grafts and native coronary arteries in a 64-year-old female patient with atypical angina pectoris. There is ostial occlusion of the venous bypass graft, which passed to the left circumflex coronary artery, as can be seen in the three-dimensional reconstruction of CT (*arrow* in **Panel A**). In axial source images and a sagittal reconstruction of CT, the occlusion (*arrow*) looks like a small outpouching of the lumen (**Panels B** and **C**). Conventional angiography confirmed the occlusion (*arrow* in **Panel D**). The left internal mammary artery (LIMA) is patent to the left anterior descending coronary artery (**Panels E** and **F**), but CT detected significant stenosis at the distal anastomosis (*arrows*) of the venous bypass graft to the posterior descending coronary artery (V to PDA, **Panel G**)

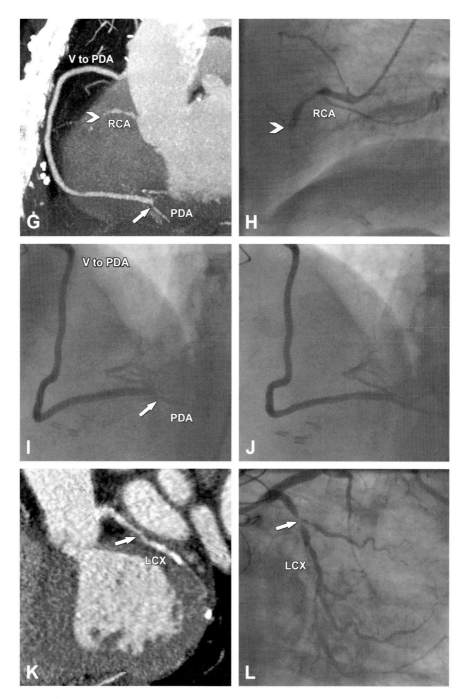

Fig. 19.23 (continued) **Panel G** is a maximum-intensity projection demonstrating the stenosis at the anastomosis to the PDA (*arrow*). The right coronary artery (RCA) is occluded at the junction of segments 1 and 2 (*arrowhead* in **Panel G**). Both the occlusion of the RCA (*arrowhead* in **Panel H**) and the stenosis at the distal anastomosis of the venous bypass graft to the posterior descending coronary artery (*arrow* in **Panel I**) were confirmed by subsequently performed conventional angiography. During the same angiographic session, percutaneous coronary stenting of the stenosis of the distal anastomosis was performed (**Panel J**). CT also found a significant stenosis (*arrow*) of the left circumflex coronary artery (LCX, **Panel K**), which was confirmed by conventional angiography (*arrow* in **Panel L**) and was also treated interventionally

19

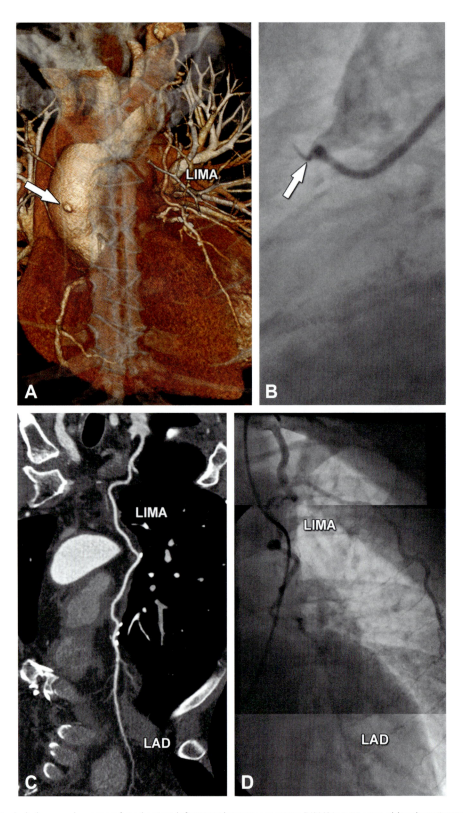

◘ **Fig. 19.24** Occluded venous bypass graft and patent left internal mammary artery (LIMA) in a 64-year-old male patient with atypical angina. Ostial occlusion of the venous bypass graft (*arrow*) that supplies the left circumflex coronary artery (**Panel A**). **Panel A** is a three-dimensional reconstruction (anterior view). This finding was confirmed by conventional coronary angiography (lateral projection, *arrow* in **Panel B**). The LIMA to the left anterior descending coronary artery (LAD) was unremarkable on both CT (curved multiplanar reformation, **Panel C**) and conventional angiography (**Panel D**)

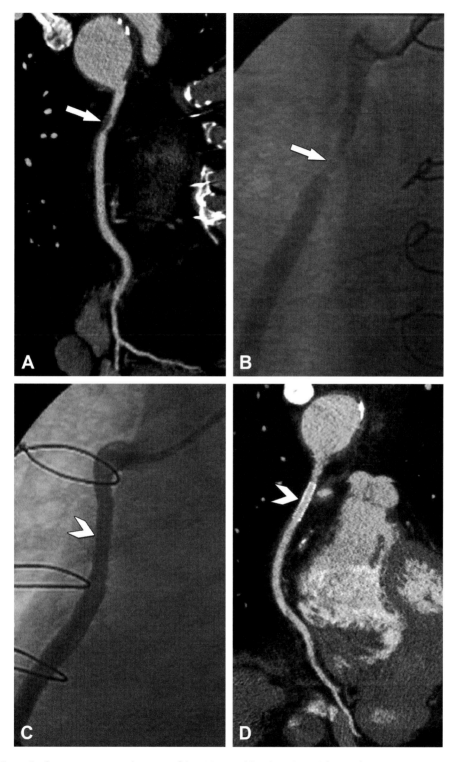

⬚ **Fig. 19.25** Stenosis of a venous coronary bypass graft in a 69-year-old male patient with typical angina pectoris. Curved multiplanar reformation of CT shows a noncalcified plaque (*arrow*) in the proximal portion of a venous bypass graft to the right coronary artery, resulting in 80% diameter stenosis (**Panel A**) as measured with digital calipers on orthogonal cross-sections. Subsequently performed conventional angiography confirmed this finding (*arrow* in **Panel B**), and during the same angiographic session, percutaneous intervention with a 4.0-mm stent was performed (*arrowhead* in **Panel C**). Follow-up CT demonstrated a patent stent without significant in-stent restenosis (*arrowhead* in **Panel D**)

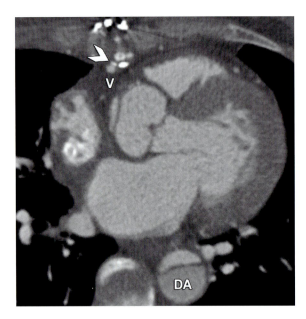

🔲 **Fig. 19.26** Prior to reoperative cardiac surgery, CT can identify important findings. In this patient, a sternal wire (*arrowhead*) is located near a venous bypass graft (V). Also, the distance from the sternum to bypasses can be easily measured using CT before reoperation. In this case, there was also a dissection of the descending aorta (DA)

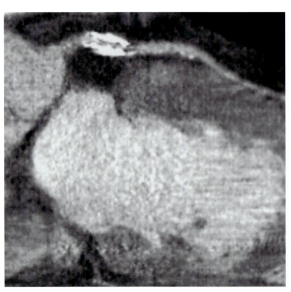

🔲 **Fig. 19.28** Nondiagnostic coronary artery stent in the proximal left anterior descending coronary artery (curved multiplanar reformation) in a 64-year-old male patient with nonanginal chest pain. Despite the large diameter of the stent (4.0 mm), the lumen was not evaluable because of motion and beam-hardening artifacts. Interestingly, stents as large as this one are implanted in only about a fifth of all cases, and the vast majority of patients receive coronary stents of 2.5 or 3.0 mm in diameter, which can be reliably evaluated by CT in only 50% of the time (Chap. 20)

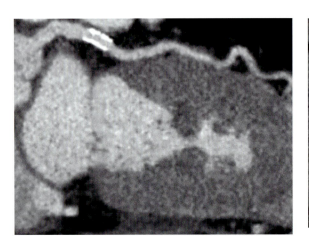

🔲 **Fig. 19.27** Patent coronary artery stent (3.5-mm diameter) with good runoff in the proximal left anterior descending coronary artery (curved multiplanar reformation) in a 58-year-old female patient presenting with typical angina pectoris

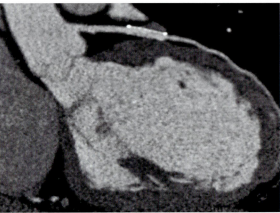

🔲 **Fig. 19.29** Patent coronary artery stent (3.0-mm diameter) in the proximal left anterior descending coronary artery (curved multiplanar reformation) in a 41-year-old male patient who was asymptomatic but at high risk (history of acute anterior myocardial infarction and stenting at the age of 36). Note the irregular vessel wall immediately distal from the stent that did not result in significant stenosis

19

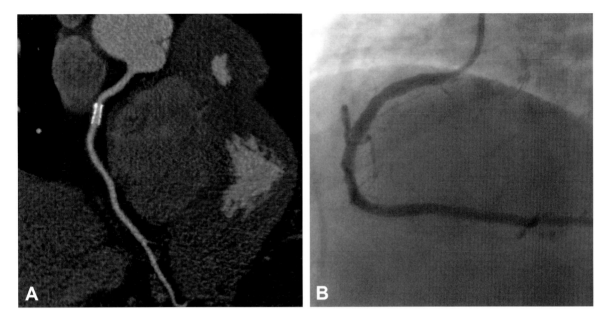

◻ **Fig. 19.30** Patent coronary artery stent (4.0 mm diameter) in the mid-right coronary artery without significant restenosis (curved multiplanar reformation, **Panel A**) in a 64-year-old male patient presenting with typical angina pectoris. There is good agreement in this large-diameter stent with conventional coronary angiography (**Panel B**)

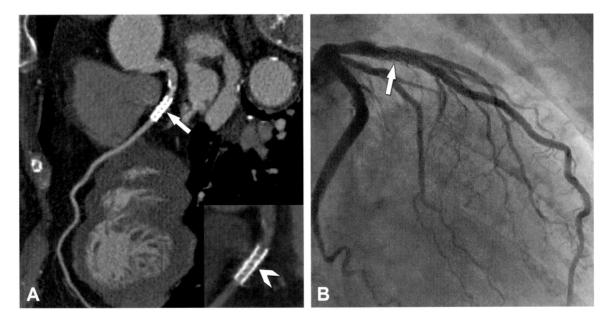

◻ **Fig. 19.31** Nondiagnostic small-diameter coronary artery stent (2.5 mm) in the proximal left anterior descending coronary artery (*arrow* in **Panel A**, curved multiplanar reformation) in an 80-year-old female patient presenting with typical angina pectoris. The runoff seems excellent but this is not a reliable sign on its own in excluding significant in-stent restenosis; enhancement may as well be caused by collateral flow that can be overlooked in nondynamic CT imaging. Even stent kernel reconstructions (inset in **Panel A**, *arrowhead*, curved multiplanar reformation) did not allow reliable exclusion of significant in-stent restenosis in this case. Conventional coronary angiography (**Panel B**) showed some neointimal proliferation (*arrow*) but no significant in-stent restenosis

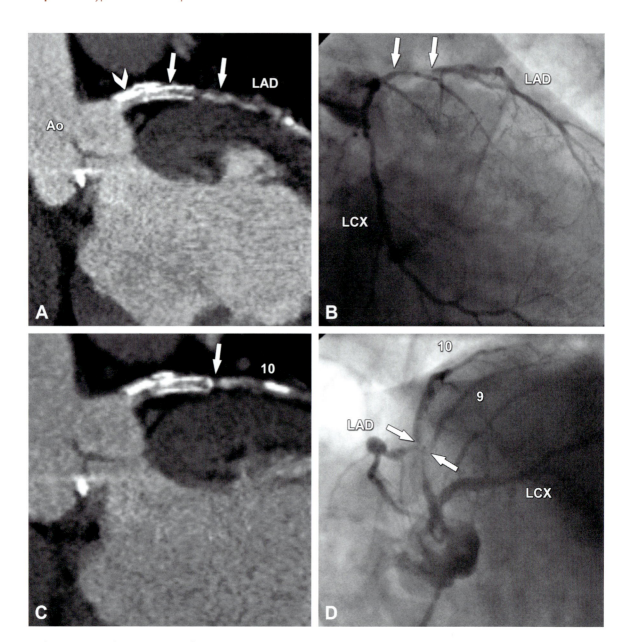

□ Fig. 19.32 Significant restenosis of a 3.0 mm diameter bare-metal stent in the proximal left anterior descending coronary artery (LAD) in a 63-year-old male with typical angina pectoris. Coronary CT angiography suggested occlusion of this stent (*arrows* in **Panel A**, curved multiplanar reformation). There was also a large calcified plaque in the left main coronary artery that did not cause significant luminal narrowing (*asterisk* in **Panel A**). In contrast, quantitative analysis of conventional coronary angiography demonstrated that there was no occlusion, but 90% in-stent restenosis had occurred (*arrows* in **Panel B**). Because of its lower spatial resolution, CT is often unable to differentiate high-grade stenosis from occlusion. Because of the location of the stent at the branchings of the first (9) and second (10) diagonal branches, a complex situation involving a trifurcation stenosis was present (*arrows* in **Panels C** and **D**). The left circumflex coronary artery (LCX) had no significant stenosis (**Panel D**)

19

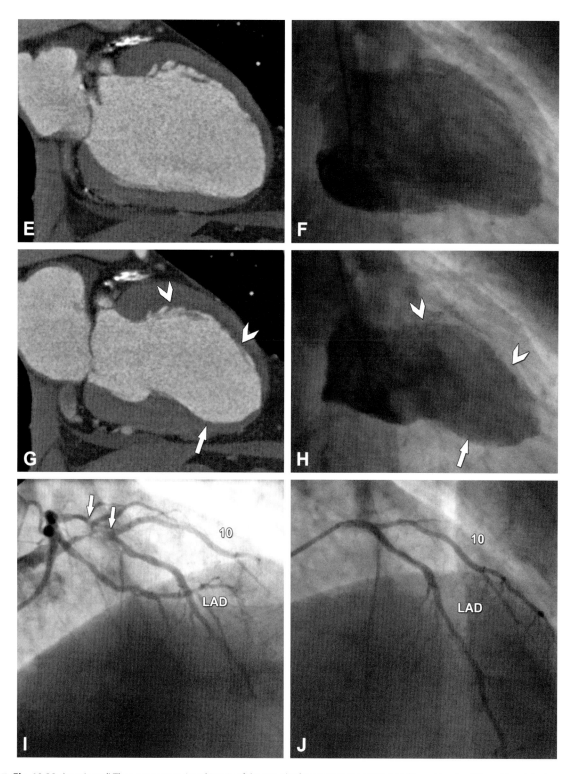

☐ **Fig. 19.32** (continued) There was extensive akinesia of the apical inferior segment (*arrow*) and hypokinesia of the midventricular and apical anterior segments (*arrowheads*) in the two-chamber view on CT (**Panels E** and **G**) and in the right anterior oblique projection by cineventriculography (**Panels F** and **H**, with **Panels E** and **F** representing end-diastole and **Panels G** and **H** representing end-systole). During the same angiographic session, successful complex percutaneous intervention of the LAD and the second diagonal branch (10) was performed (**Panels I–J**). *Ao* aorta

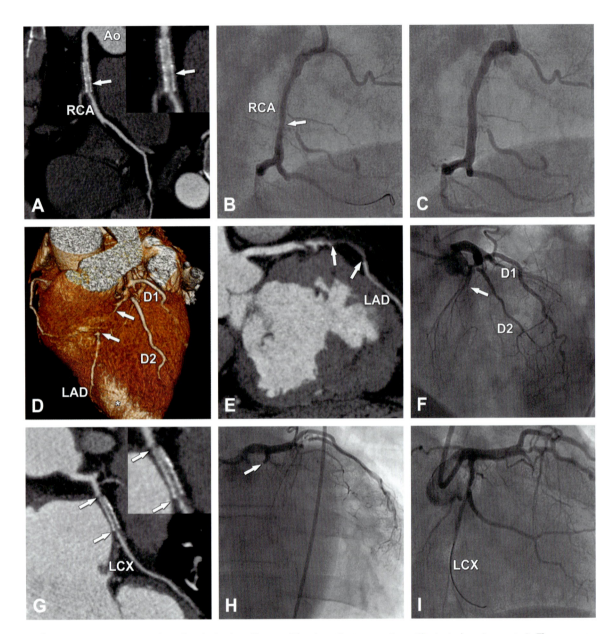

◘ **Fig. 19.33** In-stent restenosis and occlusion in a 63-year-old male patient presenting with atypical angina pectoris. The *upper row* (**Panels A–C**) shows the results for the right coronary artery (RCA), the *middle row* (**Panels D–F**) for the left anterior descending coronary artery (LAD), and the *bottom row* (**Panels G–I**) for the left circumflex coronary artery (LCX). Because of the presence of hypodense material in the distal part of the RCA stent (*arrow* in **Panel A**, curved multiplanar reformation), CT suspected significant in-stent restenosis (see inset in **Panel A** for a magnified view). Conventional angiography was initiated and confirmed a significant in-stent restenosis in the mid-segment of the RCA (*arrow* in **Panel B**). Percutaneous coronary intervention was performed during the same angiographic session (**Panel C**). CT also showed a known occlusion of the LAD (*arrows*), as depicted here in a three-dimensional volume-rendered reconstruction (**Panel D**), and a curved multiplanar reformation along the vessel (**Panel E**), which was confirmed on conventional angiography (**Panel F**). There were intracoronary LAD collaterals via septal branches that bypassed the occlusion, as seen on CT (**Panels D and E**). The LAD occlusion had resulted in apical infarction causing wall thinning (*asterisk* in **Panel D**). The second stent in the proximal left circumflex coronary artery (LCX) was filled with hypodense material (*arrows* in **Panel G**, curved multiplanar reformation), and based on coronary CT, occlusion of this stent was suspected (see inset in **Panel G** for a magnified view). Conventional angiography also confirmed stent occlusion in the proximal LCX (*arrow* in **Panel H**), and the stent was percutaneously recanalized in the same angiographic session (**Panel I**). *D1* first diagonal branch (segment 9); *D2* second diagonal branch (segment 10)

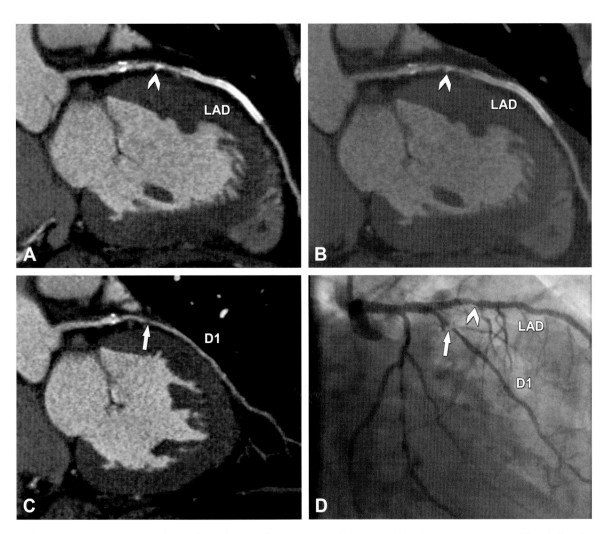

⬛ **Fig. 19.34** Importance of stent kernels for evaluation of coronary stents. This 53-year-old male patient presenting with typical angina pectoris had a history of stenting of the left anterior descending coronary artery (LAD), with two 2.5-mm diameter stents. Curved multi-planar reformation based on standard reconstruction kernel for coronary arteries did not allow reliable assessment of the stent lumen (**Panel A**). Use of stent kernels, however, showed no sign of in-stent restenosis (**Panel B**). Also, the calcified plaque (*arrowhead* in **Panels A** and **B**) was easier to assess using a stent kernel, and significant luminal diameter reduction resulting from this plaque was excluded (**Panel B**). However, a 90% diameter stenosis (*arrow*) of the first diagonal branch (D1), caused by a noncalcified plaque (**Panel C**), was confirmed on conventional angiography (*arrow* in **Panel D**). Conventional coronary angiography also confirmed that the calcified plaque in the mid-LAD caused only a nonsignificant reduction in diameter (*arrowhead* in **Panel D**)

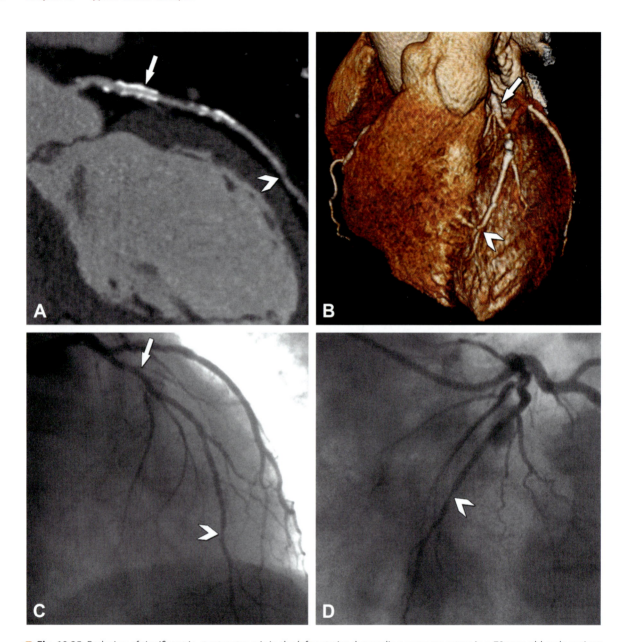

◘ **Fig. 19.35** Exclusion of significant in-stent restenosis in the left anterior descending coronary artery in a 70-year-old male patient. The 3.5-mm diameter stent was unremarkable on curved multiplanar reformation of coronary CT (*arrow* in **Panel A**), but a 60% diameter stenosis resulting from a noncalcified plaque was suspected in the distal left anterior descending artery (*arrowhead* in **Panels A** and **B**). Conventional coronary angiography confirmed the patency of the stent (*arrow* in **Panel C**), but the distal stenosis was considered on quantitative analysis to represent a 40% diameter reduction (*arrowhead* in **Panels C** and **D**). This example further illustrates the fact that there is sometimes less-than-perfect agreement between CT and conventional angiography in terms of quantifying coronary artery stenoses. Such disagreements are attributable to the three-dimensional nature of CT, which is advantageous (**Fig. 19.16**) in that it allows a more accurate assessment of diameter reduction, especially in the case of bifurcation lesions; in contrast, the relevantly higher spatial resolution of conventional angiography is a pivotal advantage of this test

19

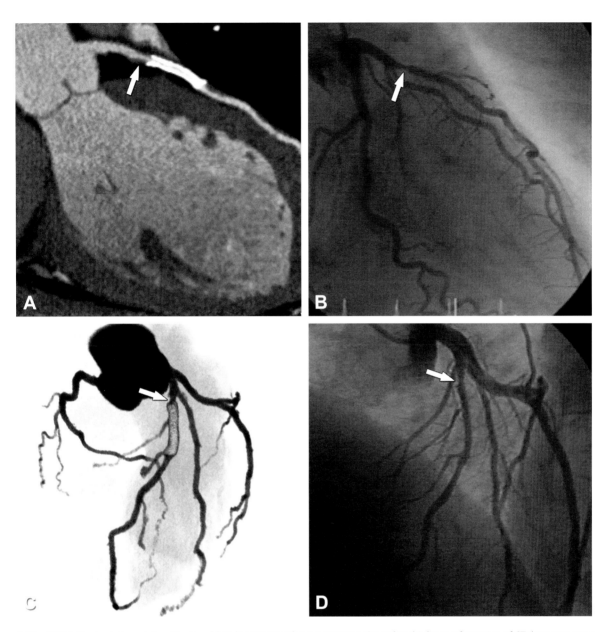

◘ Fig. 19.36 Prestent stenosis in a 45-year-old male patient without symptoms. Curved multiplanar reformation of CT demonstrates a 30% diameter reduction in the lumen immediately proximal to the stent, resulting from a noncalcified plaque (*arrow* in **Panel A**). Significant in-stent restenosis was excluded using stent kernel curved multiplanar reformations (not shown). Conventional angiography also demonstrated the 30% prestent stenosis (*arrow* in **Panel B**). Angiographic emulation of coronary CT angiography nicely demonstrated the stenosis (*arrow* in **Panel C**), with an excellent correlation with conventional angiography (*arrow* in **Panel D**). Note that the angiographic emulation of CT has the advantage of simultaneously depicting the left and right coronary artery

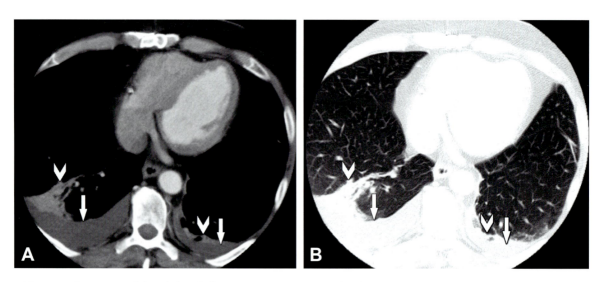

Fig. 19.37 Postoperative bilateral pleural effusion (*arrows*) in a 61-year-old male patient who underwent bypass grafting. Results are shown on large fields of view with soft tissue (**Panel A**) and lung window-level settings (**Panel B**). Note that the effusions cause (nonobstructive) atelectasis in both lower lobes (*arrowheads*)

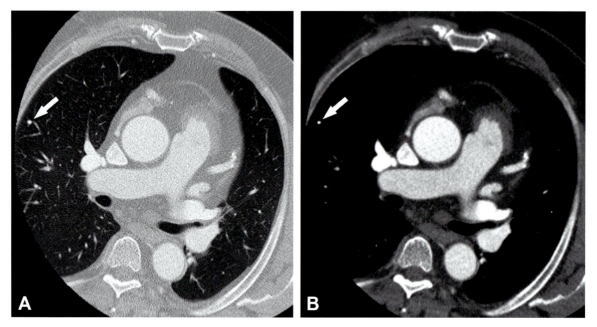

Fig. 19.38 Calcified pulmonary nodule 0.4 cm in diameter (in the size range of 0.3–0.5 cm, lesions are called "ditzels") in the middle lobe (*arrow* in **Panels A** and B) in a 61-year-old male patient without known malignancy. The appearance is characteristic for calcified granuloma that is most likely caused by a prior infection (e.g., tuberculosis, histoplasmosis)

19

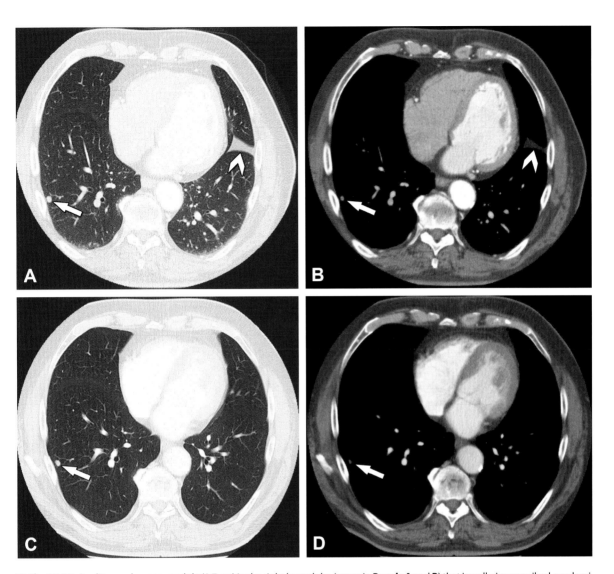

Fig. 19.39 A solitary pulmonary nodule (0.7 cm) in the right lower lobe (*arrow* in **Panels A** and **B**) that is well-circumscribed, predominantly solid, and does not contain any calcifications. There is also an effusion in the left oblique fissure (*arrowhead* in **Panels A** and **B**) Guideline-based 6-month follow-up (according to MacMahon et al. Radiology 2005) standard chest CT was performed, which showed a minor decrease in size and ruled out potential malignancy (*arrow* in **Panels C** and **D**). Differential diagnoses for such nodules include benign infectious lesions, atypical adenomatous hyperplasia, metastases, and lung cancer. Follow-up CT scans can serve to differentiate benign and malignant pulmonary nodules in indeterminate cases

Fig. 19.40 Cavernous lung lesion in the right lower lobe (*arrow*) in a 56-year-old male patient presenting with atypical angina pectoris, who was referred to rule out coronary artery stenoses. There were no significant coronary stenoses, and the nodule with a thin-walled cavity was found on the large fields of view only and was suspected to be due to tuberculosis. Transthoracic biopsy, however, was initiated and revealed a lung carcinoma. Note that because a medium-size scan field of view (320 mm) was chosen for acquisition (to allow using a small focus spot), the reconstruction field of view cannot be larger than 320 mm, and thus the carcinoma is only partially visible

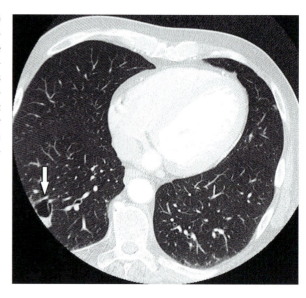

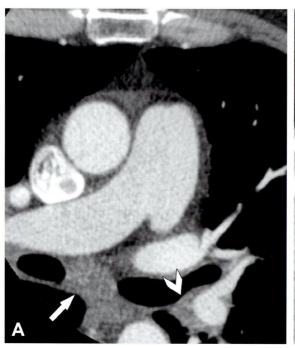

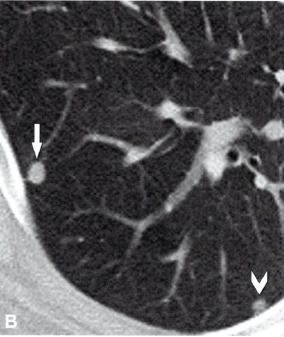

Fig. 19.41 Infracarinal 2 × 1.5 cm mediastinal lymph node (*arrow*) and peribronchial thickening (*arrowhead* in **Panel A**) in a 48-year-old male patient. Pulmonary nodules (*arrow*) and pleural-based opacities were also visible (*arrowhead* in **Panel B**). The final diagnosis was pulmonary sarcoidosis. Common differential diagnoses of mediastinal lymph nodes include lymph node metastases, lymphoma, sarcoidosis, amyloidosis, and silicosis

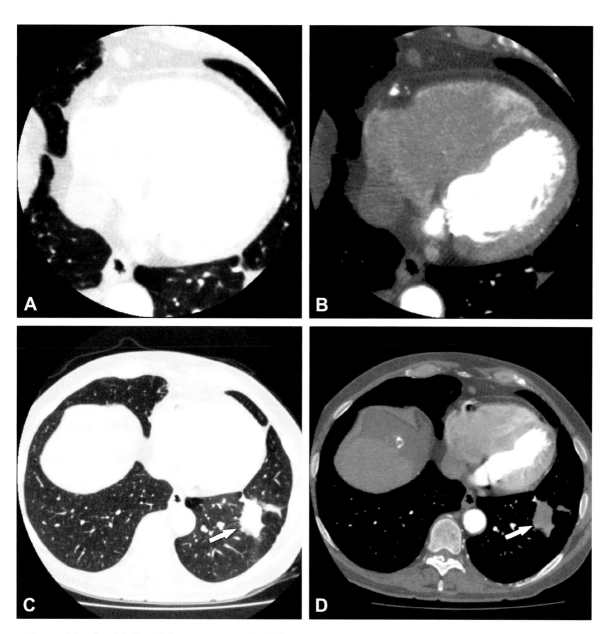

◻ **Fig. 19.42** Incidental finding of a lung carcinoma in the left lower lobe not recognized on dedicated small reconstruction fields of view for coronary artery evaluation (**Panels A** and **B**) but visible on the large fields of view with a 320 mm size (*arrow* in **Panels C** and **D**) The *left column* represents lung window-level settings, and the *right column* soft tissue window-level settings. The irregular 2.5 cm mass in the left lower lobe was spiculated and had pleural tails (**Panels C** and **D**), highly suspicious of malignancy. Both bronchoalveolar lavage and transbronchial biopsies were negative (no malignant cells found). However, transthoracic CT-guided lung biopsy resulted in a diagnosis of nonsmall cell lung carcinoma. A positron-emission tomography scan showed no signs of metastasis, and the patient underwent lobectomy of the left lower lobe with partial lingula resection. The final diagnosis was adenocarcinoma, with spread into the lingula and visceral pleura. There were free margins after resection, and no peribronchial metastases (complete resection of a pT2N0M0 tumor). This case underlines how important it is to always reconstruct the lungs on large fields so as to avoid overlooking any pathology. Coronary CT angiography was performed in this 72-year-old female patient before renal transplantation for renal failure resulting from polycystic kidney disease. Note the partially imaged liver cyst with calcification in association with polycystic kidney disease. Images courtesy of L. Kroft

■ **Fig. 19.43** Large hiatal hernia in an 82-year-old male patient (*arrow*). Such hernias can cause chest pain mimicking angina pectoris, and proton pump inhibitors may reduce the symptoms of reflux. The displaced esophagus is located posteriorly (*arrowhead*) to this "upside-down" stomach

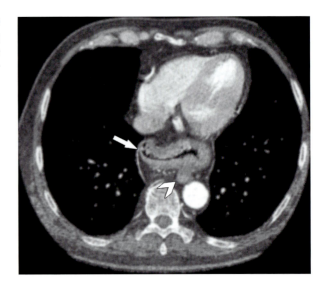

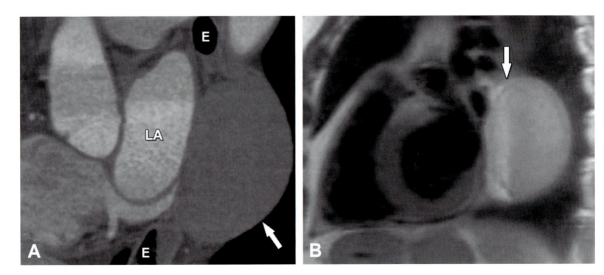

■ **Fig. 19.44** Mediastinal cystic lesion on cardiac CT in a 72-year-old man who presented with dyspnea and atypical angina pectoris (*arrow* in **Panel A**, sagittal reformation). An oval hypoattenuating 8-cm mediastinal tumor was found posterior to the left atrium (LA). The differential diagnosis in this situation included a pericardial, bronchogenic, or lymphatic cyst, or less likely, a lymphoma or a malignant tumor arising from a different origin (e.g., the esophagus, E). Magnetic resonance imaging was performed for further clarification (**Panel B**) and demonstrated a fluid level (*arrow*). Thus, the lesion was assumed to most likely represent a benign cyst, e.g., of lymphatic origin (lipid-water level) or originating from the pericardium. This case highlights the importance of the availability of different modalities for clarification of noncardiac findings in cardiac CT

19

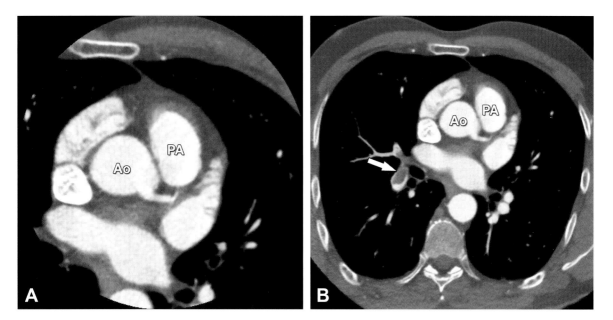

☐ Fig. 19.45 Unexpected pulmonary embolism in a 39-year-old male patient that was not seen on dedicated small reconstruction fields of view for coronary artery evaluation (**Panel A**) but was visible on the large fields of view with 320-mm size (*arrow* in **Panel B**). Note the filling defect in the interlobar pulmonary artery, which was only seen on large-field reconstruction (*arrow* in **Panel B**). Extensive pulmonary embolism was found in the right middle and lower lobes at maximum reconstruction fields-of-view. The patient had to be readmitted for medical treatment of this complication. Coronary CT angiography was performed for evaluation of scar tissue and/or complications after right ventricular radiofrequency ablation therapy of an arrhythmia focus. This case again demonstrates that large fields of view should always be reconstructed and evaluated. *Ao* aorta; *PA* pulmonary artery. Images courtesy of L. Kroft

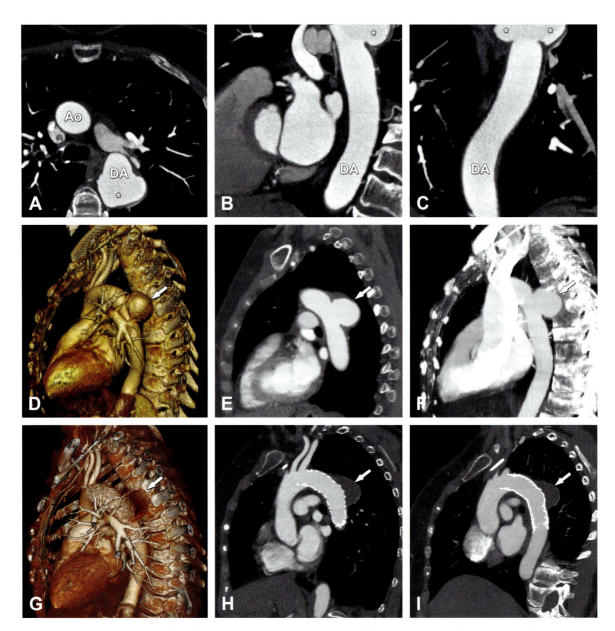

Fig. 19.46 Saccular aneurysm of the descending thoracic aorta in a 65-year-old female patient. On the most cranial slices of coronary CT angiography, a focal excentric dilatation (4.3 cm, *asterisks* in **Panels A–C**) of the descending aorta (DA) is partially visible. **Panel A** represents an axial source image, and **Panels B** and **C** represent double-oblique sagittal and coronal slices. Because of this extracardiac finding, CT angiography of the thoracic and abdominal aorta was subsequently performed. This test confirmed the focal saccular aneurysm, which did not extend to the aortic arch (*arrow* in **Panels D–F**, lateral views). Percutaneous interventional treatment with stenting was performed, and follow-up CT scans showed that the stent excluded the aneurysm well, resulting in thrombosis and exclusion from perfusion of the aneurysm (*arrow* in **Panels G–I**, lateral views). The suprarenal location and the absence of atherosclerosis in other vascular territories indicate that this was most likely a mycotic aneurysm. *Ao* aorta

19

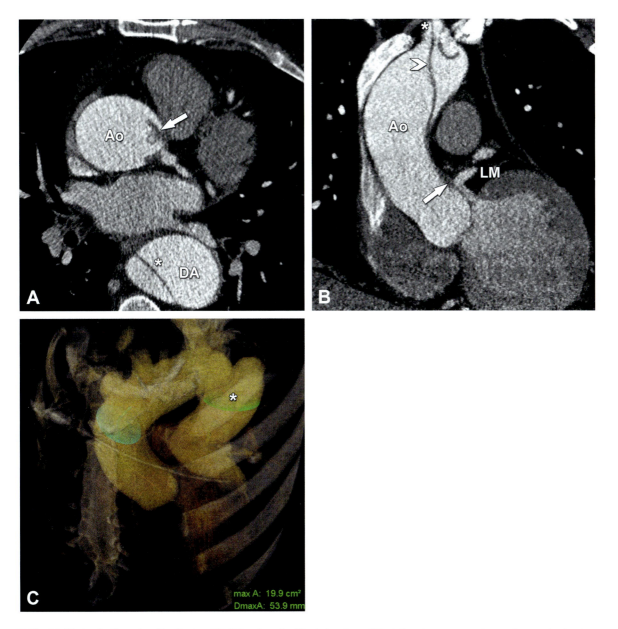

Fig. 19.47 Aortic dissection (Stanford and DeBakey type I) with obstruction of the left main coronary artery ostium and extension into the descending aorta (DA) in a 48-year-old male patient presenting with acute thoracic back pain. Axial source images (**Panel A**) and double-oblique coronal images (**Panel B**) demonstrate the dissection membrane in the ascending aorta (*arrowhead* in **Panel B**) and descending aorta (*asterisk* in **Panel A**). The dissection extends into the innominate artery (brachiocephalic trunk, *asterisk* in **Panel B**) and obstructs the left main coronary ostium (LM, *arrow* in **Panels A** and **B**). Automatic measurement of the inner diameters of the thoracic aorta was performed (**Panel C**) and revealed a maximum diameter of 5.4 cm (descending aortic aneurysm). The advantage of this comprehensive ECG-synchronized CT imaging approach is that the coronary arteries can be simultaneously evaluated. Emergency aortic repair and bypass grafting (left internal mammary artery to the left anterior descending and venous bypass graft to the left circumflex) was performed

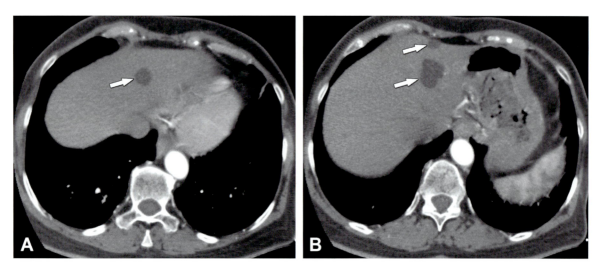

◘ **Fig. 19.48** Incidental finding of multiple (up to 2.5 cm) liver cysts (*arrows* in **Panels A** and **B**) in a 66-year-old female patient who underwent coronary CT angiography that excluded significant coronary artery stenoses. Differentiating liver cysts from low-density metastases or liver tumors can be difficult (**Figs. 19.49** and **19.50**) because only the purely arterial phase of liver perfusion is available with coronary CT. Thus, dedicated liver imaging, e.g., using ultrasound, is recommended whenever liver lesions that are suspicious for malignancy or not seen on prior imaging are detected

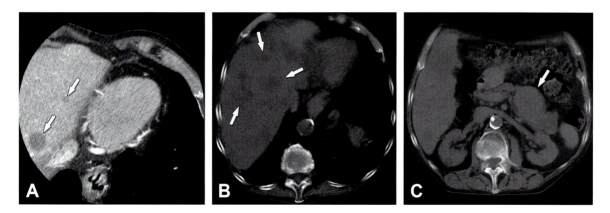

◘ **Fig. 19.49** Primarily misinterpreted hepatic metastases. Two round, well-circumscribed hypo-attenuating hepatic lesions were seen on the basal slices of a cardiac CT scan (*arrows* in **Panel A**) in a 78-year-old male patient who was referred for analysis of atypical chest pain. These lesions were reported and thus the referring physician, who had done an ultrasound in this patient a few years ago, recognized that these were new. Thus, abdominal CT (**Panels B** and **C**) was performed for further analysis, confirming that these lesions had already increased size in the short interval since the cardiac CT scan and revealing many more ill-defined lesions (a few of them are marked with *arrows* in **Panel B**), compatible with metastases. Also, a large pancreatic tumor was diagnosed (*arrow* in **Panel C**). Imaging was limited to unenhanced CT because of renal dysfunction. The patient's condition rapidly deteriorated and he died within 2 months. Pancreatic cancer was confirmed at autopsy. From Dewey et al. Eur Radiol 2007

19

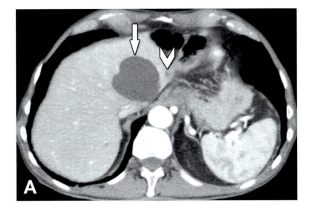

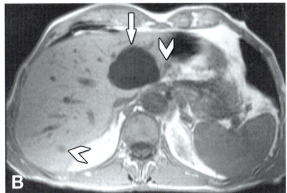

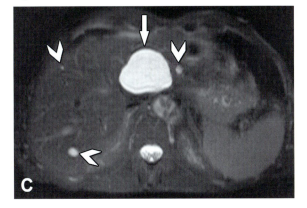

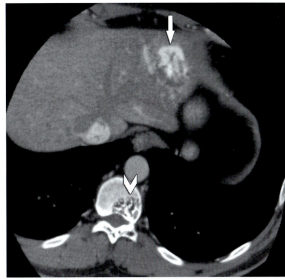

■ **Fig. 19.51** Incidental finding of a hepatic and vertebral body hemangioma in a 52-year-old male patient presenting with atypical angina pectoris. Coronary CT angiography excluded significant coronary artery stenosis and demonstrated a 3.7 cm well-marginated tumor with peripheral globular enhancement in segment II of the liver (*arrow*). Ultrasound confirmed the typical imaging findings of a hepatic hemangioma (not shown). There was also a well-marginated area in a vertebral body (*arrowhead*) with typical trabeculation pattern diagnostic for vertebral body hemangioma

■ **Fig. 19.50** Hepatic cysts confirmed on magnetic resonance imaging. Multiple hypo-attenuating lesions with the largest measuring about 5 cm were incidentally found on cardiac CT of a 76-year-old male patient (*arrow* in **Panel A**). Because of additional smaller lesions (*arrowhead* in **Panel A**) and the fact that cystic liver lesions are not always easy to analyze on the arterial phase images provided by cardiac CT (**Fig. 19.49**), this patient underwent magnetic resonance imaging with T1- (**Panel B**) and T2-weighted (**Panel C**) sequences. These clearly confirmed the benign nature of the liver lesions diagnosed as biliary cysts (*arrow* and *arrowheads* in **Panels B** and **C**)

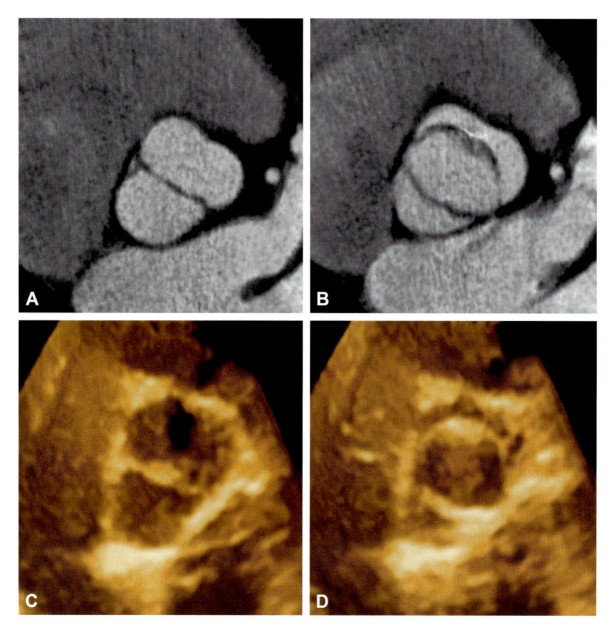

◻ **Fig. 19.52** Bicuspid aortic valve in a 48-year-old male patient. There is normal closure (**Panel A**) and opening of the aortic valve (**Panel B**) as seen with CT. CT data are shown as minimum-intensity projections. There is excellent correlation with the findings of three-dimensional transthoracic echocardiography (**Panels C** and **D**). Echocardiography images courtesy of A.C. Borges

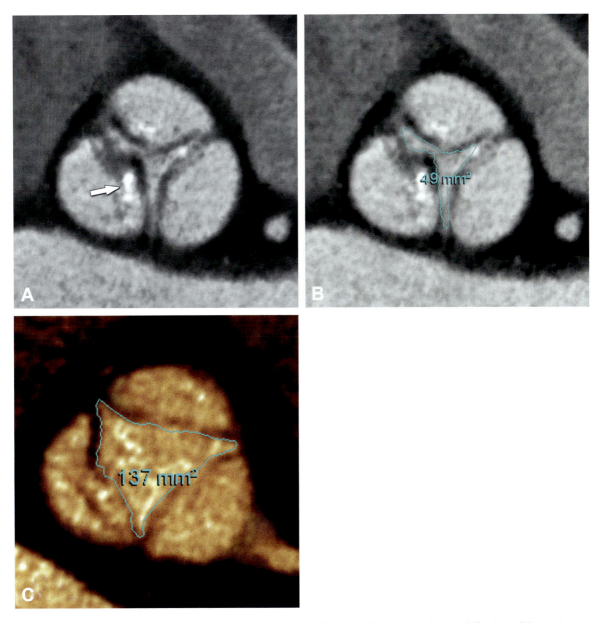

□ **Fig. 19.53** Tricuspid aortic valve in an 83-year-old female patient with stenosis. There are moderate calcifications of the aortic cusps (*arrow* in **Panel A**) that lead to severe (<1.0 cm^2) stenosis of the valve during systole (**Panel A**). Caliper measurement of the aortic valve area during systole (**Panel B**) shows a valve area of 0.49 cm^2. After surgical replacement of the valve, there is marked increase in the systolic aortic valve area (**Panel C**). Mild and moderate aortic valve stenoses are represented by aortic valve areas of >1.5 cm^2 and 1.0–1.5 cm^2, respectively. CT data are shown as minimum-intensity projections

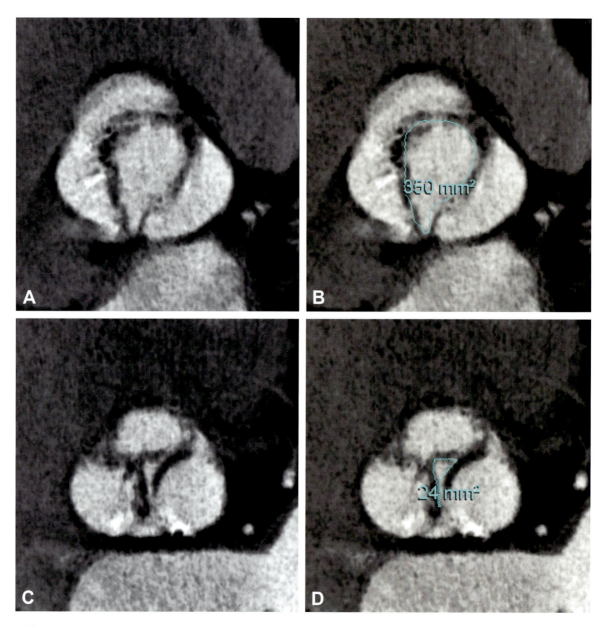

■ **Fig. 19.54** Tricuspid aortic valve with regurgitation in a 48-year-old male patient. **Panels A** and **B** show results of systole with normal opening of the valve cusps, while **Panels C** and **D** show the aortic regurgitation area during diastole (0.24 cm²). The right column shows the caliper measurements of the aortic valve area. CT data are shown as minimum-intensity projections

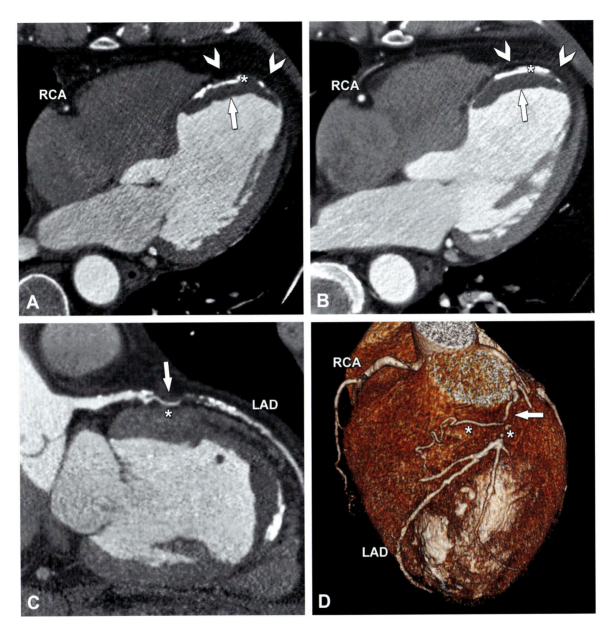

■ **Fig. 19.55** Left ventricular apical aneurysm with thrombus in a 79-year-old male patient with a history of anterior myocardial infarction 19 years ago, who had suspected thrombus on transthoracic echocardiography. There is a left ventricular crescent-filling defect (*arrow* in **Panel A**), representing an apical thrombus. The thrombus is due to stasis of blood in the akinetic apical aneurysm resulting from chronic myocardial infarction. The myocardial infarct has resulted in myocardial calcification (*asterisk* in **Panel A**) and fatty degeneration (*arrowheads* in **Panel A**). The fatty changes in the myocardium are seen as densities similar to those of the pericardial fat. **Panel A** is a four-chamber view of the left ventricle obtained with a 0.5 mm slice thickness. For comparison, the findings are also shown as a 5 mm thin-slab maximum-intensity projection in the four-chamber view (**Panel B**) The myocardial infarction was the result of an occlusion of the left anterior descending coronary artery (LAD, *arrow* in **Panels C** and **D**). Left-to-left collaterals (*asterisks* in **Panels C** and **D**) bypass the occlusion. Nevertheless, a large infarction with an apical aneurysm and thrombus formation eventually occurred in this patient. *RCA* right coronary artery

⬛ **Fig. 19.56** Left atrial thrombus in a 65-year-old male patient presenting 6 months after arterial (A) and venous (V) bypass grafting. The thrombus (*arrow*) is seen in the left atrial appendage (LAA) on axial (**Panel A**), coronal (**Panel B**), and sagittal images (**Panel C**). The patient also has a cardiac defibrillator (*asterisk* in **Panels A**–C). The left pulmonic pericardial recess (*arrowhead*) is seen in **Panel A** and can be differentiated from thrombotic material because it has lower density. Adding a late phase (2 min after contrast agent injection) increases confidence in the use of cardiac CT in the diagnosis of a trial thrombi. *Ao* aorta; *LA* left atrium; *LV* left ventricle

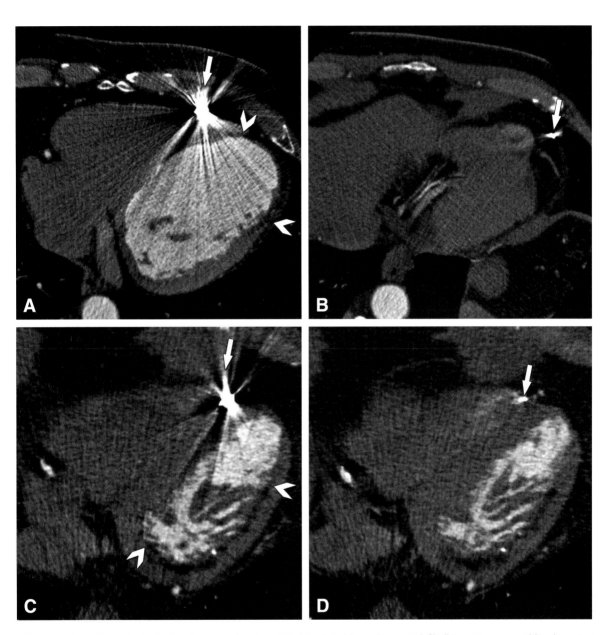

Fig. 19.57 Right ventricular lead perforation of an automated implantable cardioverter defibrillator in a 57-year-old male patient who had pacemaker dysfunction on testing. In **Panel A**, the lead is still in the right ventricle (*arrow*), and an apical infarction (*arrowheads*) is visible. A few slices further caudally, the tip of the lead can be seen penetrating into the pericardial cavity (*arrow* in **Panel B**) For comparison, the same anatomical regions are shown in a different 67-year-old male patient presenting with typical angina pectoris (**Panels C** and **D**). This patient has an inferolateral myocardial infarction (*arrowheads* in **Panel C**), and the tip of the lead is located within the right ventricle (*arrow* in **Panel D**)

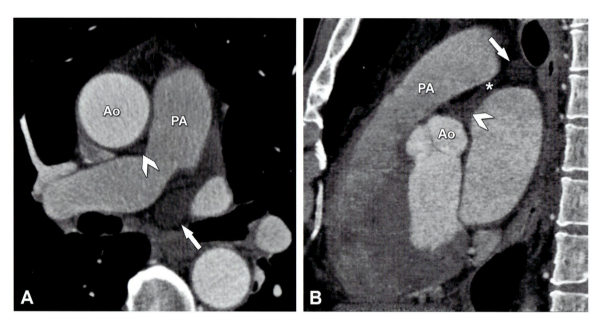

■ **Fig. 19.58** Pericardial recesses and sinuses need to be differentiated from effusions, lymph nodes, and dissections. **Panels A** and **B** show an example of a left pulmonic pericardial recess (*arrow*) in the groove inferior to the left pulmonary artery (PA). This recess commonly communicates (*asterisk* in **Panel B**) with the transverse pericardial sinus (*arrowhead* in **Panel B**), which is located posterior to the ascending aorta (Ao). Also communicating with the transverse sinus is the superior aortic recess (*arrowhead* in **Panel A**). The posterior pericardial recess (not shown) is also sometimes seen and is located posterior to the right pulmonary artery as part of the oblique pericardial sinus. The typical location and CT appearance (density of water, well-marginated, tapered configuration) allow pericardial recesses to be distinguished from mediastinal lymphadenopathy, pericardial effusions, and aortic dissection

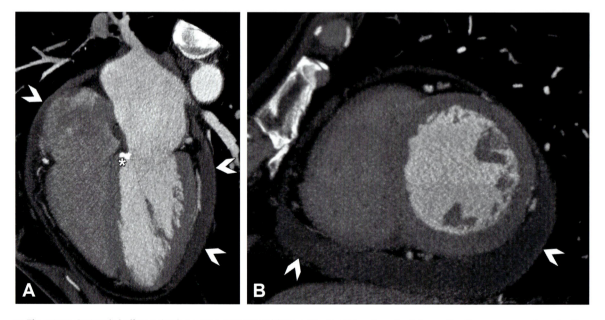

■ **Fig. 19.59** Pericardial effusion (with a 2 cm posterior width) in a 61-year-old male patient 6 months after coronary artery stenting. Both the four-chamber view (**Panel A**) and the cardiac short-axis view (**Panel B**) show the large pericardial effusion (*arrowheads*). There is a small mitral valve annulus calcification (*asterisk* in **Panel A**), another noncoronary cardiac finding. CT data are shown as maximum-intensity projections

Fig. 19.60 Circumferential calcification of the pericardium (*arrows*) in a four-chamber view. Such calcifications typically cause constrictive pericarditis, which can be associated with elevated right cardiac pressures, dyspnea, exercise intolerance, and even ascites. Most pericardial calcifications have an infectious etiology (e.g., tuberculosis, histoplasmosis)

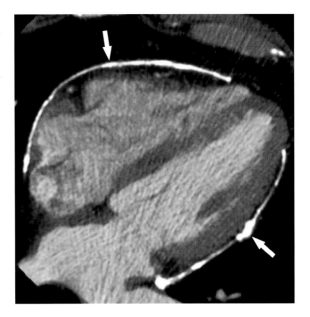

Results of Clinical Studies

M. Dewey

Abstract

This chapter summarizes the diagnostic performance of cardiac CT.

20.1   Coronary Arteries

Noninvasive coronary angiography using multislice CT as a means of ruling out significant stenoses in patients with low-to-intermediate likelihood of disease is the foremost clinical application of this test. Numerous single and multicenter studies have addressed the diagnostic performance of CT in detecting stenoses of the native coronary vessels, and we have summarized the results in terms of per-patient sensitivity and specificity in **Fig. 20.1**. Please note that the negative predictive value of CT is 95% in this analysis (data not shown in the figure) and represents the major advantage of this test (Chaps. 5 and 6).

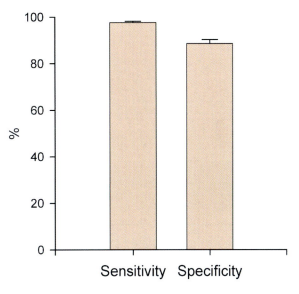

◘ **Fig. 20.1** Per-patient diagnostic performance (sensitivity, specificity, and nondiagnostic rate) of coronary CT angiography in native coronary vessels, when compared with conventional coronary angiography as the reference (gold) standard. Results were obtained using all published studies on this topic. Error bars represent 95% confidence intervals. Please note that because this figure represents per-patient results, direct comparison with the following figures (per-graft and per-stent results) is not possible

M. Dewey, *Cardiac CT*,
DOI: 10.1007/978-3-642-14022-8_23, © Springer-Verlag Berlin Heidelberg 2011

20.2   Coronary Artery Bypasses

Assessing coronary arterial and venous bypass grafts is an important application of CT in some patients (e.g., patients with recurrent chest pain and equivocal stress results). Numerous single-center studies have addressed the diagnostic performance of CT in coronary artery bypass grafts, and we have summarized the results as per-graft sensitivity and specificity in **Figs. 20.2** and **20.3**.

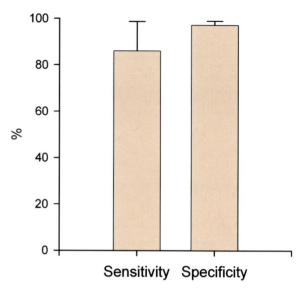

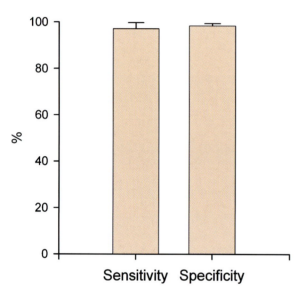

Fig. 20.2 Per-graft diagnostic performance (sensitivity, specificity) of coronary CT angiography in detecting coronary artery bypass graft occlusion, when compared with conventional coronary angiography as the reference (gold) standard. Results were obtained using all published studies on this topic. Error bars represent 95% confidence intervals

Fig. 20.3 Per-graft diagnostic performance (sensitivity, specificity) of coronary CT angiography in detecting coronary artery bypass graft stenosis, when compared with conventional coronary angiography as the reference (gold) standard. Results were obtained using all published studies on this topic. Error bars represent 95% confidence intervals

20

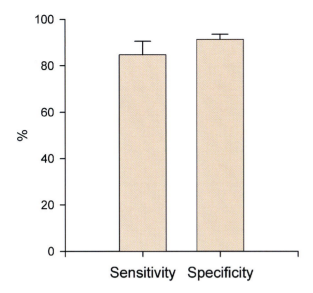

Fig. 20.4 Diagnostic performance (sensitivity and specificity) of coronary CT angiography in detecting coronary artery in-stent restenoses, when compared with conventional coronary angiography as the reference (gold) standard. Results were obtained using all published studies on this topic. Please note that patients with overall nonassessable image quality had to be excluded from this summary, as most studies did not provide detailed information about how many stents were present in these patients. Moreover, in patients with overall acceptable image quality, the per-stent nondiagnostic rate was 15%. Error bars represent 95% confidence intervals

20.3   Coronary Artery Stents

The successful detection of coronary artery stent stenoses with CT is limited when compared with assessment of the native vessels using current technology. Sufficient image quality and accuracy are, in general, achieved only for large stents (at least 3.5-mm diameter). In the case of smaller stents, only about 50% of cases are evaluable. Numerous single-center studies and one multicenter study have addressed the diagnostic performance of CT in detecting in-stent restenoses, and we have summarized the results as per-stent sensitivity and specificity in **Fig. 20.4**. Please note that the positive predictive value is only 70% in this analysis (data not shown in the figure), a major limitation of CT for coronary stent evaluation.

20.4   Cardiac Function

Global and regional cardiac function can easily be assessed using the same data that have been acquired for coronary CT angiography. Because it has considerable influence on patient management (Chap. 11), left ventricular function should be evaluated in all patients undergoing cardiac CT (Chap. 15). We have summarized the accuracy of CT in determining left ventricular ejection in **Fig. 20.5**.

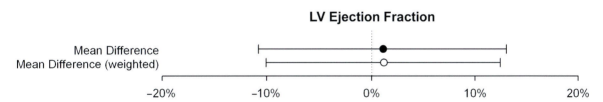

Fig. 20.5 Bland-Altman analysis of the accuracy of CT in determining left ventricular ejection fraction, vs. magnetic resonance imaging as the reference standard. Results are shown as unweighted and weighted (according to study size) mean values and limits of agreement (±95% confidence intervals). The limits of agreement indicate the expected maximum difference between CT and the reference standard and are approximately ±12%. The agreement between cineventriculography and echocardiography and the reference standard is significantly lower than that of CT, as shown in head-to-head comparisons. There is a slight underestimation of the ejection fraction by CT (as identified by the mean of approximately + 2%)

Outlook

M. Dewey

Abstract

This chapter discusses anticipated technical and clinical developments with regard to CT.

21.1   Technical Developments

There is an exponential growth in cardiac CT research. Technical developments expected in the near future are summarized in **List 21.1**.

> **List 21.1. The foremost upcoming technical developments**
>
> 1. Single heartbeat whole-heart CT
> 2. Multisource CT, potentially further improving temporal resolution
> 3. Further reduction in gantry rotation times
> 4. Further reduction in slice collimation

21.1.1   Single Heart Beat Whole-Heart CT

Both 320-row CT scanners (with wide-area detectors, Chap. 10a, **Fig. 21.1**) and second-generation dual-source CT with fast prospective spiral acquisition (Chap. 10b) are able to scan the entire heart during a single heart beat (**Fig. 21.2**). Thus, this technology greatly reduces the scan time for coronary angiography from 8 to 10 s for 64-row CT to less than 1 s in patients with low and stable heart rates. This improvement significantly reduces the likelihood of both ECG and breathing-related motion artifacts and thus improves image quality (**Fig. 21.3**). Moreover, prospective acquisition covering the entire heart without oversampling and overranging reduces the effective dose by a factor of 3–10 to an average of less than 1–5 mSv for coronary angiography in patients with low and stable heart rates. These improvements have a great potential to contribute to the widespread clinical application of

M. Dewey, *Cardiac CT*,

DOI: 10.1007/978-3-642-14022-8_24, © Springer-Verlag Berlin Heidelberg 2011

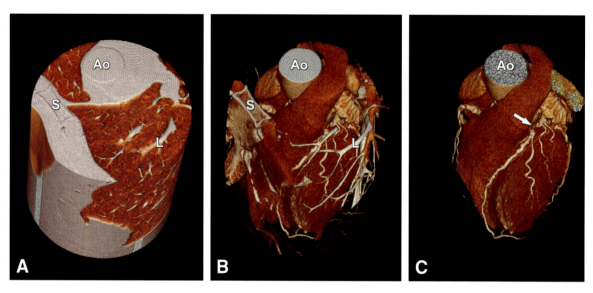

Fig. 21.1 Cardiac imaging with volume CT using 320 simultaneous detector rows shows the cylindrical appearance of the volume, which was prospectively scanned within a single heartbeat (**Panel A**). After changing the window-level settings of this three-dimensional reconstruction, the lung veins (*L*) become evaluable (**Panel B**). Using automatic segmentation tools (**Panel C**) the heart and coronary vessels are isolated, and a significant stenosis becomes visible in the left anterior descending coronary artery (*arrow*). *Ao* aorta; *S* sternum

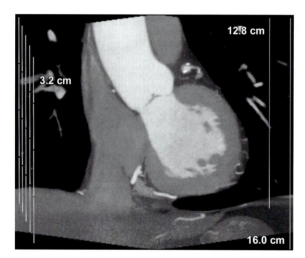

Fig. 21.2 Scanning of the entire heart in one rotation with 320-row CT and a coverage of 16.0 cm (superimposed on a coronal maximum-intensity projection of the left ventricle and aorta), compared with conventional coverage using 64-row CT with 3.2-cm detector width (left side of image, based on a pitch of 0.2). Please note that the angle of the X-ray beam using 320 simultaneous detector rows is 15.2°. Thus, the volume acquired with a single X-ray shot looks like a cylinder bounded by two circular cones (**Fig. 21.1**)

cardiac CT. Nevertheless, these scanners are not yet as widely available as previous scanner generations.

The amount of contrast agent required is further reduced with single heart beat whole-heart CT. However, a drawback of the 320-row volume scanner is that the increased width of the detector (by a factor of 5) to some degree increases scattered radiation, and therefore image noise. To compensate for this scatter, the tube current has to be slightly increased from that of 64-row CT. Nevertheless, image quality is improved with volume CT, and radiation exposure can be significantly reduced, as with the fast prospective spiral acquisition using dual-source CT. One important advantage of the prospective 320-row volume acquisition is that it may provide more flexibility when extrasystoles occur (Chap. 8) and in patients with atrial fibrillation (**Fig. 21.4**).

21.1.2 Multisource Scanning

Dual-source CT has been available for some time now and has been of great value in improving temporal resolution and reducing the dependency on heart rate. It is expected that further technical developments will lead to the availability of clinical multisource CT scanners, which could further reduce the length of the image reconstruction windows within the RR interval. In this way, coronary CT angiography could become fully independent of heart rate. However, scattered radiation also increases when more X-ray tubes are used.

Despite cost issues, it is, therefore, likely that the concepts of wide-area detector and multisource CT will eventually be merged within a single CT scanner, making the advantages of both approaches available for patient care.

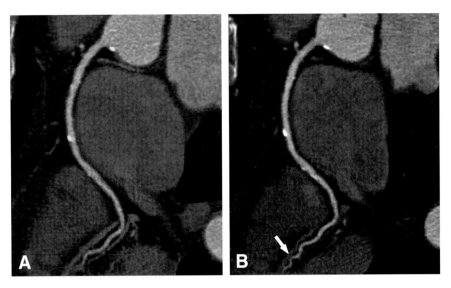

□ Fig. 21.3 Comparison of image quality obtained with 64-row CT and 320-row CT using curved multiplanar reformations along the right coronary artery (**Panels A** and **B**). There is a tendency for longer vessel segments (*arrow*) visualized with 320-row CT

21.1.3   Better Temporal Resolution

Further reducing the gantry rotation time (to below the currently achieved 270–350 ms) is an obvious approach to improving temporal resolution and reducing heart rate dependency. However, our ability to shorten the rotation time is limited by the dramatic increase in centrifugal forces that occurs as the rotation time is reduced. For instance, at a 400-ms rotation time, the relative centrifugal force is 18–20 g, which already requires considerable centripetal force to counteract. However, at 200 ms (equal to an image acquisition window of 100 ms with halfscan reconstruction), the relative centrifugal forces rise to 74–80 g because they are equal to the square of the velocity. New technologies such as an air-bearing CT gantry and faster data transfer systems might alleviate this problem and make it feasible to reduce the rotation time to 200 ms or even shorter. However, it is not very likely that a reduction in the rotation time alone will be pursued as a strategy for further improving temporal resolution. Instead, it is much more likely that the three concepts of (1) multisource scanning, (2) adaptive multisegment reconstruction, and (3) shortening the gantry rotation time will be developed further and combined in some fashion to improve temporal resolution.

21.1.4   Better Spatial Resolution

The current slice collimation of coronary CT angiography (between 0.5 and 0.75 mm) limits its application to small structures such as coronary plaque and its internal makeup. Thus, thinner slice collimation (e.g., of 0.2–0.3 mm) or better in-plane resolution (Chap. 10c) have the potential to improve the assessment of plaques and stents and facilitate the quantification of stenoses by coronary CT angiography (**Fig. 21.5**). However, reducing the slice collimation by a factor of 2 requires the radiation exposure to be increased by a factor of 2 (if the same detector technology is used) to keep the image quality constant. Thus, improvements in spatial resolution are not easily achieved using the current technology, and further developments (e.g., detector material) are necessary for clinical applications if one does not wish to increase radiation exposure again.

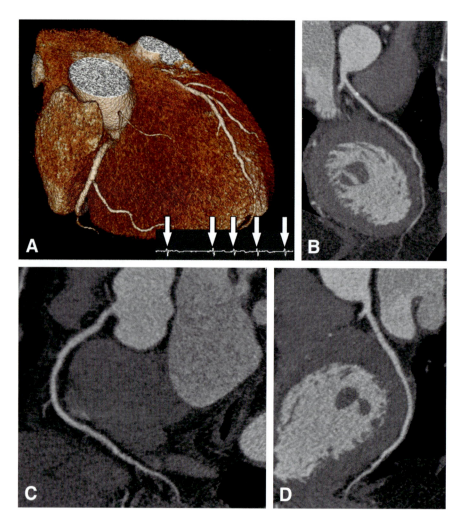

■ **Fig. 21.4** Normal coronary arteries in 320-row CT in a patient with atrial fibrillation. **Panel A** shows the three-dimensional reconstruction and the ECG strip with atrial fibrillation (*arrows* in the inset). **Panels B**, **C**, and **D** show curved multiplanar reformations along the left anterior descending, right, and left circumflex coronary artery, respectively, without significant diameter reduction. There is a small artifact in the mid-RCA, but otherwise image quality is very good. Images were acquired during one heartbeat with arrhythmia control using volume CT covering the entire heart in a single gantry rotation

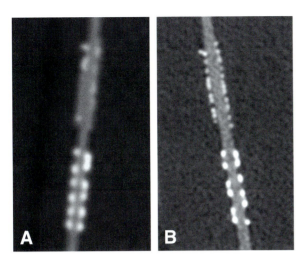

◨ **Fig. 21.5** Advantages of high-resolution (fine-cell detector) CT with a ~0.3-mm slice thickness for coronary stent imaging. Multiplanar reformations along a coronary stent with 2.5-mm inner diameter (in a phantom) obtained using 0.625-mm slice collimation and cell width (**Panel A**), and high-resolution CT with 0.3-mm slice collimation and cell width using a 0.3×0.3-mm focus size tube (**Panel B**). The opacified lumen within the small stent is more clearly seen, with fewer blooming artifacts, using the thinner slice collimation. Images courtesy of Sachio Kuribayashi. Department of Radiology, Keio University School of Medicine

21.2   Clinical Developments

The expected upcoming clinical developments are summarized in **List 21.2**.

List 21.2. The foremost upcoming clinical developments

1. Reliable coronary artery stent imaging
2. Myocardial perfusion and viability imaging
3. Imaging and follow-up of coronary plaques after medical interventions
4. Application of CT to asymptomatic high-risk patients

21.2.1   Coronary Stent Imaging

The technical innovations described above may make possible the reliable assessment of coronary artery stents for the presence of restenoses. For this purpose, it will be instrumental to add the fourth dimension to our analysis and to reduce motion artifacts that are related to ECG irregularities or patients' limited breath-hold capacity. Also, better spatially localized and temporally resolved quantitative measurements of the inner diameter of coronary stents will be pivotal to our efforts to broaden the clinical use of CT and extend it to the follow-up of patients who have undergone percutaneous coronary stent placement.

21.2.2 Myocardial Perfusion and Viability Imaging

Another advantage of volume CT and second-generation dual-source CT is that a fourth dimension, time, can be added, making it possible to assess myocardial perfusion and coronary blood flow ("dynamic volume CT"). With this new option, CT might to some extent replace conventional approaches involving myocardial perfusion imaging, while additionally providing information about the hemodynamic relevance of coronary stenosis (**Fig. 21.6**). Similar to magnetic resonance imaging, CT can detect late contrast enhancement in the myocardium as a marker of infarction ("viability imaging," **Fig. 21.7**). Nevertheless, the required additional contrast agent injection and radiation exposure seriously limit the use of CT for myocardial viability imaging.

21.2.3 Coronary Plaque Quantification and Characterization

One of the greatest potential advantages of coronary CT angiography is its ability to noninvasively determine the volume, characteristics, and composition of coronary artery plaques (Chap. 14). Since most acute coronary

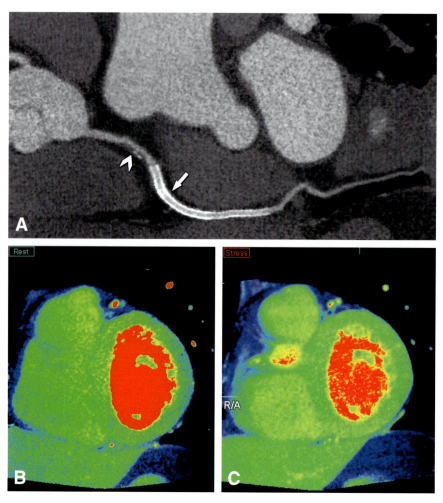

Fig. 21.6 Usefulness of myocardial perfusion imaging using 320-row volume CT in a 67-year-old female patient with atypical symptoms 3 years after stenting of the right coronary artery. Coronary CT angiography shows mostly noncalcified plaque immediately proximal to the stents (*arrowhead* in **Panel A**, curved multiplanar reformation). No significant in-stent restenosis can be identified;, however, the small size of the stents (*arrow*, 3 mm diameter) precludes reliable exclusion of significant stenosis. Myocardial perfusion analysis during rest (**Panel B**) and stress (**Panel C**) rules out significant defects

21

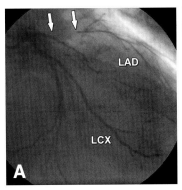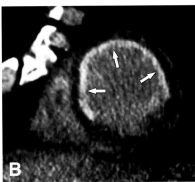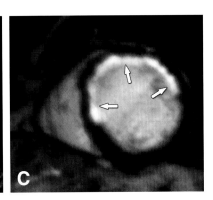

Fig. 21.7 Myocardial viability assessment using CT in a 74-year-old male patient who underwent stenting of a left anterior descending (LAD) coronary artery stenosis 2 years earlier. He was now re-admitted to the hospital for recurrent angina. Conventional coronary angiography showed proximal LAD occlusion (*arrows* in **Panel A**) with distal filling via collateral vessels arising from the left circumflex coronary artery (LCX). Prospectively ECG-triggered CT immediately following cardiac catheterization (without additional intravenous contrast agent) revealed subendocardial late enhancement (*arrows* in **Panel B**) in the anteroseptal, anterior, and anterolateral segments of the left ventricular wall. These findings were confirmed by delayed contrast-enhanced MR imaging (*arrows* in **Panel C**). Images courtesy of Andreas Mahnken, Aachen, Germany

events arise from plaques that cause only a minimal percent stenosis, it is of importance to identify plaque characteristics that are unambiguously associated with a higher risk in individual patients and would be expected to trigger intense medical treatment and preventive measures. However, characteristics such as positive remodeling, noncalcified components, and spotty calcifications, which are more likely to lead to acute evens, have not yet been shown to be useful in directing further medial treatment in order to result in better clinical outcomes.

Although it competes with intravascular ultrasound, CT is also a potential candidate for following up coronary artery plaques after initiation of certain medical therapies. Thus, if further large studies demonstrate its clinical validity and measuring accuracy, coronary CT angiography could become the foremost diagnostic surrogate parameter and test for analyzing the outcome of new drugs in terms of regression of coronary plaques.

21.2.4 Asymptomatic High-Risk Patients

Since 50% of men and 64% of women who die suddenly of coronary heart disease were previously asymptomatic, it is obvious that an ongoing search is necessary to identify parameters that reliably predict such coronary events. The identification of coronary plaques and stenoses in these patients might help optimize further

treatment. However, it must be borne in mind that no evidence exists that revascularization of coronary stenoses in asymptomatic patients improves outcomes. Given the radiation dose reduction possible with prospectively triggered acquisition, CT may be used for screening asymptomatic high-risk patients in the future if the clinical usefulness for this indication can be proven. However, large-scale randomized trials that analyze hard and soft events are required before a final decision can be made. Until then, cardiac CT is clearly not indicated in asymptomatic patients for routine clinical screening.

Recommended Reading

1 Burgstahler C, Brodoefel H, Schroeder S (2009) Cardiac CT in 2009. Minerva Cardioangiol 57:495–509

2 Choi SI, George RT, Schuleri KH, Chun EJ, Lima JA, Lardo AC (2009) Recent developments in wide-detector cardiac computed tomography. Int J Cardiovasc Imaging 25(Suppl 1):23–29

3 Dewey M, de Vries H, de Vries L, Haas D, Leidecker C (2010) The present and future of cardiac CT in research and clinical practice: moderated discussion and scientific debate with representatives from the four main vendors. Rofo 182:313–321

4 Flohr TG, Leng S, Yu L et al (2009) Dual-source spiral CT with pitch up to 3.2 and 75 ms temporal resolution: image reconstruction and assessment of image quality. Med Phys 36:5641–5653

5 Flohr TG, Raupach R, Bruder H (2009) Cardiac CT: how much can temporal resolution, spatial resolution, and volume coverage be improved? J Cardiovasc Comput Tomogr 3:143–152

6 Gaztanaga J, Garcia MJ (2009) New noninvasive imaging technologies in coronary artery disease. Curr Cardiol Rep 11:252–257

7   George RT, Ichihara T, Lima JA, Lardo AC (2010) A method for reconstructing the arterial input function during helical CT: implications for myocardial perfusion distribution imaging. Radiology 255(2):396–404

8   Itagaki MW, Suh RD, Goldin JG (2009) Cardiac CT research: exponential growth. Radiology 252:468–476

9   Kalra MK, Brady TJ (2008) Current status and future directions in technical developments of cardiac computed tomography. J Cardiovasc Comput Tomogr 2:71–80

10 Krombach GA, Niendorf T, Gunther RW, Mahnken AH (2007) Characterization of myocardial viability using MR and CT imaging. Eur Radiol 17:1433–1444

Index

M. Dewey, *Cardiac CT*,
DOI: 10.1007/978-3-642-14022-8, © Springer-Verlag Berlin Heidelberg 2011

Printing and Binding: Stürtz GmbH, Würzburg